THE
PREMATURE
MENOPAUSE
BOOK

Avon Books are available at special quantity discounts for bulk purchases for sales promotions, premiums, fund raising or educational use. Special books, or book excerpts, can also be created to fit specific needs.

For details write or telephone the office of the Director of Special Markets, Avon Books, Inc., Dept. FP, 1350 Avenue of the Americas, New York, New York 10019, 1-800-238-0658.

THE PREMATURE MENOPAUSE BOOK

WHEN THE "CHANGE OF LIFE" COMES TOO EARLY

KATHRYN PETRAS

Foreword by MICHELLE WARREN, M.D.

WHOLE CARE

AN AVON BOOK

The information contained in THE PREMATURE MENOPAUSE BOOK is not intended to replace the care prescribed by your physician. Always consult your physician
before beginning a new health regimen or altering any course of treatment set up by
your doctor.

AVON BOOKS, INC.
1350 Avenue of the Americas
New York, New York 10019

Copyright © 1999 by Kathryn Petras
Back cover author photograph by Roger LeMoine
Published by arrangement with the author
Library of Congress Catalog Card Number: 99-94866
ISBN: 0-380-80541-3
www.avonbooks.com/wholecare

First WholeCare Printing: July 1999

WHOLECARE TRADEMARK REG. U.S. PAT. OFF. AND IN OTHER COUNTRIES, MARCA REGISTRADA,
HECHO EN U.S.A.

Printed in the U.S.A.

OPM   10 9 8 7 6 5 4 3 2

ACKNOWLEDGMENTS

This book wouldn't have been possible without the help of many people, among them: Kris Dahl, Sean Desmond, Ann McKay Thoroman, Sarah Durand, and, of course, the Early Pausers, the wonderful group of women who shared their stories to help other women dealing with premature menopause, who have helped me every step of the way in coping with my own diagnosis, and who have offered such great comfort, advice, and camaraderie—especially Amy, Bryana, Cathy, Cheryl, Iris, Jodi, JoAnn, Karen, Sally, both Staceys, Steph, and Susan. You can't imagine how grateful I am to have met you all and how thankful I am for your contributions to this book and, on a more personal level, for being there.

Thanks also to my ever-supportive friends and family and, of course, my husband, Mitch, for dealing with me through the night sweats, mood swings and hot flashes—not to mention my constant discussion of the whys and wherefores of premature menopause.

And a special thanks to Dr. Michelle Warren for her inspiring work in hormonal disorders and menopause.

CONTENTS

FOREWORD

Premature menopause is a devastating diagnosis. Telling a patient that she has lost her ability to conceive and that this is most likely a permanent affliction is very much like telling someone she has cancer or a fatal disease. A piece of her life has been lost, a piece on which she had hoped to build her future. The tears and the shock are predictable and the doctor often feels helpless. Most cases are of unknown origin. One of the most frequent questions I am asked is "Where can I read about this?"

Kathryn Petras's book is a timely and much needed answer to this question. The medical literature is often too esoteric for the layman. Premature menopause or primary ovarian failure is a condition covered mainly in specialty journals or textbooks and the material is incomprehensible. The symptoms of menopause are very frightening, especially the night sweats, flushing, moodiness and fatigue. This book covers symptoms in detail as well as their response to treatment.

There is much that can be done to prevent the effects of aging due to estrogen loss and in fact this is imperative particularly for young women. The more a person knows about a condition the more she will make an effort to take care of herself and explore options for staying healthy. These options are well covered in this well-researched book. *The Premature Menopause Book* also covers what is known about this disease in a concise and easy-to-understand format. Hopefully the future will offer more answers and perhaps even cures or prevention, but at the present time this volume represents the most comprehensive source of information for women with this problem. This book is also an answer to a doctor's prayer: I will at last have an answer when asked about reading material.

—Michelle P. Warren, M.D.
Medical Director, Center for Menopause,
Hormonal Disorders and Women's Health;
Professor of Medicine and Obstetrics and Gynecology at
Columbia University, College of Physicians and Surgeons;
Wyeth Professor in Women's Health

A Personal Note from a Woman Going Through Menopause Years Before She Expected To

It was a sunny day in New York City. I was in a cab going downtown on Seventh Avenue. Outside Madison Square Garden there was a huge crowd. Traffic was bumper to bumper. Radio talk show host Howard Stern was holding an outdoor concert to promote his new movie. The street was filled with screaming teenagers and young adults.

But I was completely oblivious. Those people out there, the ones laughing and yelling, were in another world. They were still young and happy. I felt I had moved years beyond them in one day, and in many ways, I had. . . . I was just returning from a visit with a reproductive endocrinologist; for the third time in two months, I had been told I was in menopause—and this time, there was no question about it. I had celebrated my 38th birthday and I felt like I was 58.

I was in menopause.

I kept repeating it to myself. I was trying to make it real to me even though it already was all too real. I was only 38 and I was menopausal. And I was devastated.

It had all started years ago—but I didn't know it at the time. I had trouble sleeping. I would wake up in the middle of the night drenched in sweat. I would get odd episodes of sweating during the day as well. I used to joke about it. I would call it "hot flashes" and laugh, sure that what I was experiencing had something to do with stress or with allergies or maybe thyroid problems, but not menopause, of course. I skipped a few periods every now and then but, again, figured it was due to stress. It hadn't been an easy few years for me. I had recently ended an unhappy long-term relationship and was starting a new life. At the same time, my writing career was taking off—so work was getting more and more crazy. It seemed only logical to me that my body would exhibit strange symptoms. My gynecologist agreed and told me to try to relax.

But the sweating got worse and worse. My pillow would be soaking every morning; my clothes would get damp dozens of times every day. And I hadn't had a period in three months. Worried that my family's history of thyroid disease was showing itself in me, I finally went to my general practitioner for testing. But when I explained my so-logical hypothesis to the doctor, he didn't agree. It sounded like menopause, he said. I, of course, thought that was ridiculous. He took some blood, and said he would run a few tests and get back to me with the verdict.

I remember going home and laughing about it. Menopause? At age 38? It was insane. The doctor would see my blood tests and realize it was thyroid-related and that would be that.

Of course, it wasn't. I called my doctor three days later for the results of the blood test. "You're in menopause," he said. "Your FSH level is 35, which means you're perimenopausal." I had no idea what he was talking about. I didn't know what FSH meant, what perimenopausal meant. This all meant nothing to me. There must have been a mistake, I kept thinking. So right after I hung up the phone, I called another doctor—a gynecologist this time.

I sat across the desk from him, explained what had happened, and was relieved when he agreed with me. Maybe I had been exercising too much, or perhaps something else was wrong with me. As for the blood test I had taken that showed me in menopause, well, perhaps it was wrong. He would give me another blood test, then once menopause was ruled out, we could try some other tests. Again, I remember being convinced that the test would prove that I was fine. But when I called, he sounded upset. It definitely was menopause, or actually premature ovarian failure, he explained. My FSH levels were even higher than last time. I asked what normal FSH levels were. 15. And what were mine? 65. I tried to stay calm. I made some bad joke about how I had always been an overachiever. I told him that I was fine, I had expected this, and I made an appointment to see him in a few months.

Then I hung up the phone and started crying.

I think I cried, on and off, for three months. I cried when I realized I would never see the child I had finally planned to have, the child that was part of me and part of my husband. I cried when I saw babies on television or on the street. I even cried when I saw tampon ads and realized I wouldn't be needing them any longer. I cried because I felt suddenly old, definitely unsexy, and completely *different*.

In between the crying, I went to a fertility center and to my mother's endocrinologist, hoping that somehow this had all been a terrible mistake. I was excited when my period suddenly returned—convinced that my body had "cured" itself—but tests proved that I was wrong. Having my period didn't mean I was suddenly not menopausal at all.

Finally I realized it was time to stop crying and start coping. This wasn't going to go away. I had to move on, accept it and learn all I could.

I went on-line and searched for anything on premature ovarian failure and premature menopause. I didn't find all that much—a few studies written in medicalese about fragile X carriers and gonadotropins and such, two or three magazine articles that mentioned premature menopause in one or two lines, and information on menopause in general with a passing reference to premature menopause. I read any book I could about menopause—and again, found little information specifically about premature menopause, aside from an occasional mention.

It was an odd feeling. I had finally planned to have children, yet here I was reading up on menopause: books that talked about the empty-nest syndrome, when I hadn't even begun a family; uplifting articles and chapters about how it was possible to keep the sizzle in your sex life even though you were middle-aged . . . but I *wasn't* middle-aged.

I also started reading infertility books, hoping to get information about my chances for having a child. But again, premature menopause was mentioned only in passing—usually in a brief comment about how it was an irreversible condition that required donor eggs for pregnancy.

I spent hours wading through scientific journals, medical articles, and abstracts. I posted inquires on Internet infertility and menopause message boards looking for any information I could about premature menopause. I had so many questions . . . and I couldn't find the answers. Why had this happened to me? What could I do about it? Was it reversible? What were my chances for getting pregnant? And I found hundreds of other women with my condition—all asking the same questions.

That's when I realized that there wasn't anything out there for women like me. So, ultimately, I decided to write *this* book—the book I was looking for.

WHY WE NEED THIS BOOK

In all honesty many of the books available about menopause in general are excellent. But there's a big problem with these books where those of us with premature menopause are concerned: they're not about *us*. They're written for an older woman. Yet we confront a different set of problems and challenges from the average woman in menopause.

Going through premature menopause is no walk in the park. Because we're in menopause so many years before the norm, we're facing specific emotional and physical issues. We have to deal with the psychological baggage that comes with knowing our reproductive system has effectively shut down early, and with the fact that we can no longer have children naturally.

And we have to cope with the physical symptoms—and very real potential long-term health consequences—that come with premature menopause.

It's no wonder, then, that when you learn that you're in premature menopause, you're filled with concerns, worries, and questions. But, as I mentioned before, it is very difficult to find support, information, and answers. Even many doctors don't have much information on premature menopause.

But we need information and answers. We need to understand often complicated medical studies looking into the causes of—and possible reversals of—premature menopause. We need to know where to go for more information. We need to know the questions to ask our doctors—who all too often treat us simply as if we were older women in menopause, even though our cases are quite different. We need to know what to look for—and to look out for—in selecting among different treatment options.

And this is where *The Premature Menopause Book* can help.

Menopause isn't a disease, but it is a lifelong condition—something we have to deal with now and for the rest of our lives. So *The Premature Menopause Book* tells you what is happening to you now, and what can or will happen to you later. It offers support and supplies information, and answers the questions that inevitably arise when you learn you are in premature menopause. Most importantly, it gives you the tools you need to take control of your body and your medical situation—to ask the right questions of your doctor and to evaluate the medical alternatives open to you. In other words, it gives you the tools to be *empowered*.

And because it's written by a woman in premature menopause, not a doctor, it addresses our concerns head-on. Unlike someone who has dealt with patients with this condition, but not the condition itself, I truly understand what premature menopause is like because I've gone through it. I've had to deal with the unpleasant surprise of the diagnosis, the hot flashes and physical changes, the emotional ups and downs, and the readjustment of my self-image. Most important, I've had to deal with an incredible lack of information about this condition. So, as a *writer* with premature menopause, I hope in this book to answer the many questions I had—without preaching and without pushing a particular point of view. Just the facts, ma'am, as they say.

Actually, this is something I feel very strongly about. I believe that as adult women we are entitled to make our own decisions based upon knowledge. The key, of course, is having access to that knowledge. When I was first diagnosed, my gynecologist immediately wrote out a prescription for Premarin and Provera and told me to get it filled. When I asked why I needed it, he just said that I would be a fool not to take it. End of story. (And end of going to him as a patient!) That wasn't exactly the answer I wanted! I wanted to know *why*. I wanted to know if there were alternatives. And I wanted to be certain that he understood my particular situation. I had read that women in menopause didn't necessarily need hormone replacement therapy, and I wanted to know if the same studies applied to women in premature menopause. (This is covered in Chapter 5, which explores the positives and negatives of HRT as they specifically apply to women who are prematurely menopausal.) But when I tried to read the medical information I was able to find on the Internet, I found it was virtually incomprehensible to a layperson.

The Premature Menopause Book, then, allows you to be your own advocate and determine your own course of action by giving you both the information and the resources to make an educated decision. In addition, I've included resource listings because I know how often you may want more information or contact with other women in premature menopause. This includes listings of new clinical research and trials, menopause specialists, associations, medical centers, support groups, and more.

To sum it up, *The Premature Menopause Book* is the only central source of information—and inspiration—that deals with our devastating condition. It is written specifically *for* women going through premature menopause *by* a woman going through premature menopause, with information on health and emotional issues, answers to frequently asked questions, discussion of up-to-date research, and more.

HOW TO USE THIS BOOK

Because the process of understanding, accepting, and living with premature menopause is a step-by-step process, *The Premature Menopause Book* goes through premature menopause step by step, from a basic explanation in Chapter 1 of what premature menopause is and what causes it, to an exploration in Chapter 3 of long-term consequences, such as osteoporosis and heart disease, and what you can do about them, through coping with the emotional impact of the diagnosis (Chapter 4), through the possibilities of pregnancy with premature menopause (Chapter 8). It includes an extensive look at hormone replacement therapy, as well as herbs, vitamins, minerals, and other natural sources. *The Premature Menopause Book* covers the basics—dealing with uncomfortable symptoms like hot flashes—and special situations you may run into—such as coping with the problems premature menopause often causes in your romantic life.

Throughout the book, you'll notice bold-faced passages. These are words from other women, as well as myself—and, to me, one of the most crucial parts of the book.

When I first was diagnosed with premature menopause, I felt very alone. Regardless of how hard they tried, my family and friends couldn't completely understand what I was going through. Finally I met a group of wonderful women on the Internet, women who, like me, found themselves going through menopause years before they ever expected it. We formed a support group, the Early Pausers, to share stories, trade tips on different treatments, and, most important, to remind each other that there *were* other women out there like us—other women we could complain to, laugh with, even cry with. Many of the Early Pausers' stories are in this book. In fact, if I could choose what I consider the most important feature of this book, I think I would point to these personal stories. They give voice to the common fears, the worries, the concerns of those of us going through premature menopause. They also express ways to cope, the necessity of retaining a sense of humor, and the importance of putting things into perspective. In this sense, they are testimony to the resilience of the human spirit.

Above all, though, they remind all of us going through premature menopause that we're not alone.

I think that was the most difficult thing for me to deal with when I first heard I was in menopause at age 38: that feeling that no one could understand what I was going through. And I hope that this book and my personal insights and those of other women in premature menopause help you the way the support of others has helped me.

Ultimately, that's what this book is all about—support. I realize just how tough it is living with premature menopause, and I want to offer resources, information, and advice to help other women with my condition.

A FEW FINAL THOUGHTS

I hope this book helps you cope in general, and helps you realize that premature menopause isn't premature aging. Having lived with the diagnosis for over a year now and having spoken with hundreds of other women in premature menopause, I can safely say that you *do* adjust to the idea that you are in menopause prematurely. You have ups and downs about it (I know I did, and still do sometimes), but it becomes easier to cope with as time goes on.

I finally realized that all premature menopause meant was that my reproductive ability was gone. Yes, I was going through "the change," as menopause is sometimes called. But that didn't mean *I* had changed.

Remember, you're still the same you. Yes, you're stuck coping with a condition that you normally wouldn't have dealt with for 20 years. But you're not old! Your ovaries just are responding as if they were older. I know when I was first diagnosed, I felt instantly old and generally undesirable. But it finally hit me that nothing about me had changed but my reproductive system. I'm a lot more than my reproductive system—and so are you!

Chapter 1

When Menopause Comes Early

You're Not Too Young . . .

Like most women, I knew about menopause, of course. It was something that usually happened to women in their fifties. It meant hot flashes, no more periods, an end to your reproductive years. It was a natural part of a woman's life that was far in the future. And it didn't have anything to do with me, since I was still much too young.

That's what I thought—but I was wrong.

At the age of 38, I learned I was going through menopause. In fact, I was *well* into menopause. Menopause: the cycle in a woman's life when her ovaries stop producing eggs, when her periods begin to stop, when her hormone levels shift. Menopause: something that typically happens at about the age of 51.

It didn't make sense to me. Menopause was something that happened to older women, women who have already had a full life; who are perhaps dealing with the empty-nest syndrome; whose children are in college; women who *expect* to be going through menopause. It was something my mother was going through. It definitely wasn't anything I had thought could happen to anyone in their thirties, let alone me. I was still trying to have a child. I wasn't old. Me in menopause?

But menopause can and does happen to millions of women well before the "normal" age. According to recent medical studies, approximately eight out of every 100 American women of childbearing years—about 3.9 million women—go through natural menopause before the age of 40. A similarly high number enter menopause early due to surgery (removal of the uterus and/or ovaries) or chemotherapy or radiation treatment for cancer.

Lately there has been a rise in diagnoses of premature menopause. Some doctors believe it's being detected more often because so many women have put off having children until their thirties. Others think there could be a link between high stress or environmental toxins and premature menopause. And other doctors point to the increase in cancer treatments that often cause premature menopause.

Premature menopause, then, isn't nearly as rare as you might think. All things considered, it's a relatively common condition, but one with uncommon consequences.

Regardless of the cause, the effect on your life is immense: You're in your twenties or thirties—still a relatively young woman by most standards—and you're facing something that usually would have happened decades down the road. You're dealing with the physical effects of menopause—hot flashes, mood swings, anxiety—and you're dealing with the *emotional* side effects of entering menopause so many years earlier than normal—feeling out of synch with your peers, coping with the depression that comes when you realize your reproductive years are over before you ever dreamed they would be. It's a double whammy: your body is going through immense changes, and your psyche, your self-image, is rocked. And unlike older women who go through menopause at the "normal" time, you're completely unprepared. Premature menopause usually comes completely out of the blue.

Last summer I was having what I thought were hot flashes. My friends all thought I was off my rocker—"No way, it's just the heat." The summers here average 110°, so I figured maybe they were right. By September and three skipped periods, I was having full-blown hot flashes,

mood swings so bad I could not even stand myself, and night sweats. When I called the doctor's office, they said it would be two months before I could get an appointment. I then insisted on a blood test to check the hormones. By the time I saw the doctor in mid-December, I had the results, which showed I was postmenopausal. What I thought would be a ten-year process when I was 50 turned out to be over before I knew it.
—Cheryl, age 36

No matter what other people may say or think, going through premature menopause is different from going through normal menopause. I've had several heated debates on this topic with older women in menopause. They argue that it's the same thing, because they too are coping with the hot flashes and other physical symptoms as well as the moodiness and other emotional symptoms. Of course, they are right to some degree—there are, most definitely, overlaps between our experiences. But I remain convinced that there is a significant difference, and many doctors and studies agree with me.

First, the physical consequences of premature menopause are greater than those for normal menopause. Think about it—when you go through premature menopause, your body is experiencing a change *before* it is normally expected. In fact, you may be going through this change *20 or more years ahead of time*. Twenty years is no insignificant number when it comes to crucial hormone levels. When you go through menopause, your estrogen levels drop. So, since the "normal" age for menopause is 51, when you go through premature menopause, this means your body may be deprived of estrogen for 20 years or so. As a result, you're at a much greater risk for weaker bones and, at the worst, osteoporosis. Making matters even more critical, according to a recent National Institute of Child Health and Human Development study, women with premature menopause are at an increased risk of bone loss compared with normal menopausal women—and their bone loss occurs much more rapidly. Similarly, because estrogen helps protect against heart disease, having low levels of estrogen at an early age increases your risks for elevated blood pressure and heart disease.

These are two of the reasons that many doctors stress how important it is for women with premature menopause to begin taking care of their condition *immediately*—through hormone replacement therapy (HRT), alternative methods, changes in diet and exercise, and more. In fact, many of those who don't usually advocate hormone replacement therapy for the older menopausal woman believe that hormone replacement therapy is crucial for women with premature menopause, and explain that the well-documented risk of HRT-induced breast cancer doesn't necessarily apply to women in premature menopause. The reason? When you take HRT because of premature menopause, you are replacing what your ovaries *should be making normally, but aren't*. This means that the standard arguments for and against HRT are different for the woman in premature menopause. (Chapter 5 takes a close look at the pros and cons of HRT for the prematurely menopausal woman.) There are other physical differences as well. When you go through premature menopause, you are more prone to hot flashes—and *worse* hot flashes. Weight gain in your midsection is more noticeable, and probably due more to hormone changes than to aging.

Then, as I mentioned before, there is the emotional fallout of premature menopause. It's a very difficult concept to come to grips with. The ads in magazines for estrogen replacement show gray-haired older women that may remind you of your mother, but now you're in the same boat. You may have put off having children, like me, until you reached your thirties. Now you learn that you probably won't be able to have those children. Or you already have children, and you're coping with the demands of raising them at the same time that you're dealing with hot flashes, incredible fatigue, and other menopausal symptoms. Your friends complain about PMS and ask if you have a spare tampon, and you haven't had a period in years. They're worried about their biological clock, and your biological clock has stopped. You feel isolated, out of synch with your peers.

You feel *old*.

Worse, often no one will listen to you. If you do suspect menopause, everyone, from well-meaning friends to doctors, will insist that you're too young.

> **I think the hardest part is having to argue all the time. I asked the pharmacist's advice on calcium and he dismissed my concerns: "Oh, you're too young for that." Why won't anyone believe that this is *real*! Do they think I'm making it up?**
>
> **—Amy, age 35**

It all sounds frightening, to be honest, and it can be. But no matter how difficult it sometimes seems—and in the first days, it did seem incredibly difficult to me—you *can* cope with premature menopause. It doesn't have to throw your entire life into a tailspin. The key, as I've learned, is knowledge: knowing what is going on in your body, knowing what to expect, knowing what different options are open to you for treatment and management of your symptoms. Most important is knowing that you aren't alone.

This book is designed to help you make it through this unexpected change in your life step by step. The first step to take is understanding the what's and why's of premature menopause. That's what this chapter is about. It's an explanation of what premature menopause is, a brief look at how it happens and what causes it.

WHAT EXACTLY IS PREMATURE MENOPAUSE, ANYWAY?

Let's start with the most basic and sometimes most confusing question of all: What exactly is premature menopause?

Believe it or not, many books (and doctors) are a bit vague on the topic. You learn that you have premature menopause, then it's on to a discussion of hormone replacement therapy, and that's it. But you can't make decisions about hormones, or anything else for that matter, if you're not clear about what is going on with your body.

So what *is* premature menopause? Here's the obvious answer: premature menopause is menopause that occurs prematurely. But, of course, there's a little more to it than that.

Put simply, menopause is the cessation (pause) of your periods (menses). Your periods stop because your ovaries have run out of eggs, have been damaged, or have been surgically removed. You're technically considered in menopause after you haven't had a period for six months to a year. The transition period, when you begin going through the symptoms of menopause (irregular periods, hot flashes, mood swings, changes in hormone levels, and so forth), is called *perimenopause*, and usually lasts about six years, although some women have symptoms for only one year and others have them for ten years or more. Most people, though, use the word "menopause" to include the entire process leading up to and including menopause, and I'll do the same throughout this book.

The average age for women to have completed menopause is age 51, which means that most women go through this change between the ages of 47 and 53. *Premature menopause,* then, applies to those women who go through menopause well before these average ages. It is technically defined as going through menopause before the age of 40, which means that, if you're diagnosed with premature menopause, there is a very good chance that you've been having menopausal symptoms well before you hit 40. To complicate matters a bit, some women go through menopause a little earlier than the average, say in their early forties. This is often called *early menopause*. It's not a clinical term, because their menopause is still considered within the "normal" age range. But to some degree, these women who go through early menopause often share emotional fallout similar to those of us with premature menopause.

If premature menopause occurs spontaneously—that is, if you haven't had surgery, radiation treatment, or chemotherapy that led to menopause—it is often referred to as *premature ovarian failure (POF)*. This sounds devastating, but basically all it means is that your ovaries aren't working as they should. They're shutting down years, even decades, before their time. If premature menopause is a result of surgery or cancer treatments, you're facing the same situation, but for different reasons.

In other words then, premature menopause, no matter what the cause, means one simple thing: your reproductive system is no longer working the way it used to. Your body is switching from being reproductive to being nonreproductive. In effect, you've fast-forwarded to the age of 50 or so. This, in turn, affects your entire body, not to mention your psyche.

HOW YOUR REPRODUCTIVE SYSTEM WORKS AND HOW PREMATURE MENOPAUSE AFFECTS IT

To truly understand what premature menopause is and how it affects your body—and, probably more important, to be able to talk to your doctor and actually understand what she is saying, to honestly evaluate your different treatment options, and to ask the right questions—it helps to have a basic knowledge of your reproductive system and understand how the menstrual cycle works.

Like many women, my understanding of my reproductive system was somewhat vague, based mainly on those junior high films about getting your first period (films that somehow forever linked menstruation in my mind with going to the prom) and the inserts in tampon boxes with the line drawings of uteruses and fallopian tubes that I never could quite picture being part of my own body. I knew a little about PMS, ovulation, the basics. But—20-20 hindsight talking—if I had known a little more, I might have been able to understand what was happening to my body when menopause first began for me, and I would have been able to ask my doctor more penetrating questions from the very beginning.

When I first went to my general practitioner complaining about strange bouts of sweating and sleepless nights, he immediately suggested that I get my FSH level tested. FSH? I had

no idea what he was talking about. I incorrectly assumed it had
something to do with my thyroid, since that was what I thought
was causing my problems. But I now know that FSH is the
abbreviation of follicle-stimulating hormone, one of the crucial
hormones involving ovulation, and that FSH levels can signal
that a woman is going through menopause.

But FSH is only one of the hormones involved in your reproductive system. The entire menstrual cycle is based on the inter-
relation of different hormones, each having different jobs in the
whole process of getting an egg ready for possible fertilization
and implantation. And when you begin premature menopause,
it's the changing levels of those hormones that cause many of
the symptoms and the possible long-term complications.

Let's start at the very beginning, back before you were even
born. When you are still in your mother's uterus, about five
months after gestation, you start out with seven to ten million
eggs. This is the highest amount of eggs you will ever have,
because from this point on you begin losing some of these eggs,
a process that will continue throughout your reproductive life.
By the time you're born, you have about one to two million
eggs. By puberty, you're down to 400,000 eggs—which is still
a huge number! But from puberty to menopause, only about
450 or so of these eggs will actually mature and be available
for fertilization by sperm. As for those other eggs, they keep
disintegrating, the number of them keeps dwindling, so by the
time you begin menopause, you're down to only a few thou-
sand, or even only a few hundred.

During your reproductive years, from puberty to menopause,
your reproductive system revolves around helping the eggs in
your ovaries mature and travel through the fallopian tubes so
they can be fertilized. This is where different glands and hormones come into play. The key players are:

• Your *hypothalamus gland*—The part of your brain in charge
  of your entire endocrine, or glandular, system and the gland
  responsible for releasing GnRH.
• *Gonadotropin-releasing hormone* (GnRH)—In effect the master

hormone in your reproductive system, since it signals your pituitary gland to release two *other* crucial hormones, FSH and LH.

- Your *ovaries*—Probably the most important gland in your body where reproduction is concerned; your ovaries have two main jobs: manufacturing the key female hormones estrogen and progesterone, and producing eggs.
- *Follicle-stimulating hormone* (FSH)—Stimulates development of follicles (the sacs holding eggs in your ovaries).
- *Luteinizing hormone* (LH)—Causes the follicle to rupture and the egg to be released, then changes the ruptured egg sac to the *corpus luteum*, which releases progesterone.
- *Progesterone*—The pregnancy-preparation hormone (the word "progesterone" means "for pregnancy"), it is responsible for making your uterine lining more receptive to an egg and making your body in general better prepared for pregnancy by increasing your appetite, your fluid retention, and your metabolic rate. It also signals the pituitary gland to stop releasing more FSH and LH, and so prevents more follicles from growing.
- *Estrogen*—Helps prepare your uterus for possible pregnancy. It's also the hormone responsible for the development and growth of your reproductive organs and breasts, and the hormone that causes women to store fat in their hips and thighs.

All this might sound a little confusing, but it's not as complicated as you may think. Each month your body reacts to different signals from the different glands, causing the different hormones to be released in sequence. The hormones cause the eggs in your ovaries to mature, your uterus to prepare for pregnancy, one egg to be released, and certain other hormones to be released. Then, if that egg doesn't get fertilized, it's back to the beginning of the cycle once again.

How a Typical Menstrual Cycle Works

Here is a brief description of how the key players interact in a typical menstrual cycle *before* menopause:

Your menstrual cycle is usually about 28 days long and is divided into two phases: the *follicular* (or *proliferative*) *phase* and the *luteal phase*. The first half of your menstrual cycle— the *follicular phase*—usually lasts from 10 to 17 days. You enter this phase right after you've had your period. At this point, your estrogen and progesterone levels are at a low point. These low levels trigger your hypothalamus to start a new cycle by producing GnRH, which then signals your pituitary gland to release higher amounts of FSH than LH. The FSH does the job it was named for: it stimulates the growth of follicles to hold eggs, and the follicles begin maturing and producing estrogen. One egg begins to dominate and the other eggs wither away. The follicle keeps pumping out estrogen, which causes the lining of your uterus (or *endometrium*) to thicken in preparation for possible pregnancy. At this point, about 14 days into your cycle, roughly at the midpoint, your estrogen levels reach their cyclical peak. Now it's time for the LH to take over from the FSH.

This is when you enter the *luteal phase*. Your pituitary (acting on orders from the hypothalamus) stops producing FSH and instead sends out a surge of LH. The LH causes the follicle to push against the wall of the ovary and rupture. The egg is released into your fallopian tube, where it can be fertilized if and when a sperm finds it. The burst follicle transforms into the *corpus luteum* (literally, "yellow body"), which is essentially a temporary gland that has about 14 days to do its work. The corpus luteum keeps up estrogen production, but also starts manufacturing increasing amounts of progesterone. The progesterone works with estrogen to help prepare the uterus for a possible embryo—blood supply to the uterus increases, the uterine lining grows thicker, and cells that will nourish the embryo grow. If the egg *isn't* fertilized, there is no need for all of these preparations, so the corpus luteum dies. Your estrogen and progesterone levels nose-dive. Your uterine lining, which is no longer receiving hormonal signals, falls apart. The lining starts shedding, and you get your period. Once your estrogen and progesterone levels hit their monthly low, the hypothalamus begins producing GnRH, and starts the cycle from step one yet again.

What Happens to Your Cycle When Premature Menopause Begins

When you begin going through menopause prematurely, this "normal" menstrual cycle starts to change. The most important reason for this change is the most obvious one: your ovaries are running out of eggs, and those eggs you still have don't respond as readily to the hormonal signals. With fewer eggs, your production of estrogen starts dropping off, as does the monthly surge of progesterone. Your body tries to keep everything going as it always did, in spite of the change in your hormonal levels. But because your ovaries aren't working as they used to, your hypothalamus and pituitary glands go into overdrive—trying to jump-start your system by producing more and more LH and FSH. Your FSH level rises the most dramatically as the pituitary desperately tries to stimulate your follicles to ovulate. Sometimes it works. An egg responds and the cycle continues. Sometimes an egg doesn't respond, but you have enough estrogen still in your system to have *anovulatory* periods, in which no egg is released, but your uterine lining still thickens and eventually sheds.

But over time, even extremely high levels of FSH don't produce enough estrogen for eggs to mature and for your uterine lining to thicken. During this time, you may have shorter cycles; your periods may become erratic—heavy one month, light the next. You may skip periods for several months at a time, then resume them again. Finally, you stop having periods altogether. You're completely in menopause now, and ready to embark on the rest of your life!

FOLLICLE-STIMULATING HORMONE (FSH) LEVELS			
Normal Menstruating			
Follicular Phase	2.5	to	10.2
Midcycle Peak	3.4	to	33.4
Luteal Phase	1.5	to	9.1
Pregnant	0.0	to	0.2
Postmenopausal	23.0	to	116.3
LUTEINIZING HORMONE (LH) LEVELS			
Normal Menstruating			
Follicular Phase	0.8	to	25.8
Midcycle Peak	25.0	to	57.3
Luteal Phase	0.8	to	27.1
Pregnant	<1.4		
Postmenopausal	40.0	to	104.0

THE CAUSES OF PREMATURE MENOPAUSE

Why me?

That was the first question that popped into my mind when I learned I had premature ovarian failure. Then came the other questions: What had caused it? Could I have prevented it? Was it *my* fault?
—Sandra, age 29

When you first learn you are in premature menopause, the questions start coming hard and fast. And often the most confusing question of all is one of the most basic: *How did this happen to me?*

Unfortunately, many women ask this question of doctors who can't answer it. Until recently, unless there was a family history of premature menopause or a history of cancer treatment or surgery, many doctors weren't really sure why it happened. Premature menopause was one of those conditions many doctors termed ''idiopathic''—a technical-sounding term that simply means the condition has no determined cause. But with more research and more attention paid to this condition a number of factors causing premature menopause have been identified.

Why is this important to know? you may wonder. During an on-line chat of the Early Pausers chat group, a support group for younger women in menopause, one person started speculating about the cause of her premature menopause, and another woman asked why it made any difference. "We're already going through menopause," she said. "Who cares why it happened at this point?"

It was an interesting question, and I do understand where it came from. It's one thing to try to find out about a medical problem to *prevent* it. But once you already have something, does it matter why or how you got it?

I believe it does. Knowing why you are going through premature menopause might not make a huge difference once you are already in the middle of the change. It won't prevent what has already happened. But the more you understand the whys and whats of what you are going through, the better you can take control of the situation. Furthermore, knowing the cause may alert you to other potential problems or to treatment possibilities. For example, if you suspect that your premature menopause may be due to an autoimmune disorder, you can be tested to see if this is indeed the cause. If it is, you may be at risk for other autoimmune problems (such as thyroid disease) and you should be tested regularly for this. Moreover, if you want to get pregnant, you may want to look into experimental autoimmunological treatments for women in premature menopause. On the other hand, if you believe there's a hereditary basis for your premature menopause, you may want to discuss this with younger sisters or your own daughter. Finally, having an idea about what may have caused your premature menopause is yet another step in coping with what is happening to you.

Here, then, are the commonly identified causes of premature menopause, both natural and otherwise:

Autoimmune Disorder

This is a cause of premature menopause that is getting a great deal of attention in current research studies. Autoimmune-disorder-linked premature menopause was considered relatively rare in the past, but recent research indicates that it's more common than previously thought. In fact, some recent studies suggest that two-thirds of the incidents of premature menopause may be due to an autoimmune disorder.

An autoimmune disorder means that your body's immune system mistakenly attacks itself. In effect, your body senses part of itself as an invader, so it sends out antibodies to destroy this perceived threat. In the case of premature menopause, you may have antibodies to your own ovarian tissue, to your endometrium, or to one or more of the hormones regulating ovulation. These antibodies attack your reproductive system and may interfere with and ultimately destroy your ovarian function.

Women with autoimmune-caused premature menopause sometimes have or develop *other* autoimmune disorders, such as thyroiditis, hypoparathyroidism, hypoadrenalism, diabetes mellitus, rheumatoid arthritis, myasthenia gravis, and pernicious anemia. By the same token, it's also not uncommon for a woman with one of these autoimmune diseases to find herself in premature menopause. Both you and your doctor should be aware of this possibility, be alert for any symptoms, and do testing, if necessary.

In addition, if your premature menopause does not have an obvious cause such as surgery, cancer treatments, and so on, you may want to be tested for autoimmune disorder—especially if you want to get pregnant, as there are new experimental treatments available that may temporarily restart your reproductive system, allowing you to get pregnant. (This is a relatively new area in premature menopause treatment and is covered in more detail in Chapter 8.)

Surgical Menopause (Oophorectomy or Total Hysterectomy)

This is one of the most common causes of premature menopause, and often one of the most difficult to deal with, since you are coping with the fallout from surgery as well as sudden menopause.

In this case, you experience premature menopause after removal of both of the ovaries (a *bilateral oophorectomy*) or removal of the uterus, both fallopian tubes, and both ovaries (a *total hysterectomy*). Because both of your ovaries are removed, your estrogen and progesterone levels plunge, leading immediately to menopause. Because of this sudden drop, you may experience more intense symptoms than those who go into premature menopause spontaneously.

Ovarian Damage Due to Other Surgical Procedures

Usually, as long as you have at least one ovary, you can continue producing hormones and shouldn't go into premature menopause. But in some cases after a hysterectomy in which one or both ovaries are left intact, one or both of them fail—either immediately after surgery or up to a few years later. This may happen when the ovary or ovaries are damaged or otherwise affected by such procedures as cyst removal or when the surgery damages blood vessels and so interferes with blood flow to the ovaries. In this case, the follicles on the remaining ovary or ovaries slowly die out, resulting in menopause.

Similarly, some women experience premature menopause after *tubal ligation* (getting your "tubes tied," as it's commonly called). Again, this is a result of the surgery interfering with blood flow to the ovaries, causing eventual ovarian failure.

Radiation Therapy and/or Chemotherapy

With the rise in cancer treatments has come a rise in premature menopause due to these treatments. Unfortunately, the significant doses of radiation or chemotherapy used to kill cancer can also damage the ovaries, resulting in premature menopause. There are, of course, variables in the damage done and its results, including the following:

- *Age*—Usually the younger you are when you received these cancer treatments, the less likely your chances for permanent ovarian failure. Since a younger woman has more eggs, more eggs will usually survive. In this case, you may experience temporary ovarian failure but return to normal menstrual periods after treatment. If you undergo chemotherapy when you are over 30, though, you have an 80 percent chance of never getting your periods again, according to studies.
- *Duration of treatment*—In general, the longer the amount of time you underwent treatment, the more likely your chances for ovarian failure.
- *Type of drugs and dosages*—Certain drugs used in chemotherapy, especially cytotoxic drugs, affect your ovaries, stopping menstruation and otherwise disrupting normal ovarian function. These drugs include busulfan and vinblastine; and Cytoxan, chlorambucil and other alkylating agents. More specifically, research shows that approximately 50 percent of women aged 35 or younger and 80 percent of women aged 35 to 44 who have CMF chemotherapy (Cytoxan, methotrexate, fluorouracil) enter menopause as a result of the treatment. Fewer women who undergo Adriamycin chemotherapy enter menopause, but it is still not uncommon.
- *Location of radiation treatment*—If your ovaries or pelvic region in general are irradiated, your reproductive system is almost always permanently, and negatively, affected, leading you to enter premature menopause.
- *Type of cancer you were treated for*—Certain cancers are more likely to cause premature menopause than others. Obviously, cancers in your reproductive organs are the most likely to result in ovarian failure, primarily because these cancers usually result in surgery or in directed radiation. In the case of other cancers, the real key is the dosage and length of

time of treatment. The general rule of thumb: low-dose, short-term treatment tends to result in fewer cases of permanent ovarian failure.

In some cases, especially when you've received low-dose, short-term treatment, you may experience *temporary* menopause due to chemo or radiation therapy. Your ovarian function may stop working regularly, but then return to normal after four months or so. But often, even when your periods return, you remain infertile.

Tamoxifen

Tamoxifen used to be prescribed after you were diagnosed for breast cancer, and, as with other forms of chemo, you would run a risk for premature menopause as a side effect.

But recently doctors have begun prescribing tamoxifen as a preventative to women with a high risk for breast cancer, since it appears to cut breast cancer rates by about 45 percent. While the media has focused on the positive aspects of this drug (and there are many), there is an important potential side effect to tamoxifen that hasn't been played up a great deal: use of tamoxifen can send you into premature menopause. Put briefly, this occurs because tamoxifen is a SERM, or selective estrogen receptor modulator. It attaches to the estrogen receptors in your body. In plain English, it takes the place that estrogen would, and so acts as an estrogen-blocker. Since your body isn't getting the regular amount of estrogen it would naturally get, and since low estrogen levels signal your body to produce more FSH, your body may react by entering menopause prematurely.

Family History of Early Menopause

It's not a hard-and-fast rule, but most women go through menopause at about the same age their mothers did, which means that if there is a family history of premature menopause (your mother, your grandmother, your sister), there's a chance that you too will experience it. Some studies, however, seem to indicate that only about 5 percent of all women who are prematurely menopausal have a family history of this condition. So family history is not necessarily destiny but could be an early indicator if you suspect premature menopause.

Chromosomal Irregularity

Some cases of hereditary premature menopause are caused by defects on an X chromosome. It's a very clinical topic, but here's a brief idea of what happens:

Women have two X chromosomes, inherited from both their father and mother. Even though only one of these chromosomes is active, a defect on either one can cause premature menopause. This defect, sometimes called "fragile X syndrome," apparently interferes with the production of eggs. So if you are a fragile X carrier, you have fewer eggs in your ovaries, which in turn leads to an earlier menopause, generally at least six to eight years before other women. According to a study conducted in the United Kingdom, about 28 percent of women with fragile X syndrome enter menopause before the age of 40. The National Institutes of Health is currently conducting a study to determine exactly how a defective X chromosome causes premature menopause, with the hopes that this will eventually lead to treatment or prevention.

Another related form of genetically caused premature menopause is called Turner's syndrome. In this case, you're born without a second X chromosome or without part of the chromosome. Since you need two Xs for your ovaries to develop properly, a missing X or a faulty X leads to deficient ovarian development (called *ovarian dysgenesis*). Often women with Turner's syndrome never have their periods at all, since their ovaries never develop enough and don't produce ovarian estrogen. On the flip side, some women enter premature menopause because they have *three* X chromosomes—which interferes with ovarian development as well.

Viral Infections

As mentioned before, you begin developing eggs when you are still in your mother's uterus. If your mother contracts a viral infection during this time, it can affect your ovarian development, causing you to be born with lower number of eggs than you otherwise would have had. In this case, since you start with fewer eggs than most women, you run out of eggs more quickly, which results in premature menopause. Similarly, some studies theorize that a small number of women may experience premature menopause if they have had mumps and the infection spread to their ovaries.

THE FALLOUT OF MODERN LIFESTYLES: POSSIBLE CONTRIBUTORS TO PREMATURE MENOPAUSE

There are other factors that some researchers think may contribute to your chances of getting premature menopause. Unlike those mentioned above, these factors probably aren't the main cause of your premature menopause. But as more women are diagnosed with premature menopause than ever before, many doctors believe that modern lifestyle factors may be contributing to the problem.

Lifestyle Habits

Smoking is a factor that is commonly mentioned in discussions about early menopause. We all know smoking isn't good for us, and a number of studies point to smoking as a culprit in earlier menopause than normal. According to these studies, smokers tend to have lower levels of estrogen in their bloodstream. Low levels of estrogen contribute to a decline in ovarian function and, eventually, menopause. But most of these studies actually indicate that smoking will push your menopause earlier by only about two years on average. In other words, smoking may contribute to an earlier menopause than you otherwise would have had, but it probably isn't a key factor in premature menopause. (That said, it is, of course, a good idea for you to quit smoking if you currently smoke—especially since smoking may increase menopausal symptoms and may interfere with your processing of estrogen.)

Alcohol has also been linked in some studies to early menopause. Heavy drinking may contribute to interference with estrogen production and disrupted menstrual cycles. As with smoking, though, it's not a cause of premature menopause, but may help bring menopause a few years earlier than it otherwise would have.

The Stress Factor in Premature Menopause

Stress is another factor that some people think may contribute to premature menopause. But the key word here is *contribute*. When they first learn they're in premature menopause, some women (and I was one of them) immediately blame themselves and their high stress levels. "That's what caused it," they'll say. "I shouldn't have worked so hard," or "I should have relaxed more. It's my fault." But they're blaming themselves needlessly. It's simple: you don't "give" yourself premature menopause by being stressed out. You may, however, increase *symptoms* of premature menopause.

Briefly, stress affects your hypothalamus, the gland that sends signals to the pituitary gland, setting off a chain of hormonal interaction that results in the production of estrogen and progesterone. When your stress levels are high, your hypothalamus overreacts, resulting in excessive release of estrogen. In addition, stress taxes your adrenal glands. They become unable to produce enough stress-relieving hormones, so your body compensates by converting progesterone into those hormones, resulting in low progesterone levels, which, in turn, may throw your menstrual cycle off course. A number of studies have shown that under excess stress, many women miss periods. In addition, if the cause of your premature menopause is an autoimmune disorder, there is a possibility that stress has helped to trigger an autoimmune response. But even in this case, your premature menopause is an autoimmune problem—one that stress may enhance.

The bottom line, then, is a simple one: stress may make symptoms of premature menopause worse and may contribute to the underlying cause of your premature menopause, but it isn't the prime factor.

Environmental Factors

Xenobiotics—synthetic substances that mimic the effects of human hormones on the body—are substances that have been in the news for the past few years. These are chemicals (usually petrochemicals) found in or used to manufacture a wide range of products, including plastics, pesticides, clothing, soaps, computer chips, medicines, and much more. You are exposed to these chemicals not only when you wash your hair or breathe polluted air, but also when you eat pesticide-treated foods or meat or dairy products from animals who were fed pesticide-treated grain. Some researchers believe that exposure to these chemicals may interfere with normal reproductive functioning.

In the case of premature menopause, a specific subset of xenobiotics called *xenoestrogens*—synthetic chemicals that act like estrogen—might play a role in its cause. Because they mimic estrogen and are often more potent than human estrogen, they may either stimulate the hormonal response (in other words, act like a megadose of your own estrogen) or may block the estrogen receptor, thus preventing your own estrogen from doing what it is supposed to do. Studies conducted on animals and birds have indicated that a wide range of problems arise from xenoestrogens, including failed ovarian follicles and abnormal ovarian development. Some scientists have conjectured that there may be a similar effect on humans; however, a definite link between xenoestrogens and premature ovarian failure in women has yet to be proven. For the time being, the jury is still out.

Chapter 2

How Can You Be Sure You Are Going Through Premature Menopause?

The Symptoms and Signs that Can Tip You Off and the Tests You Should Ask Your Doctor For

For several years, I had episodes of sudden sweating during the day, drenching night sweats, insomnia, and up-and-down moods. I figured something was wrong with me, but the thought that it might be menopause never once occurred to me—even though, as it turns out, I was experiencing common menopausal symptoms.

I was lucky enough to have a doctor who immediately suspected premature menopause when I finally went for a check-up. So many other women aren't as lucky. . . .

When you begin going through premature menopause, your body starts sending you messages. But if you're at all like me, you may not know what those messages mean. You may think that it's all due to stress, or just have a nagging feeling that something is wrong but have no idea what the something is.

It makes sense, really: because you're young and aren't thinking about menopause, you don't put two and two together. Instead, you come up with a hundred other reasons for the symptoms you're experiencing. You missed a period? It's because you've been tense, you tell yourself. You've got insomnia? Well, there's too much on your mind. Your menstrual cycle is irregular? Maybe you just made a mistake in counting the days. You've been weepy lately? It must be PMS. You can keep coming up with reasons, but never hit on the right one.

The clues can be staring you right in the face, but if you don't know that they're clues, you can't figure out what they mean. That's what happened in my case. I had heard about hot flashes, and knew that women going through menopause often got them. But even though I was inundated with sweat dozens of times during a day, I never once realized I was having hot flashes! I thought that I was just . . . well . . . sweating for some strange reason. I didn't realize I was experiencing one of the most common symptoms of menopause. So I didn't put it together with the fact that I was also skipping periods every now and then, having trouble sleeping, and going through mood swings. Yet all of these signs—and many others—pointed directly to premature menopause.

> **For four years, I was going through such weird things. Panic attacks, hair loss, migraines, moodiness. I would go to the doctor and get sent for tests, X rays, CAT scans. Everything was normal. When I asked about the possibility of menopause, the doctor immediately said it couldn't be that. I was too young. So I believed him, kept my mouth shut, went home like a good little girl—and kept feeling rotten.**
> **—Jenny, age 37**

> I had many symptoms which I didn't know could be related to menopause or early menopause, starting in 1992 (I was aged 32) after getting pregnant while on birth control pills and having a blighted ovum. I had a D&C after miscarrying "the remains" (umbilical cord, placenta, etc.) and had a severe pelvic infection because of the "remains" not being removed immediately. My ob/gyn at the time said I had a choice when the blighted ovum was discovered in my fourth month. I could let things happen naturally or have a D&C immediately. I opted for nature taking its course, but it took another two months to do anything. By then I guess I was pretty infected . . . I had

to be admitted to the hospital for 24-hour IV antibiotics (which I think came close to destroying my immune system at that point).

Anyway, at first I thought I was just emotionally distraught over the miscarriage (though I'm not an overly emotional person and tend to think there's a positive aspect to every negative event), but I felt absolutely bizarre physically and mentally/emotionally for a few years. It took me that long to try to figure out what might be going on. I went to a myriad of doctors who never came up with a diagnosis. Every time I mentioned hormonal imbalance to one of them they patronizingly grinned and said I was too young to have hormonal problems.

—Bryana, age 38

Sometimes you may be experiencing a number of menopausal symptoms and go to your doctor wondering about menopause, only to run into a roadblock. Your doctor doesn't pick up on the clues. This happens to many women in premature menopause. They suspect something is wrong and ask their doctor if it could be menopause, only to be told: "That's impossible. You're much too young!"

This is unfortunate. As I mentioned before, you're definitely *not* too young—millions of women in their twenties and thirties go through menopause prematurely. This makes it all the more important that you be aware of the signs of premature menopause. You might not be able to count on your doctor to be aware of what may be happening with you, and you might have to ask for tests to determine if you are in premature menopause or not.

I first suspected I was in premature menopause when I was working in an ob/gyn office, listening to women in their fifties telling me their symptoms. I remember thinking, "I'm having these exact same problems!" My gyn/oc of more than nine years was not open to my thoughts. I was "stressed" and should "see a psychiatrist." Even hearing my symptoms and knowing my medical history (ovarian cancer treatment and wedge resection surgery), he was reluctant to even consider menopause. He wouldn't even order the blood tests. So, I asked the ob/gyn I was working for at the time. She had me stop my birth control pills for three months, then have an FSH and LH drawn. The results were: FSH 130, LH 69! I called my gyn/oc and he said, "Yep, you're in menopause!" Well, thank you very much!

—Steph, age 28

This chapter covers both the signs of premature menopause and the tests that can back up those signs. You now know how your hormones interact, both before and during premature menopause. Here we look at how the changes in your hormone levels affect how you feel, and how your body signals you that you are going through premature menopause—the physical and emotional symptoms you may experience as your reproductive system cycles down, and what you can do about them.

Some of these signs are obvious ones—changes in your period, hot flashes, and more; others are not as easy to pinpoint (especially the vague emotional signs), but they're just as real. You may have many of these symptoms or very few. Some women are lucky enough to go through the early stages of premature menopause with little difficulty. Others (like me) get a full onslaught of uncomfortable symptoms. Some women will notice more emotional than physical changes. It varies from woman to woman. There are a few rules of thumb, however: in general, if you are overweight, you will probably have fewer symptoms, since estrogen is produced by fat cells. If you smoke, you may often experience more or more obvious menopausal symptoms, because smoking interferes with the production of and processing of estrogen. And if you have undergone surgical menopause, usually you'll find that your symptoms are much more intense—the result of having a sudden drop in your estrogen levels as opposed to a tapering off.

But the bottom line is a simple one: listen to your body. The physical and emotional symptoms described in this chapter are telling you something. They're telling you that your hormones are shifting, that your body is changing, that, yes, you may be going through premature menopause.

The key, of course, is knowing what the signs are, knowing how to read them and knowing what you can do about them. This chapter should help you do just that.

> Learning I was in premature menopause hit me like a ton of bricks, but if I look back over the past 10 years, reviewing my difficulties getting pregnant, several surgeries for endometriosis and cysts, shortened cycles, etc., I guess it was only partly out of the blue. By the time I went to my doctor, I knew I had to be menopausal. I had never before missed a period, had missed two in a row, and I was having hot flashes at least once per hour round the clock. My doctor said that although it would be rare (I am 37), it was possible, and she would "work" with me either way.
>
> —Cathy, age 37

IS IT HOT IN HERE OR IS IT JUST ME?
HOT FLASHES, MISSED PERIODS, AND OTHER PHYSICAL SYMPTOMS OF PREMATURE MENOPAUSE

When you start going through premature menopause—probably before you even know that you're going through it—your body begins going through a number of hormonal changes that are translated into physical symptoms, ranging from the very common hot flashes to the less common (but still annoying) upset stomach or itchy, crawling skin.

> The physical symptoms I went through? Hot flashes and cold a lot of the time—temperature extremes. Dehydrated feeling, always thirsty (I'm not diabetic and have no other illnesses), lack of energy, and skin very dry, flaky, and itchy. Eyes very dry also—contact lenses uncomfortable. Periods a week early, 10 days early, heavier, a lot of abdominal

pain. Never had night sweats but had insomnia quite a bit. Fluid retention became a problem—never had before. Have had to have rings cut off fingers. . . . Fluid mostly in hands, feet and abdominal area.
                                        —Bryana, age 38

I have had night sweats, depression, migraines, lack of sex drive, sore breasts, tiredness, low energy level, mood swings, memory loss, no periods . . . I think that covers it all!
                                        —Stacey, age 30

Most of these symptoms are easy to notice if you know what you're looking for. As I mentioned before, it's easy to blame something else for the appearance of these physical signs of premature menopause in your life. Other than having a sudden stop to your periods, you can overlook these symptoms and assume they'll go away eventually. I ignored my hot flashes and night sweats for three years, and, only after I was nagged by well-meaning family members did I go to a doctor. Would it have made a difference if I had learned I was in premature menopause any earlier? Frankly, I don't know. But I *do* know that I would have been able to weigh my treatment options earlier—and I would have been able to free myself from a fair amount of discomfort. And maybe most important, I wouldn't have spent as much time worrying that something was wrong with me.

That's one of the problems with premature menopause. Your body starts doing odd things and you start thinking that you're completely falling apart, going crazy, or seriously ill.

It's not fun. But it really helps when you know that the strange things that are happening to your body aren't uncommon. They're unpleasant, yes, but they're just the effect of going through premature menopause.

To help you determine if you're entering premature menopause, here are the most common physical signs of menopause, why they happen, and some tips on how to cope with them.

One quick note about coping with these physical signs of premature menopause: you'll probably experience many of them for several years until you are completely through menopause. But there are ways to control them—most prominently, hormone replacement therapy (HRT) and alternative methods (herbs, vitamins, and nutrition). Because these topics are covered in depth in chapters 5 and 6, I haven't gone into them here. Instead, this breakdown of symptoms is designed to be more of a checklist of what you can expect when you go through premature menopause, whether you go through it naturally or surgically, and some of the simple things you can do to cope with them.

Irregular Periods

> I started missing periods—I hated that feeling of "am I pregnant?" every month. The doctor checked thyroid, blood sugar, etc. and said it was stress. I asked about the possibility of it being premature menopause, which he quickly dismissed. I was much too young and it is *very* rare (yeah, right . . . !)
> —Cheryl, age 36

Often, since you're not expecting menopause at such an early age, you won't notice that your periods are getting irregular. Sure, you're a few days late, or your flow is lighter or heavier, but since you're not thinking menopause, you can easily overlook these signals. Many women learn that they're going through premature menopause when they keep trying to get pregnant and can't—and finally go to a doctor to see what's wrong. Or you may miss a period, immediately assume that you could be pregnant, take the test and learn that you're not—and wonder why you skipped that period in the first place.

Or you may be like some women who notice that their periods are changing, but have no idea why this is suddenly happening, and assume there's something very wrong with them.

> About four years ago I started having my periods closer together. I discussed this with my doctor of 16 years and she asked me to chart them for a year. After the first year I started skipping one or two from time to time. After this happened a few times I got a little worried, since I was as regular as clockwork for years. For some reason I was convinced I had cancer or something.
>
> —Karen, age 39

A change in your menstrual cycle is one of the first signals that you're going through menopause, a signal that about 80 percent of all women experience. On average most women have about a 28-day menstrual cycle, and usually can count on having their period for about five days. But when you start going through menopause, you can't count on your cycle running normally any more.

Your periods may come more frequently, every 24 days instead of every 28, or they may come later than they used to. You may have a light period that lasts only a few days, then the next month have very heavy bleeding. Your period may last a shorter amount of time, or go on and on for what feels like an eternity. You may skip a month, then go back to normal for several months, then skip two periods in a row. In fact, when you first begin to enter menopause, often the only consistent thing about your monthly menstrual cycle is its *inconsistency*.

This inconsistency mirrors the fluctuation of hormones in your body. In the initial phases of premature menopause, your hormones are erratic, and your periods are reacting to this instability. The type of irregularity you experience is usually a tip-off to what is happening in your body:

- *Shorter cycles* (your period comes more frequently) usually signal that you are producing lower levels of estrogen during your preovulatory stage, and that your FSH levels are higher than normal. With more FSH to stimulate them, your follicles are developing faster, which shortens your cycle.
- *Extremely light periods* usually means that you aren't making enough estrogen to build up your uterine lining. It can also be a sign of an anovulatory period.

- *Extremely heavy bleeding* is also often a sign of an anovulatory period, but in this case, estrogen builds up the uterine lining at the same time as you are producing too little progesterone (since you haven't ovulated and so created a corpus luteum). Without progesterone to stop it, the uterine lining keeps building up until the estrogen production finally drops off and the lining is shed.

Very possibly, you will experience all of the above in the initial stages of premature menopause. Your cycle will vary from month to month—one month light, another month relatively normal, another month heavy.

Then, as your ovaries continue declining and as your eggs dwindle, your menstrual cycle starts cycling down. Over time, even extremely high levels of FSH don't produce enough estrogen for eggs to mature and for your uterine lining to thicken. As you get closer to menopause, your menstrual cycle usually lengthens. Periods come less frequently and there's more time between them. Then you may begin skipping periods. And eventually, in the biggest change in your menstrual cycle, you will stop having periods altogether.

One important point: you should be aware that some irregularities in your menstrual cycle may not be related to premature menopause, but could be a sign of some abnormality, including cancer, polyps, nonmalignant tumors, or fibroids (which are very common when women first begin going through menopause). If you've had a checkup and there's nothing wrong with you, then you know that irregular periods are something you'll have to get used to for a while.

HOW TO COPE

It's one thing to read about these changes with your period and another to experience them. One of the most annoying things about having irregular periods is the feeling of being out of control. In the past, you probably could count on your period coming at a set time.

Now you have no idea when it will come—or even if it will come. And when it does come, you may be flooding or barely spotting. The bad news is that there really isn't much you can do to get your irregular periods back to normal. But you can get at least a little control back:

- Since you may be dealing with this for a few years, it's a good idea to *keep tampons or sanitary napkins with you at all times,* just in case your period sneaks up on you out of nowhere. This is especially important if you've skipped periods, because you can't be sure when your cycle will suddenly start up again. I remember going to a wedding after I hadn't had a period in three months, when I suddenly I had an unwelcome surprise. Of course, I hadn't brought any protection—after three months without a period, I had assumed (incorrectly) that that was that. Well, it wasn't, and I had to spend some frantic minutes discreetly asking other female guests if they had a tampon I could use. After that, I made sure to keep carrying tampons even when I had been period-free for a few months.

- *Start keeping a menstrual calendar when you notice your cycle is getting irregular.* It sounds annoying, but it isn't as difficult as you may think. Just jot down the basic information—when your period comes, how heavy or light it is, any unusual cramping, and the like—on a calendar, date book, or a plain piece of paper. Not only will this allow you to see if there are any trends in your cycle (time between periods is getting longer, periods are shorter in duration, and so on), but also it's very helpful when you see your doctor. It's difficult to remember the specifics about the past four months of periods when you're sitting in the doctor's office. Having a calendar enables you and your doctor to better assess your condition. It may also alert your doctor that you're experiencing problems other than premature menopause.

- *Finally, if you're frequently having very heavy bleeding, you may want to talk to your doctor about some form of treatment.* Taking progesterone for the second half of your cycle often helps reduce bleeding and regularize your period. It can also help with the bloated PMS feeling you may be getting more strongly than in the past, and will prevent your endometrium (uterine lining) from building up excessively. But taking progesterone isn't risk-free and it doesn't work well for everyone, so be sure to discuss all possible side effects with your doctor. Your doctor may also prescribe a low-dose birth control pill to regularize your periods—but again, be aware of any potential side effects.

Infertility Problems

I had been trying for about three years to get pregnant . . . but it didn't happen. I went to an infertility clinic to see if they could help. I thought I would get a prescription for Clomid or one of the other fertility drugs. Instead I was told that I had premature ovarian failure—and that donor eggs were my only chance for pregnancy.

—Rita, age 34

Possibly one of the most upsetting clues that you're in premature menopause is the inability to conceive. You may still be having your period, you may still assume everything is perfectly normal—but you just can't get pregnant. Or you may be noticing irregular periods and assume there's something else wrong with you and never think it's menopause.

Many women learn that they're in premature menopause when they go to their doctor or reproductive endocrinologist to determine why they're not getting pregnant. Usually when you first ask about infertility problems, your doctor gives you a test to determine baseline levels for follicle stimulating hormone (FSH) and luteinizing hormone (LH). It's the level of your FSH that typically indicates whether you are in menopause. This test (and others) is discussed later in this chapter.

HOW TO COPE

This is one of those situations where there is little you can do on your own other than consult with a doctor—more specifically, a reproductive endocrinologist or infertility clinic—to determine the different options available to you. One thing to make clear: premature menopause doesn't necessarily mean you'll never have a child. There are options open to you, such as donor eggs or adoption. In addition, some women in premature menopause do have children with their own eggs, either spontaneously or through medical treatment. Chapter 8 discusses these different options, ranging from donor eggs to experimental autoimmunotherapy to adoption and more, and lists sources where you can find more information.

Beyond this, perhaps the best way to begin coping with possible infertility is to begin researching the different options open to you in terms of having a child on your own. I found it helpful to read up on different infertility treatments, specifically those recommended for premature menopause, so I could more easily discuss them with a doctor. (Among the most helpful Web sites with useful information are www.INCIID.org and www.fertilitext.org.) I also began reading about adoption to see what my options were in that area.

All in all, this is one of those symptoms that there is no quick fix for, but if you take the time and do a little research, you may be able to discover the right way to proceed.

Hot Flashes

> I had hot flashes so bad I used to say I could melt Antarctica just by lying on it!
> —Steph, age 28

> The hot flashes were really bad before starting the remefemin [black cohosh, an herb used for menopausal symptoms]. Sometimes they were so intense that I would almost black out.
> —Karen, age 39

You're sitting quietly reading or watching television, minding your own business, doing nothing out of the ordinary, when—boom! A heat wave rises up from your neck and shoulders, your face turns red, and sweat starts pouring. Then, just as suddenly, the heat recedes and you feel normal again. Welcome to the not-so-wonderful world of hot flashes—one of the best-known signs of menopause, and definitely one of the most annoying.

Most people have heard of hot flashes and know them as the trademark symptom of menopause. About 75 to 85 percent of American women are estimated to get hot flashes when they're in menopause. And where *premature* menopause is concerned, hot flashes tend to be even more prevalent. Many studies indicate that if you go through natural menopause before the age of 51, you have an *increased* chance of having hot flashes. It's even more common for women who have had their ovaries surgically removed—about 80 to 90 percent of these women typically get hot flashes. To make matters worse, hot flashes may be more intense physically for those of us in premature menopause (especially if your premature menopause is caused by surgery or cancer treatments) and they can definitely be more troublesome emotionally. As if it's not enough that you have to deal with the psychological blow of knowing you're in menopause prematurely, something that you didn't expect for a decade or two, you *also* have to cope with the feeling that your hot flashes are advertising the fact to everyone. When you're sitting and talking with friends, then start pouring sweat for no apparent reason, you sometimes feel as if you are wearing a sign: "Look at me! I might be young, but I'm menopausal!"

I would be teaching in front of the classroom and I could feel a hot flash coming on. It was embarrassing—all those people looking at me and I would be dripping sweat even if it was cold in the room. I kept hoping no one noticed, but I was sure they did. I mean, they'd have to be blind to have missed it.

—Anna, age 31

Like irregular periods, hot flashes are often one of the first signs you'll have that your reproductive system is changing. In fact, they may begin before you even notice any menstrual irregularities. I started having hot flashes years before anything else seemed different with my body, and they continued long after other symptoms appeared.

Usually, though, hot flashes are most apparent during the first two years, and taper off over time. Some women have hot flashes throughout their lives (don't worry, though—this is very uncommon!), but most women have them for about four years.

So what exactly *is* a hot flash, and why do we have them?

Scientists aren't exactly sure, but apparently it's all the fault of the hypothalamus, the gland that is in charge of your entire endocrine system, and also regulates your body temperature. Usually when your body starts getting too warm, the hypothalamus sends out a signal to cool down, telling your heart to pump more blood, blood vessels to dilate and let out heat, and your skin to perspire. It's your body's air-conditioning system at work, and it works very well—until you begin menopause. When you're in menopause, your estrogen production decreases, which affects the body temperature regulator in the hypothalamus. Instead of sending out the "cool down" signal when your body normally gets hot, it starts turning on the air conditioner at inappropriate times. In effect, it resets your body's thermostat, causing the cooling reaction at a lower temperature than in the past. Your body responds by going through the dilation of blood vessels and sweating in an effort to reset its thermostat back to its normal temperature. In other words, you get a hot flash.

That's the scientific side. Here's what it translates to in your body: hot flashes usually start with a hot, prickly feeling in the middle of your back. A heat wave then rises to envelop your back, chest, neck, face, and scalp. Your skin temperature can rise by up to 8 degrees. Often if you touch your skin, it actually feels hot as though you've been out in the sun. Your pulse shoots up and you start sweating as your body tries to cool itself down. Sometimes you get a flush—your face, neck, and chest turn pink or even deep red. And very often, you suddenly shift from feeling incredibly hot and sweaty to feeling very chilled, even shivering.

> **Every night I would get drenched. I would wake up in the morning with the worst case of bad hair since it had matted from all the sweating. I had circles under my eyes. Worst of all, I didn't know why I was getting these night sweats. I looked them up in a medical symptoms encyclopedia and the one thing I kept noticing was that night sweats were a sign of cancer. I actually spent a few months convinced I had cancer—which only made me have more trouble sleeping!**
> **—Elizabeth, age 29**

You may also get the nighttime version of hot flashes, *night sweats*. Technically a night sweat is the same as a hot flash—another example of your internal thermostat running amok because of reduced estrogen levels. But for me and other women I've spoken with, there was a marked difference with night sweats. When I had a hot flash during the day, the heat and sweating was restricted to the middle of my back and up. When I had night sweats, *everything* poured sweat—even my knees. Night sweats are particularly debilitating because they interfere with your sleep. You may wake up numerous times during the night feeling overheated. You toss off the covers to cool down, then have to pull them back on when the sweat passes because you're freezing. Your sheet, pillow and nightgown may get wringing wet. In fact, many women have to get up in the middle of the night to change nightgowns. And you wake up in the morning feeling as though you haven't slept at all.

As you would imagine, there's also an emotional toll to dealing with hot flashes and night sweats. Not only might you feel like you are advertising your menopausal state, but you also might find it difficult to remain psychologically cool when your body is on fire. Many of the emotional signs of menopause (which are listed later in this chapter), such as irritability, the feeling of being out of control, and extreme fatigue, are either

HOW TO COPE

The good news about hot flashes is that they can be controlled by HRT and also to varying degrees by herbs, vitamins, natural supplements, and other alternative methods, covered in chapters 5 and 6. But there are some other things you can do to help deal with these so-called "power surges."

- *Try to reduce stress*—It's not easy when you're bright red and sweating dozens of times a day, but keeping as calm as possible actually helps cut down on the number of and severity of hot flashes, while stress increases them. If you find yourself getting stressed out and feel that telltale prickly heat sensation at the back of your neck, breathe deeply, close your eyes, even try mental imagery—just try to let all your tension out, and often your hot flash will burn out more quickly.

- *Watch what you wear*—Natural fibers breathe better than synthetics, which helps when you're in the throes of a hot flash. Wear layers, so you can peel off outer garments when a hot flash hits and put them back on when you get a chill. Loose-fitting clothes also usually help your body cool off faster. And avoid restrictive clothing like turtlenecks.

- *Exercise*—A recent study indicated that aerobic exercise helps temporarily raise your estrogen levels, which in turn helps prevent hot flashes.

- *Cut back on caffeine, alcohol and spicy foods*—These have all been linked to hot flashes.

- *Stay cool at night*. Have cold water by your bed ready to drink at the first sign of a sweat. Use cotton sheets and cotton nightclothes (I found men's T-shirts to be the best—cool and absorbent!). As with your clothing, sleep under layers, so you can kick off extra bedcovers when you get hot and replace them when the chills start.

- *Splash cold water on your face or wrists when a hot flash starts*—This helps your body cool down more quickly.

tied to hot flashes or made even worse by them. And because your heart rate often increases when you're having a hot flash, it's even easy to fall into a full-fledged hot-flash-induced anxiety attack.

But no matter how unpleasant it all is, most of us going through premature menopause will have to deal with hot flashes. The severity and frequency of them, though, varies from person to person. You may get hot flashes only during the day; or only get night sweats; or you may be in for a double whammy (like me) and get both. You may get dozens of hot flashes each day or only a few—or only a few each month. About a third of all women get 10 or more a day. Some lucky women don't get full-fledged hot flashes, but just get a slightly warm feeling every now and then.

In general, though, there are a few rules of thumb: in the very early stages of premature menopause, most women start with a mildly overheated feeling as opposed to full-fledged hot flashes. Hot flashes usually worsen when you stop having your period and your estrogen levels drop. If you are in premature menopause because of surgery or cancer treatments, chances are you'll suffer with worse hot flashes because of the suddenness of your hormonal change. Smokers also tend to have worse hot flashes, probably because smoking affects estrogen production. On the plus side (no pun intended), heavier women generally have a better time with hot flashes than thin women. Aside from these specifics, however, overall hot flashes are a fact of life where premature menopause is concerned.

Vaginal Dryness and Atrophy

> I started having problems with sex. It was real painful. I felt like I had sandpaper or something in there. I didn't realize it was part of my POF. I was clueless—and very uncomfortable. It even started hurting to use a tampon.
> —Celia, age 26

This is a decidedly upsetting aspect of menopause in general, and all the more psychologically draining when you're in menopause prematurely. When your vaginal tissues begin drying and atrophying, sex becomes uncomfortable, you may be more prone to infections, your vagina is frequently itchy and easily irritated, and, on the emotional side, you may feel older. Even the words sound distressing: atrophied vagina.

Often you start noticing this symptom at the worst possible moment—when you're having sex. Suddenly it seems to take forever to get aroused, or you find yourself wincing a little bit during intercourse. You may even start getting insecure about sex in general. Unfortunately, though, this is one of those symptoms that many women often don't talk about with their friends, their mates, even their doctors, because it is so personal and a little embarrassing. But it's important to be aware that this is a common sign of menopause, not a reflection on your sex appeal, desirability, or libido.

Vaginal dryness and vaginal atrophy occur when your estrogen levels drop. Your vagina is usually very elastic, able to easily stretch for sex and childbirth. But as estrogen levels diminish, your vaginal walls get thinner and lose some of their elasticity. Your vagina becomes dryer and takes longer to become lubricated. Ultimately, it may atrophy, becoming somewhat smaller in width and length. If you experience a sudden drop in estrogen (as you do with surgical menopause), these vaginal symptoms might appear more suddenly than if you go through a natural premature menopause. Either way, though, it's a very unpleasant side effect of going through menopause— and very upsetting when you're in your twenties or thirties.

I was unlucky enough at the time to have a doctor who didn't have much of a bedside manner. He was examining me and very bluntly said: "Wow. I can tell you've been going through premature menopause for a while. Your vagina is really atrophying." As you can imagine, it was a real emotional blow to hear it put so flatly. I immediately felt like a cartoon of an old, withered crone.

Obviously, both the physical and emotional repercussions of vaginal drying and atrophy are strong. You may find it takes longer and longer to get sexually aroused. Sexual stimulation that you used to enjoy may become unpleasant instead of arousing. Intercourse can be very uncomfortable, even painful. In a worst-case scenario, your vagina may even tear during intercourse. All in all, sex may become less and less pleasurable, making you feel even worse about being in premature menopause. I remember I began thinking that, at the not-so-ripe age of 38, my days of enjoying sex were over. I was very glad when I learned that I was wrong.

That's the good news where vaginal dryness is concerned: it is one of the most treatable symptoms of menopause and it's very often completely reversible.

HOW TO COPE

When you raise your estrogen levels through HRT, your vaginal tissues generally improve dramatically. In addition to standard estrogen replacement therapy (by pills or patches) you can also use a vaginally inserted estrogen cream specifically to deal with vaginal dryness and atrophy. But there are other things you can try as well:

- *Have more sex*—It's one of the simplest and probably most fun ways of combating vaginal dryness. Regular sex helps prevent vaginal dryness. If you reach orgasm once or twice a week, either with a partner or through masturbation, you increase blood flow to your vagina and keep its muscles toned, all of which help keep the vagina in shape. In addition, some scientists believe that sex may actually help stimulate estrogen production in the adrenal glands.

- *Use a lubricant to help with dryness*—such as Astroglide, Lubrin, or K-Y jelly, or a product that enhances vaginal moisture such as Replens. You can also increase your own lubrication by having more foreplay, which gives your body time to get sexually aroused.

- *Avoid anything that can irritate or dry your vagina*—including perfumed bath oil or bubble bath and perfumed toilet papers.

- *Also avoid antihistamines and decongestants*—These are designed to help dry out mucous membranes in your respiratory system, but also will dry out mucous membranes in your vagina.

Bladder Control Problems

> I started noticing that I had to go to the bathroom more
> often than I ever had. I started waking up in the middle
> of the night with this amazing urge to pee—and I'd liter-
> ally run to the bathroom. Then I noticed that a little pee
> would slip out every now and then, like when I jogged. I
> flipped out—I thought I'd be starring in one of those June
> Allyson ads for adult diapers.
> —Cindy, age 31

This sign of menopause is connected with vaginal dryness
and atrophy—and, honestly, it sounds much worse than it is.
You're *not* going to suddenly have to start wearing Depends.
You may, however, notice that you have to urinate more frequently or with more urgency, or you may have *urinary stress
incontinence*—little leaks when you exert yourself. Again, this
is a function of lower-than-normal estrogen levels. When you're
a developing embryo, your bladder and urethra are formed from
the same tissues as your vagina. So, just as your vagina loses
muscular tone and elasticity when estrogen production lags,
your lower urinary tract does as well. The lining of your urethra
becomes thinner, and the surrounding muscles become weaker.
As a result, when you place stress on your bladder through
coughing, sneezing, laughing, or strenuous exercising, you may
release a tiny bit of urine. And it is usually only a tiny amount,
so there's no need to imagine a real disaster.

If you're experiencing severe urinary incontinence, though,
do see a doctor. A small degree of bladder control difficulty is
common in the early stages of menopause, but a greater degree
of difficulty can be indicative of another problem—one that may
require drugs or even surgery. If it's mild, however, chances are
it's connected with your depleted estrogen. Even so, though,
it's probably wise to check with your doctor to be sure there
is no other cause. Frequent urination may be a sign of bladder
infection or diabetes, for example. All in all, it's a good idea
just to be sure that what you're experiencing is just another
sign of menopause and not something else.

HOW TO COPE

Since bladder control problems are often a result of low estrogen levels, taking estrogen generally helps and may completely reverse any symptoms. But there are other things you can do:

- *Try Kegel exercises*—exercises specially designed to help strengthen the muscles around the vagina and bladder opening. An added bonus: since Kegels help your vaginal as well as your bladder muscles, they also can improve your sex life. Start by locating the pubococcygeal muscle (which is tougher to pronounce than it is to find!). This is the muscle on your pelvic floor that stops the flow of urine when you squeeze it. So the simplest way to find it is to try stopping your flow of urine while urinating *without* using your abdominals or buttocks muscle. Concentrate, and you should feel a definite squeezing/tightening sensation deep inside your pelvic region. If you're not sure if you've used the right muscle, put your finger in your vagina and try again—if your vagina tightens around your finger, you've found it.

  Once you've located the muscle, squeeze and release 10 times slowly. You can do these quickly or slowly—it doesn't make any difference. The key is to focus and be sure you squeeze as tightly as possible and relax as much as possible, and repeat these ten muscle squeezes at least *five* times a day. Over time, you should build up the number of repetitions to 15 to 20 squeezes each time or do the 10 squeezes up to 10 times a day. You should make Kegels a habit. Do them when you're reading, watching TV, standing on line, wherever. No one can see you do them, so you can exercise anywhere, anytime.

- *Cut back on caffeine and alcohol*—Both make you urinate more frequently.

Insomnia/Disrupted Sleep

> I don't think I had a good night's sleep in over a year. I don't know how many nights I would lie there, looking at the ceiling and wishing I were asleep.
> —Jenny, age 37

> I am the insomnia queen! I wake up every night at about three o'clock, and that's it. Even when I manage to fall back asleep for a few hours, I feel like I stayed up and partied all night.
> —Sarah, age 28

If you're waking up a lot at night, tossing and turning, and generally suffering with insomnia, it might be connected with menopause. When you begin going through menopause, you may find that your sleep is less and less restful—when you sleep at all. In the past, doctors believed that interrupted sleep was a consequence of night sweats, but recent studies indicate that you can also have problems with sleep that aren't connected to hot flashes. Typically, the frequency of insomnia doubles from the amount you may have had before you entered premature menopause. And research also indicates that women begin to experience restless sleep as many as five to seven years before entering menopause. Again, though, the problem is recognizing that the insomnia you're suffering from has its roots in changes in your hormone levels.

I noticed sleep problems shortly after I had hot flashes, but before I had night sweats, and I attributed my insomnia to stress. The problem is when you're getting terrible sleep, you *do* wind up getting more stressed, not to mention moodier and more irritable—all of which are also menopausal symptoms—since you're not getting enough REM sleep (the deepest, most rejuvenating type of sleep). It sometimes winds up being a vicious circle—you can't sleep, so you get more stressed out, which makes you less able to sleep, and so on.

HOW TO COPE

As with many of the other symptoms, HRT and alternative therapies often work well. In addition, disturbed sleep patterns often level off after a few years. But, of course, you probably don't want to wait a few years. You may want to try the usual tips for getting better sleep:

- *Drink an herbal tea such as chamomile before going to bed.*

- *Other herbs such as valerian are natural sedatives that may help—* A recent double-blind study found that nine out of 10 people using valerian reported better sleep. But valerian may increase the effects of other sedatives, so as with any herbal or medicinal remedy, you should check with a doctor before trying it.

- *Avoid caffeine, alcohol and other stimulants before bedtime—*And avoid strenuous exercise close to your bedtime.

- *Keep your bedroom cool.*

Palpitations

My chest was heaving, my heart was going a hundred miles a minute—and I thought I was having a heart attack or something. I went to the doctor, had an EKG, then an echocardiogram, and my heart was fine. But it kept happening. I didn't know what was wrong with me.
—Suzy, age 37

It's a frightening sensation that may happen at the same time as a hot flash or by itself: for no obvious reason, your heart suddenly starts pounding, racing faster and faster. You can be sitting calmly or lying in bed just before going to sleep, and it comes out of nowhere. Sometimes it makes you so nervous that it can blow up in to a full-fledged panic attack. And if you don't know that you're going through premature menopause and that palpitations are often a sign of menopause, you can think there's something seriously wrong with you.

But palpitations are another not-so-fun sign of menopause—and one that many women experience. Do keep in mind, though, that they may signal something else, such as hyperthyroidism or mitral valve prolapse, so don't automatically write off palpitations as a sign of premature menopause. Talk to your doctor to rule out any other, possibly more serious, conditions.

If you get a clean bill of health, there's a good chance that the palpitations are connected with your premature menopause. This is one of those symptoms, though, that some doctors don't associate with menopause, so don't be surprised if your doctor tells you that it must be stress (that catchall condition) causing your heart troubles. If you've had palpitations in the past, they may get worse when you begin going through menopause.

HOW TO COPE

- *The best thing to do is probably the hardest thing to do: calm down*—Don't get nervous when you get palpitations, since that often makes them worse.

- *In general, try to keep stress at a minimum*—(I know this is easier said than done when you're going through premature menopause, but if it's at all possible, it's a very good idea.) Palpitations often occur when you're stressed out or when you need sleep, so anything you can do to relax will help.

- *Try relaxation techniques when palpitations hit*—Such as deep breathing, imagery, and so on (see Relaxation Techniques below).

- *If you smoke, consider quitting*—Smoking often exacerbates palpitations.

- *Limit the amounts of alcohol and caffeine you consume.*

RELAXATION TECHNIQUES

The following techniques can help you control stress, which will help fight palpitations and other symptoms exacerbated by stress.

Meditation and Mental Imagery. A proven stress-buster—many scientific studies show that regular meditators have lower blood pressure, better heart function, and are much calmer. Regular meditators react better to stress as measured by stress chemicals like norepinephrine in their blood.

You don't have to become a yogi to learn how to meditate effectively. Just sit quietly with your back erect, eyes closed, and hands on your lap. You may want to touch your thumb to your index finger, but it's not necessary. Now begin breathing slowly and deeply through your nose, inhaling slowly, then exhaling. Count your breaths or quietly repeat a word to yourself—it can be a religious word or phrase, depending on your religion, or even a nonsense word that sounds relaxing. Focus on emptying your mind of all thoughts. Some people find that creating a mental picture in their minds works better. They close their eyes and imagine themselves on a beach, or by a lake or wherever. If unwanted thoughts and worries come into your mind, don't force them out, just let them gently float away and resume concentrating on your breathing and the word or image in your mind. After about twenty minutes or so, gradually come out of this state, sit with your eyes closed for a few minutes, and then get up. Do this once or twice every day, preferably at the same time. Make it a habit!

For many people, the first few times meditating are unsatisfying, but if you persist, you'll probably find that emptying your mind becomes easier and easier, and that you're calmer and more relaxed, even under the worst stresses.

Deep Breathing. Ever notice that when you become nervous or scared, you start breathing more rapidly? In fact, some people under stress breathe so rapidly that they have a panic attack and hyperventilate. Deep-breathing techniques work on the opposite principle—if you learn to breathe slowly and deeply, you can reverse your panics and fears.

Deep-breathing exercises are similar to, or often identical to, meditation. Sit (or lie) quietly, and breathe through your nose. Breathe deeply, pulling air deep into your lungs, then exhale just as deeply, emptying as much air as possible. Some people call this *belly-breathing* because it feels as if air is coming from deep inside your stomach. Continue to do this slowly for 10 to 20 minutes. As with meditation, you'll find that regular deep breathing makes you calmer. And you'll find yourself breathing more deeply at other times as well, creating better health.

Muscle Relaxation: An excellent way of reducing tension. Either sit or lie down. Beginning from your head (or feet), work on tensing and then relaxing each muscle in your body. Tense for a count of 10, then relax, then move on to the next muscle. As with other techniques, try to do this regularly.

Emergency Techniques: Any of these techniques can be used for a quick stress reliever when you suddenly feel overwhelmed at work or at home. Or if you're out in public and suddenly confronted by a rude store clerk or an angry driver, instead of getting angry, try this: count to 10, breathing slowly and steadily. It's amazing how this simple technique can give you the right perspective in a stressful situation.

Weight Gain

> I noticed weight gain in the beginning. I gained approximately 35 pounds. I am small-boned and typically slender. I was devastated and confused. My eating and exercise habits hadn't changed, yet my body did.
> —Steph, age 28

I went through a similar scenario to Steph's. I had always exercised religiously and hadn't changed my eating habits, so I couldn't figure out where this new little tummy had sprouted from. Then I noticed my waistline begin to disappear. I looked thicker. My body seemed to be changing its shape right before my eyes. It never occurred to me that this had anything to do with the hot flashes or the skipped periods. I just thought I was getting fatter—and nothing seemed to help.

I didn't know then that weight gain—specifically a thickening in your middle—is another sign of changing hormones. While a number of books and doctors claim that menopause has nothing to do with weight gain—that weight gain occurs in menopausal women because they're older and their metabolism is slowing down—other studies indicate that hormone levels are tied to weight gain and redistribution of fat.

This makes sense, since when you're going through premature menopause, you're not middle-aged, so what you're getting isn't middle-aged spread. It's *menopause* spread, for lack of a better term. According to some studies, this occurs for two reasons: first, your progesterone levels are decreasing, and progesterone increases your metabolic rate. So with lower progesterone levels, you have a slower metabolic rate. Second, estrogen is produced and stored in fat cells. So as your estrogen levels drop, your body tries to increase its estrogen by upping its fat cells. Finally, with a drop in female hormones, your body starts mimicking male fat distribution—an apple shape rather than a pear. In other words, you put more weight on in your abdomen than in the past. This accounts for the mysteriously shrinking waistline.

Weight gain with redistribution of fat is one of those signs of premature menopause that is very easy to overlook. Since it happens over a period of time, you might not notice your body shape changing. But if you haven't changed your eating or exercise habits and you've been noticing a new, fatter you, chances are it's related to your hormones.

HOW TO COPE

Yet again, you'll notice a change if you opt for HRT or other natural alternatives. In addition, changes in diet and exercise can help rev up your body's metabolic rate. These are covered in Chapter 9.

Changes in Your Skin: Wrinkling and Loss of Muscle Tone

My skin grew so dry, I noticed wrinkling by age 33 on
my face, hands, and inside of my forearms.
—Bryana, age 38

In my case, I didn't even notice it was happening. But slowly, over time, I would look in the mirror and think I was starting to look different. My facial skin was drier. Little lines around my eyes and mouth were more noticeable. And I looked somehow worn, as though my skin was getting thinner and thinner.

It wasn't in my head, although I sometimes thought it was. When your estrogen levels drop, your collagen production usually slows down as well. And, as you know from reading all the ads for moisturizers and facial creams, collagen is responsible for keeping our skin toned, fresh-looking, and resilient. So when you start running low on collagen, it shows in your skin. It gets thinner, drier, flakier, less youthful-looking.

This is another of those symptoms of menopause that makes you feel older before your time, and in this case, it's clear why. You may *look* a little older than you used to. Worst, this sign often shows up early in menopause. Like bone loss, which occurs rapidly in the first few years of menopause, collagen loss is most rapid at the beginning of menopause as well. According to studies, premature menopause leads to more rapid bone loss than menopause that occurs at the normal age, so it's possible that premature menopause also leads to more rapid collagen loss. The bottom line is, well, *more* lines.

HOW TO COPE

Since this change in your skin occurs because of low estrogen levels, when you take estrogen, you will see a swift improvement. Other than hormone replacement, though, there isn't a lot you can do. Using moisturizers helps somewhat by temporarily plumping up the top layer of skin, but the effect is short-lived. And regardless of advertising claims about "collagen-enriched" creams and so forth, remember that to really work on your skin, collagen must come from within, not be applied from without.

Headaches

I always suffered from terrible headaches. But right about the time I noticed the other changes—the different periods, some hot flashes, etc.—I started getting headaches more often, especially around my period. They got so bad, I had to start taking a prescription for migraines.
—Sherry, age 29

During the early stages of menopause, you may find that you're getting more and worse headaches. This is often caused by your dropping estrogen levels. Many women with regular menstrual cycles get headaches just before their periods or at ovulation. These headaches, sometimes called "menstrual migraines," occur when estrogen levels plunge during the menstrual cycle. So when your body begins slowing down its production of estrogen due to premature menopause, you may start getting these hormonally induced headaches. This can also happen when your progesterone levels are too high in relation to your estrogen levels—a common hormone scenario for women at the beginning of menopause. Generally, these headaches diminish once your hormone levels stabilize.

HOW TO COPE

If your headaches are caused by low estrogen, it follows that taking estrogen may take care of them. But if you suffer from migraines, HRT may actually increase your symptoms. This is covered in Chapter 5.

• *Try standard over-the-counter remedies*—Anti-inflammatories like aspirin or anti-inflammatories/antiprostaglandins like ibuprofen.

- *Certain herbs such as feverfew are also supposed to help*—Recent studies indicate that feverfew is effective for migraines and other headaches; however, as with any herbal or medicinal remedy, it is wise to check with a doctor before using them. In the case of feverfew, be sure to look for products that guarantee at least 0.2 percent of "parthenolide" (the active ingredient) on their label.

- *If the headaches are crippling, talk to your doctor about taking a prescription antimigraine medication*—If you are getting very bad migraines, your only course of action may be taking prescription drugs that specifically help with these intense headaches. Discuss this with your doctor to see if you could benefit from such medication.

Other Physical Signs You May Notice

The following symptoms are less obvious and less common, but still are often signs of premature menopause:

- *Breast Tenderness*—Similar to the feeling you get just before your period; your breasts may feel swollen and tender to the touch. This can last for days or weeks, and unlike the normal breast tenderness from PMS, getting your period often doesn't help relieve this discomfort.
- *Gastrointestinal Distress and Nausea*—Gas, indigestion, heartburn, and a green feeling that comes and goes, and often seems to have no relation to what you've eaten.
- *Tingling or Itchy Skin*—This may feel like the "creepy-crawlies," as if bugs were walking all over you, a burning sensation like an insect sting, or just supersensitivity.
- *"Buzzing" in Your Head*—An electrical feeling that zaps through your head, often occurs with hot flashes. You may also feel this shock sensation under your skin.
- *Bloatedness*—A puffy, bloated feeling that seems to come out of nowhere. Usually you'll notice bouts of this; you'll be fine for a while, then bloated, then okay again. Unlike PMS bloating, this bloating often doesn't diminish after a period.

- *Dizziness/Lightheadedness*—Sometimes comes with hot flashes, sometimes comes for no apparent reason. This may happen due to a higher progesterone level in relation to your estrogen levels.
- *Sore Joints/Muscles*—Similar to flu symptoms or arthritis, this often is connected to estrogen deficiency.
- *Hair Loss or Thinning*—Connected to estrogen deficiency, since the hair follicles need estrogen; some women notice this before any other sign because it is so obvious. You'll notice hair in your brush, your hair may also get drier and more brittle, or you'll notice a thinning or loss of pubic hair.
- *Increase in Facial Hair*—The flip side to the above, you may notice hair growth on your chin, upper lip, abdomen, or chest. This hair is often coarser or darker, as well, and happens when your estrogen levels decrease and your male hormones have a greater effect, or in reaction to high levels of LH.
- *Changes in Body Odor*
- *Dry Mouth and Other Oral Symptoms*—Caused by drying of the mucous membranes due to low estrogen; can include a bitter taste in your mouth and bad breath. You also may notice drying in your eyes and nostrils.

AM I GOING CRAZY?: MOOD SWINGS, "BRAIN FOG," AND OTHER EMOTIONAL SYMPTOMS

I think the worst thing, though, was the night fears. I could not go to sleep at night for hours because I just knew that I was never going to wake up if I did. I never told anyone about this because I thought I was going insane. Then I read somewhere that this sometimes happens with men, and I felt a little better about it. I remember going to my GP and breaking down crying. I told him that I was so tired of feeling bad. I told him about not sleeping and the panic attacks that would make my heart race like crazy. He was great. The first thing he said was:

"You are not going crazy." He told me that all of these things are very real and not just in my head. He assured me that they are normal symptoms.
—Karen, age 39

The emotional symptoms of premature menopause aren't as clear-cut as the physical ones. If you don't know that you're going through menopause prematurely, you may start wondering just what is going on. You're crying about nothing—and it's not the normal time for PMS. You're moodier than you ever used to be. You snap at your husband or your children about the littlest thing, then can't understand why you blew up. And you're more forgetful than you've ever been.

Well, you're not losing your mind. You're not slipping into clinical depression and you're not becoming a witch. What you're experiencing are common emotional signs of menopause.

Many may be related to the physical symptoms you may also be experiencing, such as hot flashes or insomnia. Others may seem to just spring out of nowhere. But they are all a consequence of the changing hormones in your body.

When you think about it, it makes sense that you would experience emotional symptoms when you enter menopause. Research has proven that many women go through mood swings and depression before their periods. So if you can get PMS from hormone swings during your normal menstrual cycle, it follows logically that changes in your hormones due to menopause would also cause emotional symptoms. Add to this the fact that your hormones are making your body go through numerous stressful physical changes, and it's no wonder you may find yourself being unusually moody, irritable, or forgetful.

Unfortunately, some people—even some doctors—may just shrug off these emotional symptoms and say that they're a function of daily stress or that you're exaggerating. But these symptoms are most definitely real for many women when they go through menopause.

Recent research indicates that the emotional symptoms of menopause are related to something called MAO (the enzyme *monoamine oxidase).* When your estrogen levels sink, levels of MAO increase and break down neurotransmitters in your brain, specifically serotonin, which is a mood leveler and elevator. In other words, then, as your estrogen levels drop and MAO levels rise, your brain becomes more prone to depression and moodiness, among other emotional symptoms. Following, then, is a brief rundown of the symptoms you may be experiencing as a result of premature menopause.

> **The mental/emotional symptoms I've had: trouble concentrating (focusing), extremely PMS-y (hated everyone's guts half the month!), wimpy feeling (shortage of confidence in myself, which I never had!), started crying very easily, depressed feelings and anxiety. . . .**
>
> **—Bryana, age 38**

Mood Swings/Sudden Tears/Depression

> **I remember waking up in the morning, feeling completely normal. Then something would set me off—sometimes it was thinking about the fact that I wouldn't be able to have a child, but other times it was nothing at all. My husband would say "good morning," and the tears would start flowing.**
>
> **—Lynda, age 34**

The weepies, supersensitivity, crying jags—whatever you call them, they are a sign of menopause and are often very irritating to deal with. Mood swings are very common for women in menopause. It's like constantly having PMS. You can feel great one moment, then be crying about nothing the next. If you don't know you're in premature menopause, you wonder what is going on. There seems to be no rhyme or reason to your moods. If you *do* know you are in premature menopause, often you are so devastated by the diagnosis that you are depressed to begin with. So not only do you have a tendency to cry, you have a reason to as well.

The culprits? Lack of sleep due to night sweats, and the draining nature of hot flashes. In addition, low estrogen levels contribute to moodiness. For this reason, this symptom is often worse for women in premature menopause due to surgery or cancer therapy, because the estrogen drop is so sudden.

In addition to or sometimes instead of mood swings, you may notice that you're always vaguely depressed. This isn't clinical depression, but a general "blah" feeling. Your energy levels lag, your get-up-and-go is definitely gone, and you can't shake the blues. Again, this seems to be connected to low estrogen levels, not to mention lack of sleep due to night sweats, and the general debilitation of hot flashes. (Note: Some women go into clinical depression, however, marked by such symptoms as exhaustion, suicidal thoughts and change in eating habits. For more information see page 124.)

If you don't know that you're entering premature menopause, it's easy to assume that you're falling into clinical depression, and in many cases, a doctor may prescribe an antidepressant. This is often more medication than you need, since your emotional symptoms aren't due to depression but to hormone levels.

One important point: contrary to past belief, menopause, premature or otherwise, probably doesn't cause clinical depression. Yes, you may get depressed because you are suddenly plunged into menopause years before you expected it, but menopause itself doesn't automatically mean you will be sent into a tailspin of clinical depression. (Chapter 4 covers the emotional fallout of premature menopause and looks at different coping strategies that should help you deal with it.) For this reason, it's important that you determine the cause of your depression. If you're feeling just a little depressed, estrogen will probably be enough to pull you out of your slump. If you're feeling very depressed, and it seems to be completely unrelated to insomnia or hot flashes, then perhaps you should explore other treatments with your doctor.

HOW TO COPE

Moodiness is never a simple thing to deal with, but there are some things you can try that may help. As you would expect, both HRT and natural alternatives can help you level out your mood swings, as do diet and exercise. In addition, you can try the following:

- *Put things into perspective*—Yes, you may feel miserable, but remember that you often feel good and that what you're going through now won't last forever. Try to focus on the positive—the important, enduring things in your life.

- *Don't fight your feelings but go with the flow*—It sounds trite, but it does help to relax. Talking with others—friends, a support group, even a therapist if you feel it necessary—may help.

- *Analyze what sets you off*—You may be able to avoid situations or triggers that make you depressed or upset, or at least understand why you feel the way you do.

- *Exercise*—It's a natural way of releasing tension and raising your spirits. When you exercise, your body releases endorphins, which act like a natural upper. In addition, you'll feel better about how you look, and may reduce physical symptoms as well.

- *Cut back on caffeine and sugar*—Both are stimulants and can make your mood swings more intense. Yes, you'll feel up for a while, but you'll crash when their effects wear off.

- *The herb St. John's Wort may ease depression and level your mood swings*—This herb has recently been the subject of a number of studies and has been proven to reduce some forms of depression. Even better, it appears to have few side effects. Speak to your doctor, though, if you are considering taking it.

- *If your quality of life is severely impaired by moodiness, ask your doctor about prescription antidepressants such as Prozac, Paxil, or Zoloft*—Antidepressants are strong drugs so, of course, it makes sense to use them only if truly necessary. Discuss your different options with your doctor if you feel that you are unable to function well due to moodiness and depression.

"Brain Fog"—Memory Lapses and Loss of Concentration

> I buy Post-it notes by the case, and now every room in
> my house and my car has them stuck everywhere, but
> then I forget what they all mean if I don't write down
> every little detail!
>
> —Marianne, age 40

It sounds funny, but it's actually a little frightening: you
suddenly can't remember the simplest things. You walk into
another room to get something, and stand there wondering just
what it was you were supposed to get. You forget appointments,
phone numbers, names. You feel generally "out of it."

It's easy to think something is drastically wrong with you
when this happens. You're in your twenties and thirties and
you feel as though you're suffering from Alzheimer's. Yet
again, though, what you're experiencing is a sign of menopause.

Studies on this aspect of menopause are uncommon, but those
that have been conducted have determined that low estrogen
levels do seem to have a relationship with short-term memory
loss. The good news? First, there's no effect on long-term memory. Second, these studies show that this short-term memory
loss is improved with hormone replacement therapy and often
disappears after menopause even without HRT.

Brain fog and memory loss can also be related to lack of sleep,
so if you're having night sweats and suffering with insomnia,
chances are you'll also periodically suffer from bouts of them.

HOW TO COPE

- *Don't panic*—The more nervous you are about forgetting things,
  the more you're inclined to forget things.

- *Become a list-maker*—It sounds simple, but it does work.

- *Try to get better sleep*—This might be tough to do if you're suffering
  from night sweats and hot flashes, but better sleep will definitely help
  your concentrative powers and memory ability.

Loss of Libido

> Sex? What's that? Seriously, I haven't been interested in
> sex for a while now. My poor husband . . . I feel sorry
> for him, but I can't get my engine running these days.
> —Marilyn, age 34

This psychological fallout from premature menopause may
be due to two factors. First, it may be caused by decreased
hormone levels—both estrogen and testosterone. Second, you
may find your libido dwindling to nothing because of vaginal
dryness and atrophy. If sex has become uncomfortable and it
takes forever for you to get stimulated, it's easy for you to start
losing interest. Finally, it may happen because of the psychological ramifications of learning that you're in menopause so many
years before you expected.

My sex drive lagged after I was diagnosed with premature menopause, and I assumed it happened because I was depressed about
the diagnosis. But it did resurge, and in retrospect I suspect I went
through the decreased libido because I was upset about the premature menopause and felt old and undesirable, but also because of
my vaginal atrophy. It had been so unpleasant for me that I had
been avoiding it. But once my vaginal tissues were back to normal
due to HRT, and once I had come to grips with the fact that I
was in menopause prematurely, my sex drive perked up again.

HOW TO COPE

In general, it's safe to say that you can easily regain your lost libido.
Usually HRT helps—either regular estrogen and progesterone replacement, or added testosterone as well—This is covered in Chapter
5. In other cases, it's more a matter of time and the acceptance of
your prematurely menopausal situation. Chapter 4, which looks into
the emotional fallout of premature menopause, discusses this issue
at greater length.

In addition, since low libido may be connected with vaginal atrophy, see the suggestions on page 49.

Other Emotional Signs

Some of these other emotional symptoms are related to the others, but for the sake of clarity, they are detailed here.

- *Anxiety*—Feeling ill at ease; sometimes verges on a panic attack or a generalized feeling of "doom"; usually a sign of a chronic sleep disturbance probably due to hot flashes and night sweats.
- *Irritability*—General crankiness that often occurs with lack of good sleep and with changing hormone levels.
- *Extreme fatigue/low energy levels*—Often connected with depression and mood swings; usually occurs as a result of interrupted sleep due to night sweats; also happens with severe, frequent hot flashes.
- *Confusion/lack of concentration*—Again, usually associated with lack of REM sleep, but may also occur as an offshoot of depression.
- *Feeling emotionally detached*—Disconnected, feeling "out of it," as though people and events don't affect you.
- *Food cravings*—Almost like pregnancy or PMS, you find yourself craving certain foods, often carbohydrates, as your body attempts to revive lagging energy.

DIAGNOSTIC TESTS TO DETERMINE IF YOU ARE GOING THROUGH PREMATURE MENOPAUSE

So you think you might be experiencing premature menopause. You've noticed a number of the physical and emotional symptoms, and you suspect menopause might be at the heart of the matter. Now what? How can you be sure that what is happening to you is menopause and not something else? The only way to be sure, as you would expect, is to see your doctor.

Even then, you may run into problems. If your doctor has the knee-jerk reaction that a woman in her twenties or thirties is too young for menopause, you may wind up being misdiagnosed as suffering from anything from stress (the old catchall) to absolutely nothing—the "it's all in your head" diagnosis. This is why it is important for you to know what tests to ask for and what those tests mean.

FSH Blood Level Measurement

This is the key test to determine whether or not you are in menopause. A sample of your blood is taken to measure the levels of FSH in your blood. Because your FSH levels rise when your ovaries stop producing enough estrogen, high FSH levels can signal that your body is entering menopause. FSH levels above 10 to 12 mIU/ml (milli international units per milliliter) indicate that your ovaries are starting to fail. In other words, this means that you are in *perimenopause,* the beginning stages of menopause when you notice physical symptoms, but before you have stopped having a period for a year. Higher FSH levels of about 35 to 40 are usually taken to signal menopause. You may even be getting periods with your FSH levels this high, but it still is a sign that your body isn't producing enough estrogen to maintain regular ovarian function.

If you have stopped having your period, you can get your FSH levels tested at any time. If, however, you are still having a period but suspect menopause because of other symptoms, you should get your blood tested on the third day of your cycle. In addition, many doctors advise having this test more than once if you're still having your period, because there is a slim chance that high FSH levels are temporary. Especially if you're experiencing no other menopausal symptoms, you may be in temporary menopause—an uncommon condition, but one that does happen. Many doctors recommend that you wait a few months and take the FSH test again, or go through other tests to determine your hormonal profile.

In addition, it's important to realize that your FSH levels can and do fluctuate. In my case, they kept going up for a long time. For example, when I first had my FSH levels checked, I hadn't had a period in three months and had a level of 35. I went to another doctor just a month later to double-check whether or not I was actually in premature menopause, and tested at a level of 65. About a month after that, I began getting my period again and thought my body had miraculously snapped back to normal. I went to a reproductive endocrinologist to check about my options where pregnancy was concerned and had blood taken on the third day of my cycle to test. This time my FSH was tested at a whopping 158—basically off the charts where FSH is concerned! In fact, according to several charts in different books, my FSH levels were those of an untreated 80-year-old woman. This is when I realized that charts don't always tell you the whole truth. Obviously, at the age of 38 I was no 80-year-old, yet my FSH levels were high enough to signal that I was technically in ovarian failure in spite of my periods.

Yet again, this hammers home the unfortunate fact that you may indeed be in premature menopause even if you're having periods. Once your FSH levels have reached a certain height for a period of time, it's highly unlikely that they'll drop back to premenopausal levels. In my case, even after my FSH was tested at over 150, I had apparently normal periods for eight months. Then when I was retested, hoping that somehow my body had snapped back to normal, I learned that my FSH level had dropped, but only to 126. Since my FSH levels had been well above 35 for over a year, I finally accepted that I was in menopause.

FSH TEST LEVELS			
	(units per milliliter)		
Normal Menstruating			
Follicular Phase	2.5	to	10.2
Midcycle Peak	3.4	to	33.4
Luteal Phase	1.5	to	9.1
Pregnant	0.0	to	0.2
Postmenopausal	23.0	to	116.3

Estrogen Levels

You may also want to get a serum estradiol concentration test, which measures the amount of estradiol—the primary human estrogen—in your blood. In this case, the doctor is looking to see if your estrogen levels are lower than normal, which is again a signal of ovarian failure or, in other words, premature menopause. Generally, if your estradiol levels are below 36 picograms per milliliter (pg/ml), you are considered menopausal. If your estradiol levels are lower than 50 pg/ml, you may still be having a period but may also be experiencing symptoms of low estrogen, including hot flashes, vaginal dryness, and sleep difficulties.

ESTRADIOL LEVELS	
	(units per milliliter)
Nonmenopausal:	
Follicular Phase	24–138
Luteal Phase	19–164
Periovulatory	107–402
Postmenopausal:	
No HRT	<36
With HRT	18–361

Sometimes your doctor will also test the blood level of the other major human estrogens, estrone and estriol. Again, low levels generally indicate menopause.

Other Ovarian Hormones

It's not necessary to determine whether you are definitely menopausal or not, but depending on your symptoms, you or your doctor may also want to test your levels of the other major ovarian hormones: testosterone, progesterone, and LH.

Low testosterone levels—less than 30 nanograms per milliliter (ng/ml)—are usually tied to a low libido. As for progesterone, menopausal levels are about 0.03 to 0.3 ng/ml. By way of comparison, premenopausal women will have progesterone levels of about 7 to 38 ng/ml during their luteal phase.

Thyroid Tests

Many doctors will also recommend that you have your thyroid tested when you suspect menopause. This makes sense for two reasons. First, many women in premature menopause are also at a higher risk for thyroid problems. Second, many symptoms of thyroid disease overlap with menopausal symptoms. In fact, thyroid diseases often interfere with menstruation. Testing your thyroid, then, will help determine whether you are in premature menopause, or instead have thyroid disease. In this case, your doctor will probably check your thyroxine and thyrotropin levels.

Salivary Hormone Tests

Some doctors recommend saliva testing to measure hormone levels. This isn't as widely used as blood testing, but advocates claim that it is quicker, less expensive, and reliable. With salivary testing, your doctor takes samples of your saliva to see the levels of hormones you are producing and to determine if you have any deficiencies. You can also order kits to test your hormone levels at home. If you do choose to do this, though, be sure to go over any results with your doctor.

Vaginal Acidity Test

This test is currently under research, but may become yet another way of determining whether you are in menopause. With the vaginal acidity test, pH paper measures the acidity on your vagina. Nonmenopausal women usually have a vaginal pH level of about 4.5. However, when your estrogen levels drop, your vagina has less lactobacillus bacteria—the "good" bacteria that helps prevent the "bad" bacteria from growing. The bad bacteria, then, flourishes, raising the acidity level of your vagina. A vaginal pH level of 6.0 to 7.5 in a woman without a vaginal infection generally points to low estrogen production and to menopause.

Ultrasound

In some cases, your doctor may perform high-resolution ovarian ultrasound to view your ovaries. This will determine whether you still have any eggs and follicles. However, generally this information doesn't help that much. According to a British study, up to two-thirds of women diagnosed with premature ovarian failure do indeed have remaining follicles. The problem is that even when eggs are detected, attempts to stimulate ovulation through hormones have been relatively unsuccessful. However, ultrasound may make sense if you are in the early stages of premature menopause and are intending to pursue an agressive fertility program. For more information on this, see Chapter 8.

A CHECKLIST OF THE COMMON SIGNS AND SYMPTOMS OF MENOPAUSE

Physical Signs
Irregular periods
 (changes in frequency, duration, skipped periods, etc.)
Hot flashes and night sweats
Vaginal dryness
Bladder control problems
Insomnia/disrupted sleep
Palpitations
Weight gain (especially around your waist and abdomen)
Skin changes (dryness, thinning look)
Headaches
Breast tenderness
Gastrointestinal distress and nausea

Tingling or itchy skin
"Buzzing" in your head, "electric shock" sensation
Bloating
Dizziness/light-headedness
Sore joints/muscles
Hair loss or thinning
Increase in facial hair
Changes in body odor
Dry mouth and other oral symptoms

Emotional Signs
Irritability
Mood swings
Lowered libido
Anxiety
"Brain fog" (difficulty concentrating, confusion)
Memory lapses
Irritability
Extreme fatigue/low energy levels
Confusion/lack of concentration
Feeling emotionally detached

Chapter 3

What's Going on
with Your Body Now?
(and What *Will* Happen?)

> When I was diagnosed with premature menopause, I understood the basic ramifications: my ovaries weren't working as they should, and I was essentially infertile. Beyond that, though, I had no idea what to expect. What did menopause really mean other than no more periods? What was going to happen to me?

Discovering you are in premature menopause is a difficult concept to comprehend on many levels, but possibly one of the toughest things to come to grips with is the long-term implications of the diagnosis.

To paraphrase the diamond advertisement, menopause is forever. It isn't curable. It doesn't suddenly go away. It's a condition, not a disease. And it's a condition that you will be living with for the rest of your life. This is why it is so important to understand what being in menopause so early does and will do to your body.

When you go through premature menopause, usually you immediately notice the hot flashes or the change in your periods. But there is more happening to your body than the obvious symptoms. Yes, your changing hormone levels are wreaking havoc with your personal temperature system and your moods.

But behind the scenes, other things are happening. Low estrogen levels are affecting your bones, your heart, and your cholesterol levels.

Your body, in effect, is behaving as if you are much older than you are. Because of a lack of estrogen, you are facing the health risks most women don't face until they are in their fifties and later.

In fact—and this is very important—many doctors now believe that those of us with premature menopause may face a higher risk of bone loss and heart disease than women who go through menopause at the normal age, because our bodies will have low estrogen levels for a longer amount of time. This is one of the key differences between premature menopause and normal menopause, and one of the key reasons it is vital to explore the long-term consequences of premature menopause and the ways you can lessen potential problems.

> **I'm only 36. I've always been healthy—I'm a runner, I take vitamins, eat well. But now I've learned that my cholesterol is up, my blood pressure is up, and I haven't changed my lifestyle at all. It's all because of menopause, the doctor told me. All I know is that it's really a shock. I could handle the hot flashes. But having something like this suddenly happen to me—it's frightening.**
> **—Anita, age 36**

It *is* often frightening, especially because the signals that your body is at risk for certain diseases often come with no previous warning. You feel as though your body is playing tricks on you. You can't count on it to react the way it used to. Usually when you enter premature menopause, you feel strong and healthy. You're still young and you are accustomed to being in great condition. Then you discover that, regardless of how you feel, your body is, well, different. I got a complete physical shortly after I had been diagnosed, and was amazed to see that my cholesterol had skyrocketed from 126 to 250 in spite of the fact that I had not changed my diet or exercise at all. I felt as though I had been dropped into someone else's body! I had always had relatively low cholesterol and had never worried about it; suddenly it was a health issue for me.

> **What worries me the most? Heart problems, bone loss, will my daughter have this too, will I age faster, early death? breast cancer. . . .**
> **—Stacey, age 33**

Coping with premature menopause, then, means accepting the fact that you will have to address health problems and risks you would normally associate with an older woman. It means rethinking your attitude toward your lifestyle. It means dealing with the quality-of-life issues and more potentially serious life-or-death issues. It makes *taking charge.*

This chapter is designed to make you aware of the long-term effects of going through menopause early, and how to circumvent them. It discusses osteoporosis, heart disease, hypertension, and other conditions that have been linked to premature menopause, such as thyroid diseases and diabetes. It explains what to be on guard for in the years to come—and what you can prevent.

Remember, although premature menopause is a lifelong condition, it isn't a lifetime sentence of old age. In fact, you can look at premature menopause in a positive light. Consider it a wake-up call or, perhaps more fittingly, a call to arms. Because of menopause, you will have to deal with issues ordinarily faced by an older woman. This doesn't make you automatically middle-aged, but it *can* make you better equipped to handle your middle age. You can start living healthier *now*—for a healthier tomorrow.

> **The one good thing about going through this premature menopause thing is that I'm really starting to pay attention to my health now. I realized it's about time I showed some real concern about my body and how to make it function to the best of its ability.**
> **—Sherry, age 29**

OSTEOPOROSIS

I had the bone-density scan done and I have osteopenia,
the beginning stages of osteoporosis. So that just made
my day. I feel so old and so scared. I've got twice the
risk of fracture of normal 35-year-olds. It's not that big
a deal, but it's upsetting. I do take my calcium, and we
bought a treadmill, so that should fix the problem. It's
just that I feel like such an invalid. Mostly I'm scared
and mad. I never have had anything wrong with me at
all and all of a sudden I'm literally falling apart.
—Amy, age 35

Osteoporosis—bone weakening and loss—is one of those diseases that most people automatically associate with old age.
You imagine a frail, older woman, perhaps someone with the
telltale "dowager's hump" on her back, or someone walking
carefully with a cane. You definitely don't picture yourself or
someone like you. It just isn't something you normally think
about when you are only in your twenties and thirties. But when
you have premature menopause, it is something that you *should*
start thinking about. And you should think about it even if you
think you aren't at a high risk.

To be honest with you, that's something I didn't do initially.
I knew that menopause often increased your chances for getting
osteoporosis, but I figured it wasn't really an issue for me. I
had always had strong bones. I consumed a lot of dairy products
and did a great deal of weight-bearing exercise—walking, Nor-
dic tracking, and weight lifting. So I assumed that I had nothing
to be concerned about. When I had a blood-chemistry test done,
though, I learned that my calcium levels were low—not extremely low, but low enough for me to realize that premature
menopause had already begun affecting my calcium absorption
in spite of all the right things I was doing. Premature menopause
was outweighing all the other factors. It opened my eyes and,
quite frankly, it scared me a little.

Osteoporosis is one of the most devastating effects of premature menopause. It is also one of the most insidious. You can't tell in the normal course of events that your bones are thinning and weakening. There are no overt signs. You don't suddenly shrink a few inches overnight or collapse on the street. But when you have premature menopause, chances are that your bones will lose calcium early and rapidly.

A recent study conducted by researchers at the National Institute of Child Health and Human Development (NICHD) concluded that women with premature ovarian failure face a risk of bone loss. Two-thirds of the women they studied had enough bone loss that they might be at risk for a hip fracture. Seventy-seven out of the 89 women they studied had *osteopenia*, below-normal bone density and a precursor of osteoporosis. Two of the women had full-fledged osteoporosis. And only 10 of the women in the study had normal bone density for their age. To make matters even more worrisome, about half the women in the study had their bone-density test within 18 months of their POF diagnosis, and nearly half of this group already had osteopenia. While this particular study looked only at women with POF, the outlook is similar for women who are in premature menopause due to surgery or cancer treatment. Many studies indicate that if you have your ovaries removed, you experience significant bone loss in the first two years after surgery.

If you go through premature menopause before the age of 35, you're at an even higher risk of osteoporosis, primarily because peak bone mass—the point at which your bones achieve their highest density—is typically reached at the age of 35. So premature menopause before the age of 35 may mean that your bones never attain their optimum strength, which makes it all the more troublesome when you begin losing bone mass. As for premature menopause after age 35, you may have attained peak bone mass, but you will have usually experienced significant bone loss if you haven't had periods for a long time and your estrogen levels remain low.

The implications are clear, then: when you have premature menopause, naturally or surgically, bone loss is a very real threat—and one that can occur rapidly. But—and this is an important but—osteoporosis *is* preventable. If you are aware of it now and start taking care of your bones from this point on, you will be able to turn the odds back in your favor and keep the healthy bones you would normally have at this age.

What Is Osteoporosis?

The word "osteoporosis" literally means porous bones, which is a perfect description of the illness itself. In the simplest of terms, osteoporosis is a weakening of your bones that leads to bone loss.

Actually, you lose bone throughout your life, but normally the old bone you lose is replaced by new, stronger bone. In a process called *bone remodeling*, cells called "osteoclasts" remove the old bone; then cells called "osteoblasts" fill in and create new bone. As long as these types of cells are in balance, your skeletal mass remains strong. On average, your bone mass reaches its peak at the age of about 35, which is why osteoporosis isn't ordinarily an issue for women until they hit their mid-forties.

But when you go through premature menopause, osteoporosis becomes a threat. The main culprit is the drop in your estrogen levels and the small amount of testosterone that you would normally produce if you weren't in menopause. Estrogen—and to a lesser degree, testosterone—helps in the absorption of calcium and other minerals, and slows or stops bone loss. So when your hormone levels drop, the delicate balance in the bone remodeling process changes. More bone is removed than added, and you begin losing bone mass. According to some studies, you may lose 6 percent a year, possibly more if you have had surgical menopause. To make matters worse, the osteoblasts don't work as well in filling the holes made during the bone remodeling. So the new bone tissue your body builds isn't as strong and solid as in the past, but porous like a honeycomb. With these weakened, brittle bones, you run a higher chance of getting fractures, a compressed spine, and rounded back.

Are You at an Even Higher Risk for Osteoporosis?

Okay, so premature menopause is definitely a risk factor for osteoporosis. But there are other risk factors as well that, combined with premature menopause, may increase your chances of osteoporosis. Some of these are genetic risk factors, which you can do nothing about. But others are lifestyle factors and are controllable. In all cases, though, knowing the risk factors and seeing if they apply to you gives you more insight as to the possibility of your developing osteoporosis. Being in premature menopause is reason enough to get your bone density checked and to start an osteoporosis-prevention program. But if you realize you have one or more of the following factors, it is all the more important for you to begin being more bone-healthy now!

INHERITED RISK FACTORS

• *Race*—It's a simple rule of thumb: in general, the lighter (or more transparent) your skin, the higher your chances of having low bone density. Asian women tend to have the lowest bone density, followed by white women. African Americans tend to have higher bone density and slower rate of bone loss.
• *Small body build*—The smaller and more fine-boned your frame, the higher the possibility of bone loss and fracture because you start out with less bone to lose.
• *Low weight*— Being too thin, that is, below normal weight, increases your chances of osteoporosis. The reason? Fat cells produce estrogen, so the fewer the fat cells, the less the amount of estrogen you produce and have produced.
• *Family history of osteoporosis*—If your mother, grandmother, aunt, or sister has or had osteoporosis, you are at an increased risk of having it yourself. According to recent scientific studies, this may be due to an inherited ''osteoporosis gene'' that is supposed to stimulate the production of a protein that assists vitamin D's job in bone-building. If this gene is defective, you generally have poor bone density.

PAST RISK FACTORS

- *No pregnancies*—When you get pregnant, your production of estrogen increases, which helps your body absorb calcium and make stronger bones. If you've had no pregnancies, your bones haven't benefited from that estrogen surge, so they haven't gotten extra strength or density from the increase in estrogen.
- *Skipped periods for a long amount of time because of excessive weight loss or exercise*—If you stopped having periods for an extended amount of time (six months or more at one time) due to excessive exercise, anorexia, or bulimia, you stopped ovulating, which means that your estrogen levels dropped.
- *Low calcium diet (especially between the ages of one and 16)*—The formative years are important ones for your bones. If you didn't get enough calcium then, your bones may never have reached their optimal mass, so you may have entered premature menopause with less bone mass than the average woman of your age.

LIFESTYLE RISK FACTORS

- *Smoking*—Yet again, a reason to quit if you smoke. Smoking interferes with your estrogen production and usage, increasing the loss of calcium from your bones.
- *Heavy drinking*—Excessive alcohol consumption affects your estrogen production, inhibits calcium absorption, and may cut down on your liver's ability to activate vitamin D.
- *High caffeine consumption*—Caffeine acts as a diuretic, which increases the amount of calcium you lose in your urine. It may also reduce new bone creation and calcium absorption.
- *High consumption of soft drinks*— The culprit here is phosphoric acid, contained in both diet and regular soft drinks. Phosphoric acid leaches calcium from your system.
- *Use of certain medications*—Several different medications and drugs interfere with the absorption of calcium. Among

them are antacids containing aluminum, corticosteroids, certain diuretics called furosemides, bulk fiber preparations such as Metamucil, and thyroid hormone.

* *Little exercise*—Weight-bearing exercise (walking, running, etc.) builds strong bones, as does resistance training with weights. If you tend to have a sedentary lifestyle, your bones are often weak.

* *Diet too high in protein*—According to several studies, if you eat a high amount of protein, you lose a higher amount of calcium in your urine.

How Healthy Are Your Bones . . . *Really?* Bone-Density Testing

Whether or not you have any risk factors other than premature menopause (and if you're like most women, you probably do), there is one thing you should do if you want to take care of your bones now and in the future: have your bone density measured. This is the only way you can accurately determine how strong your bones are now, whether you already have osteoporosis or osteopenia, and how aggressively you need to act to maintain healthy bones.

Because bone loss can be so rapid in women with premature menopause, it is a good idea to get tested when you are first diagnosed. This way, if you've already begun losing bone, you can take measures immediately. If you haven't lost any bone yet, you have a baseline to measure against in the future and you can keep monitoring your bone density to be sure that you don't start losing bone as you stay in menopause. Your doctor should suggest that you get tested, but if he or she doesn't, be sure to ask for it. It's too important to put off. And the results of the tests can be eye-opening, to say the least.

Bone-density measurements can be taken of your heel, wrist, spine, hips, or total body. Some doctors may suggest you first get a screening test. In this case, you usually have just your wrist, arm, or heel measured, and if bone density appears low, you then get a diagnostic test—a scan of your hips, lower spine, or total body. While this method is fairly common in the treatment of regular menopausal women, it may not be the best approach if you are in premature menopause. According to a number of studies, you may have significant loss in your hips and spine even while showing normal bone density in your heel or wrist. So you could be lulling yourself into a false sense of security by having only your wrist, arm, or heel tested rather than your hips or spine—and wind up losing precious time. Since the tests aren't dangerous or complicated, and women with premature menopause are at high risk, you're best off opting for a thorough bone-density test rather than a screening. Many doctors recommend that at the least you have bone-density measurements taken of your hips rather than your spine, since spine measurements can be thrown off by medical conditions such as degenerative arthritis. At the best, you should have a total body measurement done.

There are several different types of bone density tests available. Most use a safe amount of low-dose radiation to measure the density of your bones in a relatively simple, quick, painless procedure that can make a huge difference in your long-term quality of life.

The best and most accurate test is *Dual-energy X-ray Absorptiometry (DEXA)*. This is a state-of-the-art test that is able to measure even a 1 percent loss of bone. DEXA measures bone at the hip, spine, and/or wrist. (Again, though, it makes sense to have hip and/or spine, if not the total body, tested, as opposed to just the wrist.) It's an easy procedure. You lie on an examining table fully clothed, while a scanner—a mechanical imager that looks like a wand—passes over your body, taking a picture of your bones. It's sort of like being in a huge computer scanner or photocopy machine. The amount of radiation used is minimal—about one twentieth that of a normal chest X ray—and the results are extremely precise.

The DEXA prints out a picture of your bones, showing the density, and a computer measures your density (in grams of calcium per square centimeter) and "scores" your bones. You get two different scores, a Z score and T score. The Z score compares your bone density with that of an average woman of your age and body size. The T score compares it with an "ideal average woman" who is 30 years old and at her peak bone mass. By looking at your T score, your doctor can determine what percentage of bone you've lost in comparison to the ideal mass; by looking at the Z score, how you stand against the norm for your age.

It does get a little complicated. Your score is given in terms of standard deviation from the mean. For example, if you have a decrease of one standard deviation, you have about a 10 percent bone loss. If you are more than one standard deviation below the mean peak value but less than two, you have osteopenia. And if you are 2.5 standard deviations or more below the mean, you have osteoporosis. It sounds a bit complex, but your doctor will explain the results to you in plain English, not medicalese. You will wind up with one of three diagnoses: you have healthy bones still; you have osteopenia; or you have osteoporosis. In any case, you should get retested to see if you are losing bone mass, since this test shows only whether you already have bone loss, not if you are currently losing it.

> **I had been doing weight-bearing exercise regularly since I was in my twenties. So I was surprised when I got the DEXA scan at age 35 and found there was significant bone loss in my hips and spine. That's when I decided to go on HRT. I realized I had to do something and do it quickly.**
>
> **—Anita, age 36**

The DEXA scan takes about 10 to 20 minutes and costs between $150 and $300. DEXA machines are typically found only at large medical centers. There are over 700 DEXA machines currently in use in the United States. To find a site near you, you can call the National Osteoporosis Foundation at 800–464–6700. There is one problem, though, that bears mentioning. Many insurance companies don't cover DEXA, especially for women in premature menopause, because their age doesn't seem to warrant a bone density test. Check with your insurer and be prepared to fight by showing that there is justifiable cause for getting the test. Remember, you are in a high-risk group because you have premature menopause. The DEXA isn't an unwarranted test in your case, but a prudent safeguard against a debilitating illness.

Aside from the DEXA, the other bone-density tests that are sometimes used include:

- *Dual-Photon Absorptiometry (DPA)*—Like DEXA, DPA measures bone density in your spine or hip. It is a little slower than the DEXA, though, and isn't as widely used.
- *Single-Photon Absorptiometry (SPA)*—This test measures the bone density in your arm, wrist, and/or heel, takes only about 15 minutes, and is relatively inexpensive. The big drawback with the SPA test? It doesn't measure the bone density in your pelvis or spine, both of which are often most affected by osteoporosis in women with premature menopause.
- *Peripheral Dual-Energy X-Ray Absorptiometry (pDXA)*—A mini-DEXA scan, this test is very cheap—sometimes as low as $30. But it measures only the bone density in your arm, so isn't the best bet when it comes to getting as accurate a picture of your bone health as possible.
- *Radiographic Absorptiometry*—Another test that doesn't measure your spine or hips, this test determines only bone density of your hand, using an X-ray to measure bone mass.
- *Ultrasound*—Probably the easiest test of all, this measure the bone mass of your heel bone. But again, while many studies cite a correlation between heel bone density and density of pelvis and spine, there's a chance you may get a good heel density reading while suffering from bone loss elsewhere. Many doctors recommend this test first, then, based upon the readings, decide whether you need a more complete bone-density test. Again, though, you are probably better off getting a complete DEXA to begin with. It might take more time and cost more money, but your bones are worth it!
- *CAT Scan*—Having a CAT scan to determine bone density has some definite pluses and minuses. On the plus side, a

CAT scan is extremely accurate and can measure both the total bone (the outer or *cortical* bone and the inner or *trabecular* bone) or the inner bone alone. The negatives? A CAT scan is generally much more expensive. In addition, you are exposed to much higher levels of radiation than in the other forms of bone density tests.

• *Ntx Bone Loss Assay*—This osteoporosis risk assay is a follow-up test that you would get after you've had your baseline DEXA or other X-ray test. Rather than go through follow-up DEXA, you can determine if you're still going through bone loss by taking this urine test. It's a 24-hour urine test that assesses bone loss by measuring a biological marker called Type 1 collagen in your urine and, unlike the DEXA, it's extremely simple and not nearly as expensive. The only drawback is that it's relatively new, and many doctors don't offer it or prefer the more standard DEXA. (For information on the bone loss assay, contact Metamatric Medical Research Laboratory 800–221–4640).

What You Can Do to Prevent or Halt Osteoporosis

All right—you're in premature menopause, which puts you at a greater risk for osteoporosis; you know which other risk factors apply to you; you may already have been tested and know if you've already lost bone. Now what?

> I am presently considering HRT (Estratest and Prometrium) for prevention of osteoporosis and heart disease. I have begun calcium supplements (am working up to the recommended 1200 mg) and participate in a regular exercise routine consisting of walking, free weights, and resistance equipment. I had a bone-density test, and it was simple (except for needing to have my leg strapped in a bizarre position). I learned that my bone density is average for someone my age, but that during the first three to five years of meno, I can expect a significant loss that will put me in the category of older women.
> —Cathy, age 37

The bad news is that there appears to be no definitive cure for osteoporosis. But it can be prevented, and if you have already begun losing bone, you can halt the process. In addition, many recent studies have indicated that certain hormones and medications may actually stimulate bone growth.

First, it's important to recognize that osteoporosis isn't a foregone conclusion. Yes, premature menopause greatly increases your odds of getting osteoporosis or osteopenia, but there other factors aside from estrogen loss that are also involved. For example, if you enter premature menopause with a good bone mass, you may be one of the lucky ones who don't get osteoporosis. Furthermore, if you take precautionary measures early on, there is a good chance you can avoid osteoporosis. Because bone loss appears to occur so quickly when you enter premature menopause, the key is to act fast. There are three main factors, or "bone-boosters" that can help you fight or slow osteoporosis: calcium, hormones, and exercise.

BONE BOOSTER 1: CALCIUM, YOUR BONES' BEST FRIEND

Getting enough calcium is a definite must where bone-building is concerned. As you know, calcium is vital for strong bones because it is the key ingredient in bone-building. But many of us don't get nearly enough calcium. The National Institutes of Health recommends that if you are in menopause, you should get at least 1,000 milligrams (mg) of calcium a day if you are on HRT, and 1500 mg if you aren't.

How can you get enough calcium? Start by taking a look at your daily diet and seeing if you should increase your calcium intake through the foods you eat. In general, your best bets for calcium-rich foods are nonfat or low-fat dairy products, salmon, sardines with the bones, green leafy vegetables, and tofu. One of the best things you can do for yourself to get a head start each day on meeting your calcium requirements is to have a glass of nonfat milk each morning. If you're lactose-intolerant, you can get a calcium-enriched soy milk. You might also try calcium-fortified apple or orange juices, which have about the same calcium levels as nonfat milk.

THE BEST FOOD SOURCES OF CALCIUM

Food	Serving Size	Mg of Calcium
Dairy Products		
Nonfat yogurt	1 cup	450
Low-fat yogurt	1 cup	415
Ricotta (part skim)	½ cup	335
Nonfat milk	1 cup	300
Low-fat (1 or 2%) milk	1 cup	300
Whole milk	1 cup	290
Swiss cheese	1 oz.	270
Cheddar cheese	1 oz.	205
Mozzarella (part skim)	1 oz.	200
Muenster cheese	1 oz.	200
American cheese	1 oz.	180
Feta cheese	1 oz.	140
Cottage cheese	1 cup	135
Other Foods		
Sardines (in oil with bones)	3 oz.	370
Blackstrap molasses	2 tbsps.	300
Calcium-fortified juice	1 cup	300
Figs, dried	10 medium	270
Black beans, dried	1 cup	270
Collard greens	1 cup	270
Salmon (canned with bones)	3 oz.	200
Broccoli	1 cup	170
Farina, cooked	1 cup	145
Spinach (cooked, drained)	½ cup	130
Tofu	½ cup	130
Apricots, dried	1 cup	100
Tahini	1 tbs.	85
Almonds	1 oz.	70

It's always nice to think that we're getting all we need through our diets, but, in all honesty, most of us probably aren't. As a big dairy eater, I was convinced I was getting more than enough calcium until I sat down and actually added up the milligrams I could count on getting every day. On some days I was well over 1,500 mg, but on other days, I wasn't even close.

When you're dealing with the possibility of osteoporosis, you can't afford to be casual about calcium consumption. So if you think you're not getting enough calcium in your diet each day, you have two choices in this case: either start eating calcium-rich foods like crazy, or take calcium supplements. Because those of us with premature menopause are at such a high risk for bone loss, calcium supplementation makes sense. It's easy, and you can be assured that you're getting a certain level of calcium.

It does get a little confusing, though, when it's time to choose a calcium supplement. There are so many out there, all purporting to do the same thing, but there are differences between the different forms.

Calcium citrate is the form of calcium most often recommended by doctors, chiefly because it is the most easily absorbed. This claim to fame may not apply to you, because it is older women who make less stomach acid (and so have more digestive problems), not women in their twenties and thirties, but if you have any problems with digestion or just want a calcium that isn't hard on your stomach, calcium citrate probably makes sense. There is one drawback to this type of calcium: it doesn't contain as much elemental calcium as calcium carbonate, so you have to take more tablets, which costs more. In addition, in spite of its stomach-friendly reputation, it may cause stomach upset or diarrhea. If you choose this type of calcium, you should take it between meals or just before bedtime.

Calcium Carbonate is the other most widely used form of calcium. It is not as easily absorbed as calcium citrate, but is the most concentrated form of calcium, with 40 percent elemental calcium (which also makes it the cheapest!). A side benefit is that it's also an antacid. On the negative side, though, it can cause constipation and bloating. If you take this, it's a good idea to drink more water than usual, and take it in two or more doses, rather than all at one time. You may also want to chew it to make it easily absorbed into your system. Unlike calcium citrate, you should take this with meals.

Like calcium carbonate, *calcium lactate, calcium gluconate,* and *calcium phosphate* are less concentrated forms of calcium (containing about 15 percent elemental calcium), and are similar to calcium citrate in terms of absorbability and lack of side effects. But they usually cost more than calcium citrate—as much as three to 10 times more—so you're better off avoiding these and opting for another form of calcium.

Calcium supplements made of *bone meal* and *dolomite* are high in elemental calcium, but are not a good choice as they may contain lead and other toxic metals.

Finally, there are *calcium-based antacids*—products such as Tums and Rolaids Calcium Rich, which are probably one of the cheapest ways of getting calcium. Many women like them because you can chew them instead of swallowing. If you opt for this form of calcium, you should take them between meals. And be sure to read the label carefully. You don't want to get an antacid that includes aluminum because that will leach calcium from your system.

Whichever form you choose, there are certain rules of thumb where calcium supplements are concerned:

- It is a good idea to take your calcium twice a day, instead of in one dose, because your body can absorb only 600 mg of calcium at a time.
- Do not take calcium with iron, because it interferes with its absorption.
- Be sure that your calcium is actually doing what you're paying for by putting your tablets through this simple absorbability test. Drop one tablet in a small glass or bowl with white vinegar and stir it every few minutes. After 15 minutes to half an hour has passed, the pill should have disintegrated. If it hasn't dissolved in the vinegar, it won't dissolve in your stomach either, making it essentially useless. In this case, you should get another brand or try another form.
- You should be aware that, where calcium is concerned, you

can get too much of a good thing. Over 2,000 mg a day of calcium may pose problems for your kidneys. So if you have had kidney stones or have a family history of them, talk to your doctor before taking calcium supplements.

CALCIUM HELPERS AND CALCUIM ROBBERS

To make calcium work well, you need other vitamins and minerals to help it along. Some of these are available in combination with calcium, others are in multivitamins or trace mineral compounds, or you can take them individually. Where you get them isn't really the issue; the key is to be sure you *are* getting them to get the most out of your calcium intake. The calcium helpers, then are:

Vitamin D, which is essential for helping your body absorb calcium. While you can get vitamin D from the sun, it's not considered the best way, because you can't be sure you're getting enough (and it's tough to get if you live in a very cloudy area or use sunscreen). In fact, according to a recent study, vitamin D deficiency is much more common than previously thought. Most interestingly, 37 percent of the women in the study who had low vitamin D levels reported that they were consuming at least the minimum requirement of vitamin D. Since vitamin D is so vital in the fight against osteoporosis, it's probably best to take supplementation to be sure you're getting what you need. Most doctors agree that you need 400 IUs for maximum benefit, and can safely take up to 800 IUs daily. But more than this amount is toxic, so be sure not to overdo it.

Magnesium, which is very commonly found in calcium supplements, is also crucial for optimum skeletal health. Generally, you should take a dosage equal to half of the calcium dosage you're taking.

Vitamin K is another key player where bone health is concerned. Most women, however, get enough vitamin K through their diet because it's found in many vegetables.

You also need the following minerals: *boron* (which is also commonly included in many calcium supplements), *copper*, zinc, manganese, and silicon (all of which are usually included in multivitamins or multimineral tablets).

There is one other step you need to take to be sure you're getting the most out of your calcium: avoiding calcium "robbers." You may think you're getting enough calcium because you're eating the right things, but you might be excreting a great deal of it, winding up with too little calcium after all. As mentioned earlier in this section, there are a number of culprits. Too much sugar, salt, and caffeine increases the amount of calcium you excrete in your urine. Excessive alcohol consumption (three drinks a day or more) can interfere with calcium absorption and your body's usage of vitamin D. Too much phosphorus (which is found in soft drinks, processed foods, and red meat) and excess protein also increase calcium excretion.

DAILY VITAMIN REGIMEN TO FIGHT OSTEOPOROSIS

Here are the vitamins and minerals you need to help keep your bones healthy. Remember, the amounts listed are totals that you can reach through diet in addition to supplements:

Calcium:	1,200 to 1,500 mg (preferably in two or more doses)
Vitamin D:	400 IUs
Magnesium:	usually about 200 to 750 IUs, depending on how much calcium you take
Boron:	3 to 5 mg
Vitamin K, copper, zinc, manganese, silicon:	trace amounts (available in most multivitamin or multimineral supplements)

BONE BOOSTER 2: HORMONE REPLACEMENT THERAPY AND OTHER DRUG TREATMENTS

Hormone replacement therapy is one of the tried-and-true methods of preventing bone loss, and quite probably one of the best things you can do for your bones if you're in premature menopause. HRT is discussed at length in Chapter 5, but here, briefly, is why it makes sense where osteoporosis is concerned.

Studies have shown that replacing the estrogen you lose when you go through menopause helps slow bone loss. In fact, some indicate that replacing estrogen through HRT cuts your risk of fractures by 50 percent. If you take estrogen in addition to calcium supplements, you're helping your bones even more. According to recent clinical trials, the combination of estrogen and calcium is greater than the sum of each alone. By taking both estrogen and calcium over a one-year period, women had an average increase of bone mass in the arm two and a half times greater than with estrogen alone.

So estrogen and calcium are definitely a winning team for your bones. But estrogen isn't the only hormone that helps fight osteoporosis. Recent research has found that natural progesterone actually may build new bone. Progesterone apparently begins the bone-building process again at the same time that it helps stop ongoing bone loss. Synthetic progesterone, or *progestin*, has only some of the benefits of natural progesterone and also has more side effects, which is why many doctors recommend natural progesterone instead.

Another hormone, testosterone, which our ovaries make in a very small amount even after menopause, also appears to both slow bone loss and help build bone density. Testosterone is usually especially low in women who have had surgical menopause, because they have no ovaries. Recent studies have indicated that a combination of estrogen and testosterone therapy in surgically menopausal women showed a significant increase in their spinal bone mineral density. Researchers believe that women with natural premature menopause could also benefit from testosterone supplementation. As of this writing, the

NICHD was planning to test a patch that supplies small amounts of testosterone to see if this, in conjunction with estrogen, will help prevent bone loss in women with premature menopause.

NONHORMONAL MEDICATIONS THAT TREAT OSTEOPOROSIS

While estrogen and other hormones are probably the best way to treat and prevent osteoporosis in women with premature menopause, there are other treatments available that may make sense for you if you can't (or won't) take estrogen.

First, let's take a look at one of the newer treatments that has been in the news in the past few years: *Fosomax.* This non-hormonal drug is a biophosphonate designed to prevent osteoporosis. It is probably not as good a choice as HRT for a number of reasons. First, many doctors won't prescribe both HRT and Fosomax, since there have been no studies yet demonstrating long-term effects. In addition, once you start Fosomax, it is recommended that you keep using it for the rest of your life. So if there is a chance you will take HRT, Fosomax may not be a good choice. Second, Fosomax does have a serious side effect—it can severely damage your esophagus. Because of this, you must sit or stand for at least a half hour after taking it, and not lie down. Third, while Fosomax does increase bone mass, some researchers believe that the bone it builds is different from normal human bone. It is more brittle, which may actually increase chances of fractures. Other studies have indicated that this claim is false and that the bone is good. So this is another case in which the evidence is unclear. All in all, it may be best to steer clear of this medication if you don't need the extra boost to fight osteoporosis.

That said, it may be a different story if you already have significant bone loss. Some doctors prescribe both Fosomax and HRT to women in premature menopause who are already showing osteopenia or osteoporosis, in a double effort to build bone mass. One recent study found that combining Fosomax with HRT increased bone mineral density from two to five times more than in women who were on HRT alone. So, since premature menopause often leads to rapid bone loss, it's possible that combining HRT and Fosomax may be an advantage. The drawback, of course, is the lack of knowledge about long-term effects. But this could possibly be outweighed by the improvement in your bone density. Frankly, it's a difficult choice. If you are interested in taking Fosomax, or if your doctor recommends it because of your risk factors or bone loss, be sure to ask your doctor about all side effects, interactions with other drugs, and possible long-term effects. As with any drug, especially a new one, it is best to learn all you can before you start taking it—just to be safe.

Etidronate is another biophosphonate like Fosomax, but less potent. It slows the resorption of bone by halting the activity of the osteoclasts and also increases bone density. Studies have shown that you can get an even higher bone density by combining etidronate with estrogen than by taking either one alone. Also on the plus side, there are few side effects with etidronate, but its bone-resorption power is not as strong as that of Fosomax.

You may also have heard about *raloxifene* (sold under the brand name *Evista*). This, too, is a nonhormonal drug designed to fight osteoporosis, but actually is more like tamoxifen (the breast cancer drug) in many ways. Like tamoxifen, raloxifene is a SERM (selective estrogen receptor modulator), which blocks estrogen receptors and takes the place of estrogen. Since it is an estrogen replacement, you take this in place of estrogen. On the plus side, tests have shown that raloxifene is successful in preventing osteoporosis, offers some cardiovascular benefits, and may also help protect against breast cancer. But there are negatives: because you take this instead of estrogen, you don't get any relief from hot flashes. In fact, hot flashes are a common side effect of raloxifene, in addition to leg cramps and, though less commonly, blood clots in the legs. Furthermore, you don't get all the benefits of replacing the estrogen you've lost. Taking raloxifene, then, probably makes sense only if you can't take HRT for some reason—perhaps a history of stroke or a family history of breast cancer. Your best bet is to talk to your doctor about this drug to determine if it makes sense for you.

Calcitonin, a hormone produced by the thyroid, fights osteoporosis by blocking the osteoclasts that eat bone, and so stimulating new bone growth. Research on this drug (available as a nasal spray) has shown that over time you may get a 5 to 20 percent increase in bone mass. That's the good news. Now for the bad news: it has major side effects, including nausea, vomiting, loss of appetite, diarrhea, frequent urination, and flushing.

Calcitrol, which is what vitamin D is converted to in your body, is another treatment used for osteoporosis that appears to increase calcium absorption. One study showed that patients taking calcitrol had up to 75 percent fewer fractures than those not taking it. However, further studies are still necessary to determine how well calcitrol can work in osteoporosis prevention.

In late 1998, a new drug, *tibolone,* was studied for its effect on osteoporosis—and it appeared to be very promising. A study conducted in London, England found that patients taking 2.5 mg of tibolone plus 800 mg of calcuim for two years had a 6.9 percent increase in their spinal bone mass and a 4.5 percent increase in their neck bone mass, as compared with 2.7 percent and 1.4 percent increases for women taking only the calcuim. There's a downside, however. Tibolone causes a number of unpleasant side effects including breast tenderness, weight gain, bloating, irregular vaginal bleeding, and irritability.

Another new osteoporosis drug, *ALX1-11,* was also undergoing tests in late 1998—and results showed that it was a significant help in increasing bone mineral density. ALX1-11 is a synthetic form of human parathyroid hormone, and trails indicated that women taking it showed a rapid increase in bone mass and density (particularly at higher doses). And the increase was higher than that produced by other osteoporosis treatments currently available. Even better, rather than just prevent bone loss, it actually stimulated new bone growth. Expect to see more information coming out about this drug as studies continue.

Finally, there's *sodium fluoride*—the same fluoride that

makes teeth strong. Initial tests of large doses of fluoride to fight osteoporosis didn't work all that well. Even though bone formation increased, the bone was prone to fractures, and the treatment caused stomach upset, anemia, ulcers, and arthritis, among other side effects. But scientists have been working on a new, slower-releasing formula combining fluoride and calcium that is undergoing long-term trials. The jury is still out on this.

For all of the above drugs, it's wise to talk to your doctor to find out the pros and cons of each and to determine whether they fit into your osteoporosis-prevention plan. Chances are that if you are on HRT, you won't need any of them, since they are typically used as a replacement for HRT. However, if you can't or won't go on HRT, these osteoporosis fighters may give you what you need to stop bone loss and build stronger bones.

BONE BOOSTER 3: EXERCISE TO GET YOUR BONES (AND YOUR BODY) IN SHAPE

If you're concerned about osteoporosis, don't just sit there and worry. *Do* something!—preferably walking, running, or anything that puts stress on your skeletal system. Weight-bearing exercise is a great way of preventing bone loss and actually increasing bone mass as well. As an added bonus, it helps keep your weight down and helps minimize many menopausal symptoms. According to one study, women who exercised one hour a day only three times a week increased bone density by about 2.3 percent over one year. Those who didn't exercise at all *lost* 3.3 percent. Another study shows even more bone growth over the same time period: 5.2 percent for those who exercised, versus a 1.2 bone loss for those who didn't. While the specific findings are different, the numbers still say it all: regular exercise is a definite must where healthy bones are concerned. Many women who exercise regularly have a bone density that is 10 percent higher than those who don't.

The key, of course, is doing the right exercise—activity that puts stress on your bones. This includes aerobic activities like walking, running, jogging, stair-climbing, using a cross-country ski machine, tennis, dancing—virtually anything you do on your feet. (Swimming, because you are afloat in the water, doesn't help build bone. But exercising in water, specifically aerobic dancing or walking in water using special equipment, does, because you are putting pressure on your skeletal system and using water as a resistance.) Resistance training using weights also helps build bone. In this case, the bone under the muscle is stimulated and becomes stronger. One recent study spelled out the dramatic results: among women who had undergone surgical menopause, those who lifted weights and took estrogen had a spinal bone density increase of 8.3 percent, while the women who just took estrogen had an increase of only 1.5 percent. That's a decisive difference and should convince you that it's time to start moving!

HEART DISEASE

Virtually every study of premature menopause makes a very bald statement: women who experience premature menopause have an increased risk of heart disease compared with other women their age. Take a look at the numbers: according to recent research, women who go through menopause before the age of 35 have a two- to threefold risk of heart disease. Women who have their ovaries removed before the age of 35 have a sevenfold risk. If you're older than 35 but still younger than 40, your risk is only a bit lower—about twice the chance of developing heart disease. In fact, whether you've gone through a surgical or natural premature menopause, you're at a higher risk of heart disease than women who have gone through menopause at the average age.

These are startling figures, to say the least, and one of the key reasons it's so important to take charge of your premature menopause as soon as possible.

As with so many things that affect you when you're in premature menopause, the reason for this increased risk appears to be, again, lower amounts of estrogen. There have been several research studies exploring this link between estrogen and heart disease; however, the results have not been conclusive. As of this writing, however, most research suggests that estrogen helps protect your heart and your entire cardiovascular system. This is why although heart disease is common in women, it usually occurs 10 to 15 years later than it does in men. On average, younger women are not at a high risk for heart disease: they have estrogen working to prevent it.

But when you go through premature menopause, you're not part of the "average" group of younger women any longer. Instead, your body is thrust into the higher-risk category along with women over 50. And, in contrast to those women who are 50 and older and going through menopause, you are experiencing estrogen loss much earlier, which increases your long-term risk for heart disease. In other words, as with osteoporosis, when you are in premature menopause it's not your chronological age that matters; it's the number of years without (or with very low) estrogen that affects your health. The longer you have low estrogen, the more you increase your risk of cardiovascular disease.

According to a number of studies, it appears that estrogen protects your heart by decreasing LDL (low-density lipoprotein, the "bad" cholesterol) and increasing HDL (high-density lipoprotein, the "good" cholesterol). This keeps atherosclerotic plaque from sticking to arteries. It also reduces one form of LDL cholesterol called LP(a), which can cause stroke at high levels. Finally, it helps keep your blood vessels elastic, so they can expand when necessary to allow for increased blood flow.

But when you have an estrogen deficiency, your cardiovascular system starts working less smoothly—literally. When your circulating cholesterol changes to higher levels of the bad cholesterol and lower ones of the good, the platelets in your blood get sticky. They build up on your artery walls, clogging them up and interfering with blood flow. This can lead to heart attack or heart disease in general. In addition, the lower estrogen makes your blood vessels more rigid and more likely to constrict. As a result, you can wind up with high blood pressure, which also can result in heart disease.

It's not a great scenario, but it doesn't have to happen. Premature menopause doesn't necessarily equal heart disease. The key is getting heart-smart now.

Are You at an Even Higher Risk for Heart Disease? Other Risk Factors to Be Aware Of

Of course, there are risk factors other than premature menopause that can contribute to heart disease. Since premature menopause increases the risks to such a great degree, you should be aware of these others factors so that, if possible, you can adjust your lifestyle accordingly. This is one of those cases where it's definitely better to be safe than sorry!

The other risk factors that increase your chances of heart disease are:

• *Family history of heart disease*—This is probably the biggest risk factor of all, and unfortunately, one you can do nothing about. It's simple genetics: if heart disease runs in your family—particularly if someone in your immediate family developed heart disease before age 60—chances are good that you too will develop the disease.

• *High levels of LDL, the "bad" cholesterol*—If the ratio of your LDL to your total cholesterol is 4.5 or higher, you are at a higher risk of heart disease.

• *Being overweight*—There's not much to worry about if you're only a few pounds overweight. But if you are 30 percent or more above your ideal weight, then you are at an increased risk for heart disease.

• *High blood pressure*—Called the silent killer, hypertension is a sign of heart disease and can cause other conditions, including stroke or heart attack. Because it's often undetected, you should be sure to have your blood pressure checked regularly. African-American women, in particular, are at a higher risk for hypertension.

- *Diabetes*—Diabetics have a two-to-four-times greater risk of developing cardiovascular disease.
- *Smoking*—Here we go again, yet another negative where smoking is concerned. Even if you smoke very little, you've increased your chances of heart problems.
- *Little exercise*

It's a numbers game where these risks are concerned. The more of these risk factors that apply to you (especially in combination with premature menopause), the higher your chances for developing heart disease.

Getting to the Heart of the Matter: What You Can Do to Prevent Heart Disease

Okay, so that's all the bad news. But premature menopause won't necessarily lead to heart disease. You can fight back and, with diligence, keep your heart healthy. There are three main heart helpers that can put the odds back in your favor: *hormone replacement therapy, exercise,* and *diet.*

HEART HELPER 1: STRONGLY CONSIDER REPLACING THE ESTROGEN YOU'VE LOST

> I was against HRT. I wanted to control my symptoms through vitamins and herbs—it was just something I felt more comfortable with. But when I read more about the chances of heart disease and, even more, when my cholesterol started going up, I decided I'd rather take my chances with HRT than with heart problems. I guess I realized that even though I'd read negatives about HRT, the positives outweighed them for someone like me in premature menopause. I don't want to have heart disease at age 40.
>
> —Marilyn, age 34

When it comes to fighting heart disease, estrogen appears to be on your side. Yes, there has been a long-standing debate over the pros and cons of estrogen replacement therapy and some concern over the viability of different research studies. However, since 1970, over 32 studies have been conducted on the link between estrogen and heart disease. And the results seem quite conclusive: replacing estrogen results in a lower risk of heart disease—by as much as 50 percent if used for 15 years or longer; a 10 to 30 percent improvement if used for less than three years.

Researchers believe estrogen protects your heart by reversing the rise in LDL after menopause. According to one recent study of women taking estrogen, in just sixteen weeks LDL declined 13.5 percent while HDL increased 22.5 percent. Other studies have also shown that estrogen lowers fibrogen, a blood-clotting factor and helps your blood vessels respond well to overloading through stress or exercise.

There are a few negatives to take into consideration, however: if you take estrogen and a progestin (a synthetic progesterone such as the widely prescribed Provera), the progestin may block the benefits of estrogen. This is one of the reasons it probably is better to opt for a natural progesterone. In addition, according to a number of studies, estrogen increases your level of triglycerides (blood fat), which can cause clogged arteries and coronary heart disease, and can increase your risk of blood clots.

However, most doctors, even those who have argued against the use of HRT for normal menopausal women, believe that women in premature menopause would benefit from the use of HRT to prevent heart disease—at least until they reach the age of 50, the age at which their bodies would "normally" have experienced an estrogen drop.

To restate a point that I keep saying again and again: the key thing to remember here is that, unlike women who are taking estrogen in their fifties, when you're in premature menopause, you're taking it in your twenties, thirties, or forties—the years in which your body would normally have had this estrogen anyway. You're replacing what the average woman your age has, and so regaining the protection against heart disease that you would have had at this age.

All in all, then, HRT makes sense to reduce heart disease risks from premature menopause. Of course, this isn't a decision to make lightly. Your best course of action is to learn more about HRT, then make an informed decision. Chapter 5 takes a closer look at the pros and cons of hormone replacement therapy as treatment for premature menopause, and should help you make an educated choice.

If you can't or won't take HRT, you can still get the benefit of estrogen.

First, you can replace estrogen by upping your intake of *phytoestrogens,* estrogens found naturally in certain foods such as soy. A 1998 study found that phytoestrogens appear to be as effective in preventing stroke as Premarin (a commonly prescribed conjugated estrogen). The study is part of an ongoing program funded by the National Heart, Lung and Blood Institute that is exploring the benefits of soy phytoestrogens. You can get soy and other phytoestrogens through your diet, or by taking supplements such as soy isoflavones or ground flaxseed. Chapter 6 looks at the many benefits of soy and other phytoestrogen-rich foods and supplements and explains in more depth how they can work for you.

You also can look into taking *tamoxifen* or *raloxifene.* As mentioned before, both are so-called "designer estrogens," or SERMs (selective estrogen receptor modulators), that take the place of estrogen in your body. These seem to offer some cardiovascular benefits; however, they appear to be less effective than regular estrogen. A recent study of raloxifene found that it lowered LDL levels by 11 percent compared with 13 percent with HRT and LP(a) levels by 4 percent compared with 16 percent with HRT, and had no significant effect on HDL, whereas HRT raised HDL by 11 percent. Even so, some prevention is better than none, so raloxifene or tamoxifen may make sense for you if you are unable to take estrogen. Again, talk to your doctor.

HEART HELPER 2: EXERCISE

You've heard it before: regular exercise is good for your heart. It keeps your blood pressure down, increases the level of good cholesterol in your blood, helps you cope with stress, keeps your weight under control, and helps prevent diabetes—and these are only the benefits connected to your heart! It also keeps your lungs working well, tones your muscles, and builds bone. Quite a list of positives.

To get any benefit for your heart, you must exercise at least 30 minutes a day. The good news is that, contrary to what was believed in the past, you don't have to get those 30 minutes of exercise at one time. As long as you get your heart rate up for a total of 30 minutes, you're getting the protection you need. Walk up stairs instead of taking an elevator or escalator. Park farther from the mall and walk a few extra yards. Just get active!

HEART HELPER 3: STICK TO A HEALTHY DIET

Finally, start eating for your heart's sake. Take a look at Chapter 9, which covers healthy eating for women in premature menopause. Briefly, though, here's a quick list of heart-smart eating habits.

Opt for a low-fat diet that gets 20 percent or less of its daily calories from fat. Include a small amount of polyunsaturated fats (such as omega-3 fats, found in fatty fishes like salmon) and omega-6 fats (in vegetable oils), as well as monounsaturated fats. Eat more fruits and vegetables and other sources of soluble fiber. Try to get about 25 to 35 grams of fiber a day to help reduce cholesterol, protect against diabetes, and keep blood sugar levels stable. Finally, try to cut down on sugar and empty calories.

You've probably heard this advice before, but for good reason: it works!

HEART-SMARTS: SOME MORE QUICK TIPS FOR A HEALTHIER HEART

- *If you smoke, quit. If you don't smoke, don't start.*

- *Cut down on alcohol.* Yes, some studies have shown that drinking can be good for your heart, but excessive drinking is still considered a no-no.

- *Have your blood pressure and cholesterol checked.* Get regular checkups to be sure that your blood pressure and cholesterol levels stay low. If you start HRT, it makes sense to get checked at the very beginning, then three or so months later to see if the HRT is working well for you. Otherwise, you may need to readjust your treatment.

- *Try to minimize stress in your life.* It may be easier said than done, but if you can avoid getting stressed out, you help your heart. Try relaxation exercises, yoga, or anything else that keeps you calm.

- *Consider taking certain vitamins, herbs, and other supplements for your heart's sake.* Vitamin A, carotenoid complex, B-complex, calcium, copper, chromium, magnesium, manganese, selenium, zinc, and CoQ10 all appear to help your heart. In addition, studies have shown that garlic helps lower cholesterol and prevent arterial buildup.

AUTOIMMUNE DISEASES, INCLUDING DIABETES AND THYROID DISEASE

Autoimmune disorders affect more women than men; in fact, women account for about 75 to 90 percent of all cases of autoimmune disease. Moreover, it is estimated that about one in 10 of all women will develop an autoimmune disease. And if these figures aren't sobering enough, recent research has indicated that there may be a link between natural premature menopause and autoimmune disorders.

According to these studies, if your premature menopause is due to an autoimmune disorder, you are probably at a higher risk for other autoimmune disorders, including rheumatoid arthritis, myasthenia gravis, diabetes, and thyroid disease.

It's a vicious circle of sorts: often having an autoimmune disorder can result in premature menopause. For example, a 1997 study reported that women with Type 1 diabetes reach menopause at an average age of 40, compared with 50 for non-diabetic women. Researchers believe this may happen because Type 1 diabetes causes accelerated aging, which may then contribute to premature ovarian failure. The study concluded that premature menopause may be a previously unnoticed complication of diabetes.

By the same token, it's possible that your premature menopause has been caused by an undetected autoimmune disorder. Recent research has indicated that there may be a link between autoimmune-caused premature menopause and other autoimmune disorders. According to one recent study, there seemed to be a higher-than-normal association of premature ovarian failure with diabetes, specifically insulin-dependent diabetes mellitus (or IDDM) and myasthenia gravis. In addition, cellular immune abnormalities were present in the POF patients studied that were similar to those seen in women with endocrine autoimmune diseases such as Graves' disease (a form of thyroid disease IDDM, and Addison's disease). So, while not everyone with premature menopause is necessarily at increased risk for autoimmune disorders, for those who may have experienced natural premature menopause due to autoimmune causes, there is a possibility that you will develop another autoimmune disorder.

It's a serious problem and one you should most definitely be aware of, because some autoimmune disorders are incurable. Most can, however, be controlled through medication and, in some cases, surgery.

What Can You Do? The Importance of Being Tested Regularly

Unlike other long-term consequences of premature menopause, autoimmune disorders can't be treated simply by taking hormones or changing your diet. If you suspect you're at risk for autoimmune disorders—and, to repeat, you could be if your premature menopause occurred naturally, not as a result of surgery or cancer treatment—then it's wise to speak to your doctor and discuss getting tests.

The tests you may want to get include:

- *measurements of serum calcium and phosphorus* to check for hypoparathyroidism;
- *thyroid function and antibodies* to test for thyroid disease;
- *AM cortisol* to check for hypoadrenalism;
- *blood sugar levels* to check for diabetes.

In addition, depending upon your symptoms and your family history, you may want to get periodically tested for lupus and rheumatoid arthritis.

Often the key to controlling and living with an autoimmune disorder is catching it in time, before it has a chance to attack your body for an extended period of time. This is why it is vital to be tested periodically, especially if you have a family history of autoimmune disease. With autoimmune disease, it's better to be one step ahead.

Chapter 4

Why Me?

Dealing with the Emotional Realities of Premature Menopause

I'm not sure what was worse: the immediate shock of learning I was in premature menopause, or the low-grade depression that I slumped into in the weeks afterward. I think I was numb for a day or two, then the reality hit me like a wall. I kept trying to push my emotions aside, telling myself I could handle it, that it wasn't that bad. But I couldn't stop the grief about being suddenly infertile, the fears about my health, and all the questions that kept rattling around in my head: Was I still sexy? Was I old? Was I attractive? Was I still a real woman? I didn't feel like me any more . . .

It sounds odd, maybe, that something can shake your self-image so much. But premature menopause can and does. Most women who learn that they are in premature menopause go through a very difficult time emotionally. It's a devastating experience. Often you feel as if someone or something had died. And, in many ways, something *has* died: your youth, or, at least, your image of it.

When you know that you are in premature menopause, you suddenly feel older, different from your peers. You feel as though you have been cheated out of the normal possibilities

of life. In your twenties or thirties, you are unable to fulfill the
"normal" reproductive capacity women have.

You're plunged into a completely different mind-set from the
one you had before premature menopause. Your body is out of
control and you are helpless to change what is happening.
You're angry, upset, and numb. But, somehow, you have to
keep going.

It isn't easy. I know this through my own experiences and
through talking with so many other women coping with premature menopause.

Premature menopause brings with it a wrenching emotional
change along with the physical. Your emotions are already affected by the shifting hormones in your body, and the reality
of your condition affects your emotions even more. A study
conducted in London found that premature menopause was associated with higher-than-average levels of depression. The single most upsetting element of premature menopause, according
to all the women surveyed, was the most basic: their loss of
reproductive capacity. It didn't make a difference if they had
children or not, or even if they had been trying to have children.
The sudden switch from fertile woman to irrevocably infertile
woman was the biggest blow of all.

I never suspected I was in premature meno—I was only
32. My doctor was very concerned and felt very bad for
me. I am still not dealing with it very well. I wanted more
children and I have a hard time understanding why this
happened to me. I am still pretty depressed about it and
it is hard when other people ask when are you having
more children? It is hard for me to see friends who are
pregnant but I know I need to be happy for them. Right
now, both of my sisters-in-law are pregnant and due in
the spring and I know I have to be supportive of them,
even though I do not think they realize how painful this
is for me.

—Stacey, age 33

To make matters even more difficult, fertility is more than just the actual biological ability to have children. It symbolizes much more than this to yourself and to society. Fertility is youth, womanhood, the essence of being female. It is a substantial part of how we define ourselves as women. So when the ability to have a child is suddenly stripped from you before the normal age, you often feel less of a woman. You just don't feel whole any more.

I wouldn't have necessarily believed this if I hadn't talked to so many women who said the same thing, and if I hadn't gone through it myself. In fact, I never really realized how much the idea of being fertile was a part of my self-image. Yes, I planned to have children, but I was also a career woman, very focused on my work, and I identified myself as a writer above all. Yet when I was told that my reproductive system had essentially stopped working the right way, I was reeling. I felt I had lost a piece of myself. It wasn't only the idea that I could never have my biological child. It was also the idea that my body had stopped doing its "female" job—and had suddenly jumped ahead so many years. I was old. I had turned from a 38-year-old into an ancient crone. I felt that I had lost my fertility and my youth in one fell swoop, and there was nothing I could do about it.

Nothing I could do about it. . . . This sense of powerlessness was a very large part of my depression. Premature menopause wasn't like other health problems that I could take care of. There was no magic cure. Yes, I could treat the symptoms, but the underlying cause, the huge change in my life, was completely out of my hands. And that's where the "why me" came in. Why was I singled out? Why was I stuck with this body that wasn't working right any more? Why was I old before my time?

All of the other women I've spoken with had the same reaction. It's often even worse for women in surgical menopause, because not only have they been through major surgery, they've also literally lost something—their reproductive organs.

I didn't know until I was alert enough in the hospital that both my ovaries had to be removed. This recovery took a long time both physically and emotionally. I had to try and accept that I may not be able to have my own children. After my TAH [total abdominal hysterectomy], it was an emotional devastation. Here I was at only 27 years old and my life dream of having my own biological child was ripped away from me. This is something that I will have to live with the rest of my life and it is a very hard thing to try and accept.

—Iris, age 28

Regardless of whether the premature menopause came naturally or through surgery, and regardless of whether we were already mothers or not, we all share similar feelings of profound loss, the same grief and shock, the same pain. But, as with any life-changing event, you *can* cope. You can, with time, deal with the reality of loss. You can feel young again, like *you* again.

The most difficult thing for me emotionally was accepting my "new self," never being the mommy that I always thought I would be. At times I do feel prematurely old. I'm definitely an old soul (cancer at age 13 and POF/ premature menopause at age 21), I've had to grow up too fast, I've missed out on so much and will continue to. But I'm trying hard to be thankful for that which I do have and regain control of my life.

—Steph, age 28

To a great degree, coping with the emotional realities of premature menopause is a step-by-step process. The problems in dealing with premature menopause don't disappear overnight and, in truth, never *completely* disappear. You will have constant reminders about your condition, and some of the pain and loss will never go away. But, as with dealing with death, dealing with the loss of your young womanhood is a slow process of acceptance. You will go through bad times, but you will live through them. And after some time has passed, you can actually be stronger because of the difficult transition you have gone through. While you don't have the ability to reverse what has happened to you, you do have the power to accept the change, adjust to it, and emerge intact. I hope this chapter helps you with this journey.

> There's always change in your life—whether it's in your relationships, your job, your health, your family. And premature menopause is another change. It's another aspect of life, not one I had thought I'd be dealing with at this point, but there's nothing I can do about that. All I can do is go along with the change. It's just part of living, really.
> —Rita, age 35

RECONCILING YOURSELF TO THE CHANGE: SHOCK, GRIEF, ANGER, MOURNING, AND ACCEPTANCE

> I had been telling the doctor I thought I was going through menopause and he didn't believe me. Finally he gave me a hormone test and it proved what I had been saying all along. But even though I thought I was menopausal, when I was actually sitting there and he told me I was right, I couldn't believe it. I thought I would be ready for the bad news, but I guess I wasn't. I just sat there.
> —Diana, age 31

> When they said meno, I just went into shock. I just couldn't believe it. I was so numb I didn't know what to do or to say.
> —Amy, age 35

Shock. That's what most women in premature menopause say that they initially feel. And it is a shock to be told by a doctor that your body has begun going through such a momentous change.

"It can't be happening to me," you think. "There's got to be some sort of mistake."

Many women keep on thinking this, and go through a period of denial. I was one of them. I thought that if I ignored it, the premature menopause might go away. I couldn't or wouldn't believe that I could actually be going through menopause at age 38. So I went to different doctors, constantly hoping that one of them would tell me everything was okay and I was back to normal. Of course, this didn't happen. But along the way, I slowly began adjusting to the idea of premature menopause and admitting to myself that it had actually happened to me.

I now realize that I was giving myself one of the most important and useful coping tools I could have: *time*.

Time heals all wounds, as the old saying goes—and, in fact, it does to some degree. Time gives you the chance to readjust your outlook. You need time to get used to what is happening to you emotionally and physically and to handle the huge changes in your life.

Think about it: as I mentioned before, not only have you been hit with emotionally charged news when you first learn you're in premature menopause, but also your body is in an upheaval. Your hormones are nose-diving and surging, and your moods are riding the roller-coaster along with them. From a purely biological standpoint, then, you can't be expected to think all that clearly, and your emotional reaction to the news makes it even more difficult.

This is one of the reasons so many experts recommend not making any major decisions at the beginning. Yes, you should think about going on HRT, make sure you're getting enough calcium, and face the myriad other health issues that confront you. But you can and should take a few days or even weeks to examine the options open to you, to research the different forms of HRT, and talk to your doctor about what you believe will work best for you. Taking a little time now can save you time in the long run. If you want to have a child and have been told to try donor eggs or adoption, it's tempting to act quickly, especially since you feel as though you've already run out of time. But time is actually on your side—or rather, *taking* time is.

Our society is geared to the quick fix, but premature menopause has no instant solution. You don't need to come to grips with it overnight. You can and should allow yourself to accept slowly what is happening. Give yourself the gift of time. Allow yourself a little breathing room. Menopause isn't called "the change" for nothing. It *is* a change, a significant change, and one that is all the more wrenching when you are in your twenties or thirties and don't expect it. As with any major change, you need time to absorb its consequences fully, as well as its effects, and its actuality.

- *Take time to learn about what is happening to you*—Researching your condition is one of the best ways to begin mastering it. The more you know about premature menopause, the better you can deal with it, because you will understand what is going on with your body, what you can expect, and what your options are in terms of coping with it. Read books and articles about menopause and search the Internet for information about premature menopause, premature ovarian failure, and surgical menopause, as well as menopause in general. This is an important step not only in coming to grips with premature menopause, but also to empower you to make decisions and ask questions so you can be in charge of your body again.
- *Take time for yourself*—With any major life change, it's important to recognize that you need time for you alone. It can be as little as a few minutes every day—but setting aside any amount of personal time, especially at the very beginning of your premature menopause, helps you adjust. Your personal time can be anything that makes you happy—walking, gardening, exercising, shopping, reading, or just sitting and thinking. By spending time on yourself for yourself, you're getting reacquainted with the new you and revving up your emotional reserves so you can better handle the change in your life.

• *Take time to count your blessings*—It may sound corny, but it's great advice. Remember to appreciate the little things— a beautiful day, the flowers in your garden, a smile from a friend, a hug from your husband. Coping with premature menopause, or any big change in your life, is wrenching, so it's more important than ever to remind yourself of the good things in your life to keep your soul nourished and your spirits refreshed.

The Power of Grieving

> I started crying when the doctor told me I was in meno-pause. He looked at me as if I were crazy. "It's not like you're going to die," he said. I felt like such an ass. "That's not the point," I wanted to tell him, but I knew he wouldn't understand.
> —Sherry, age 29

Premature menopause brings with it a sense of profound loss. Whether it's for the children you will never have or for your own "normal" past, you probably will feel like grieving.

Unfortunately, you'll often have people telling you there's no need to. The problem is that there is no obvious loss. Premature menopause is a hidden, private matter, one that isn't outwardly advertised. While there are most definitely physical and emo-tional repercussions as a result of going through menopause prematurely, menopause itself often isn't something that is re-garded as a traumatic experience. Even women who are in pre-mature menopause as a result of surgery due to cancer or chemotherapy may find that people are more sympathetic toward them about the cancer, not about the resulting menopause.

People often can't understand the full impact that going through an early menopause can have on you. They can't under-stand the strange feeling of having lost a part of your life and of your identity as a woman, and can't fathom how much it can hurt. So they may act as though you have no reason to be so upset.

And often you may agree with them. There are worse things that can happen, you tell yourself—which, of course, is true. So you feel that you shouldn't grieve. Perhaps you don't want to dwell on the pain or bother your husband or friends with your sadness, or maybe you just want it all to go away (the whole denial trip). You try to put on a happy face, push aside all the negative feelings, and act as though there's nothing wrong.

But let's be completely honest, here: there *is* something wrong. No, you're not dying, as the doctor told Sherry. But something has changed irrevocably in your life, something has been lost—and grief is the natural reaction to loss.

When someone dies, we grieve. It is eminently human, and it is a way of eventually coming to grips with the hole in your life. Premature menopause is a death of a different sort. A part of you is gone forever, and the options you had before premature menopause are gone as well. One woman I spoke with put it very eloquently: she was mourning "the death of her dream children."

> The few people I told immediately suggested adoption, which made me mad. I did feel that I needed to mourn my own baby first. It felt like someone had died. But there are no support groups, no rituals to grieve the loss of a dream. I cried hourly, then daily, then weekly. No one could understand that I didn't want someone else's baby, I wanted my baby, the baby that could never be. Everywhere I looked there were pregnant women and babies, and each one felt like a knife in my heart.
> —Amy, age 35

> I find that some friends will ignore talking about their children around me. I had a coworker who became pregnant immediately after my TAH. I heard about it at work through "the grapevine" and then she found out that I knew. She told me that she was afraid to tell me and didn't know how to tell me. I appreciated that, but it was extremely difficult watching her through her nine months of pregnancy and everyone being so happy for her and

her husband. I couldn't even get her a gift, the emotional
pain was so raw for me.
                              —Iris, age 28

These are very descriptive and honest ways of putting it.
Whether or not you have children or intended to have them,
the loss of fertility is real and has powerful implications. As I
mentioned earlier, it's a symbol of femininity and of youth.
Women often say they feel "deficient" once they've gone
through premature menopause. They feel diminished, less than
they once were.

Of course, intellectually you know that you aren't deficient.
You aren't less than you were. But often, especially when you
are first in premature menopause, it doesn't matter what your
intellect tells you. What matters is what your heart says, how
you *feel*, no matter how illogical.

Because the ideas of deficiency, diminished selfhood, and
plain old loss are such difficult feelings to handle, it's vital to
go through the step of grieving. Grief is a powerful cleansing
emotion, one that allows you to accept the sadness you feel
and, in so doing, clears the way for you to move ahead with
your life. When you block your sorrow, when you refuse to
grieve if you feel the need, it won't go away. You can bury it
for a while, but eventually the grief will pop out again or under-
mine your attempts honestly and squarely to face your situation.

A reproductive endocrinologist I saw after I was first diagnosed and exploring fertility options asked me if I was sure I
was ready to make the decision about children. She then told
me about one woman who had come to her and wanted to enter
the donor egg program, believing that she had completely come
to terms with her premature ovarian failure. But once the
woman and her husband began talking seriously about the prospects with the staff psychologist, all the grief she had bottled
up about going through menopause at such a young age came
pouring out. She hadn't adequately dealt with the idea that she
would be unable to have a biological child of her own; instead
she had resolutely forbidden herself to think about it, and fo-

cused only on the possibility of having a child by donor egg. Ultimately, the fertility center told her they couldn't accept her for a donor egg procedure at that point. She had to come back in a few months, after she had worked through her mourning. Then, and only then, would they consider her ready to go ahead with a donor egg procedure.

Going through a period of grieving isn't important only if you want to explore having a child. It's important for you to get ahead with your life in general. By grieving, you can come to a new understanding of yourself and your premature menopause condition. It's a transitional emotion that enables you to face honestly what has happened to you.

Premature menopause is a serious and, yes, sad change in your life. Regardless of what others who haven't experienced it may believe, it isn't an easy thing to come to grips with. So, remember, you are *entitled* to grieve—for the children you may have wanted, for the dramatic change in your self-image, for the loss of your youth or your carefree attitude toward your health.

Grieving can be an empowering, positive act. While painful and wrenching, admitting your loss and sorrow to yourself is a step toward accepting that loss and moving onward.

- *Don't be afraid to let yourself go a little*—No, you shouldn't constantly wallow in your grief, but you should allow yourself to feel as upset as you are. If you want to cry, cry. It sounds like a simplistic piece of advice, but it's one that many of us fail to follow. We're so busy keeping a stiff upper lip that when the tears do come, we're in danger of drowning in them. It's healthier and more effective to go with the flow—literally.
- *Along these lines, indulge your grief a bit*—I found it very comforting to allow myself a "sad time" every now and then. I would listen to sad music or, after my husband went to bed, I'd stay up and watch a tear-jerker movie and let myself cry my eyes out. It really helped, since I spent many days with my "public" face on—the one that was happy, adjusted, and certainly not crying at the drop of a hat. But

this way I could let the tears come out instead of bottling them up . . . and not by dwelling on my own situation. I now realize it was, in effect, a legitimate way of getting through my grief without feeling I was overdoing it.

• *Talk out your grief with your partner, friends, or family*— It's easy to swallow your sorrow and keep it inside. But often, talking about how you feel is the best way of getting in touch with your emotions. Be honest with your husband or friends. If you open up about your sense of loss, not only will they understand you better and help you deal with it, but you won't feel the added stress of having to keep up appearances.

• *If possible, talk to other women who have gone through a similar situation.*—The old saying "misery loves company" is a true one. Talking with other people who can truly understand your feeling of loss can help you feel less alone. If possible, seek out support groups for women in premature menopause. There are several on-line (see the Appendix for a listing) or you can ask your doctor if she is treating other women with the same condition. For more on support groups, see pages 129 to 132.

Depression: The Sister of Grief

> **I remember being completely out of it for a few months— totally depressed, everything seemed bleak, nothing seemed to help me snap out of it. I thought I was never going to be happy again.**
> **—Cindy, age 31**

Often you'll go through a period of grieving, only to sink into a low-level depression. You may not feel the sharp pain of loss you initially felt at learning about your premature menopause, but you definitely don't feel good. You feel emotionally flat, generally drained, and hopeless.

Again, this is a natural feeling and nothing you should feel

guilty about. Most women who go through premature menopause (or even just regular menopause) experience bouts of
tears, weepiness, and general depression, particularly at the beginning stages. Some of it is probably hormonal. Low estrogen
levels do lower endorphins in your brain, contributing to depression. And if you've gone through surgical menopause, the
chances are even higher that you will suffer from some form
of depression, possibly from the sudden, abrupt decline in
your hormones.

In addition to the physical basis for being depressed, there's
the simple emotional side of things: you are still young, but
you're in menopause and you feel old. For some women, even
the word itself is difficult to deal with.

> The "M" word. I hate it! It sounds ugly and it makes
> me feel old every time I say it!
> —Celia, age 26

The problem is that menopause is such a loaded word. Regardless of the fact that many women in menopause look as
young and vibrant as ever, it still conveys a picture of age. And
in your twenties and thirties, it's difficult to get used to applying
the word to yourself. As more and more baby boomers enter
menopause, it is beginning to lose some of its stigma, but there
still is that feeling that menopause equals old.

Premature menopause makes you feel like you've instantly
aged. You worry about things like wrinkles (which are sometimes caused by lower estrogen). You find yourself reading articles that are aimed at 50-year-old women. You can share HRT
tips with your mother. It's no wonder you feel as though you've
stepped into a completely different age group. Added to this
"old" feeling is the natural depression about losing your fertility, and the idea that your body is playing tricks on you. You
may find that you've lost interest in sex (again, a common
complaint, especially since sex can often be painful when your
estrogen levels are low, but also because you just don't feel
sexy any more—another fallout of feeling suddenly old).

All of these factors contribute to depression, and it's important to realize that, regardless of what articles and books written for women in regular menopause say, depression is a very natural and very common reaction to premature menopause. There have been several studies done showing that women undergoing surgical menopause have a higher rate of depression than those who go through a natural menopause. The reason? Researchers conjecture this may be due to the suddenness of their menopause and the feeling of loss. And this is similar to the reaction of women in premature menopause, whether surgical or natural. This major change in their life is unexpected and comes out of the blue.

And if you're in premature menopause due to surgery, you might actually have a double whammy. Not only is depression not uncommon after surgical menopause and premature menopause, but women with surgical menopause sometimes aren't afflicted by the depression until as long as two or three years after surgery.

Whatever situation you find yourself in, though, whether your premature menopause was natural or surgical, the key thing to remember is that your depression is completely natural and understandable. Don't make the mistake of blaming yourself and thinking that you're somehow being weak or whiny because you feel low. Depression is yet another of the common offshoots of premature menopause, and it's something you can cope with.

Going on HRT usually will help you fight the premature menopause blues because it raises your estrogen levels and normalizes your body, ridding you of symptoms such as night sweats and insomnia that contribute to depression. But often you'll still feel upset while trying to adjust to the new, menopausal you. You may find yourself feeling better one day, then sink back into a gray depression the next. Again, this is all part of the normal adjustment process and something that, over time, will diminish.

There are things, though, you can do to help you handle the

depression when it comes. In addition to HRT, you can try these strategies:

- *Exercise*—This is nature's own mood-lifter, and it works! Exercise raises the level of endorphins in your brain, which are natural mood elevators. In addition, exercising is a way of reclaiming power over your body, which can also lift your spirits.
- *Get involved in your hobbies or try new ones*—Sometimes losing yourself in something you enjoy can help you weather the bad times. It's not running away from your problem, but it is a way of giving yourself something else to focus on. Often engaging in an activity you love will raise your spirits, calm your mind, and feed your soul.
- *Identify "trigger" situations that send you into an emotional slump, and avoid them for a while*—This sounds like classic avoidance, but sometimes the best move you can make for yourself is to steer clear of things that upset you. Remember, it's not forever. It's just until you get an emotional footing again. So if you are already feeling down and you know that walking past a certain playground will get you even lower, don't walk past that playground. Or if you just don't think you could handle a family gathering because you don't want to explain about your menopause, don't go this time. You know your own limits, and it's fine to respect them.
- *Focus on the positive as much as possible*—Remind yourself that menopause isn't the end of you—it's the beginning of a new you. You're embarking on a new aspect of your life, one that can be as rich and fruitful as you make it.
- *If you can't shake the depression or if it seems deep and insurmountable, definitely consider seeking professional help*— Some women going through premature menopause end up in clinical depression. If you find yourself unable to cope, if you feel that your quality of life is seriously affected, or if you are chronically depressed, see a therapist or other professional. This is no time to tough this out on your own.

THE SIGNS OF MAJOR DEPRESSION

Mild depression is a common offshoot of premature menopause. But there is a big difference between mild depression and major, clinical depression. Clinical depression is a disease and requires medical treatment. Here are the common signs of clinical depression:

- You dramatically change your eating habits and eat too much or too little.

- You begin sleeping much more or much less.

- You feel extremely lethargic or very jumpy.

- You are unable to enjoy the things you used to, especially sex.

- You are always very tired and rarely have any energy.

- You find yourself slipping into feelings of self-loathing and worthlessness.

- You can't concentrate on anything and find yourself unable to make decisions.

- You think about suicide or death.

If you suffer from four or more of these symptoms for two weeks or more, you may be clinically depressed and should seek professional help.

Anger: The "It's Not Fair" Syndrome

I was in a store today and it seemed as if there were babies everywhere I looked. I saw this woman with the cutest baby, about six months old. She was holding and cuddling him. Everyone else was smiling at them. I couldn't. I didn't even want to look. It really, really made me feel totally shortchanged.

—Anne, age 37

It is difficult not to feel shortchanged when faced with premature menopause. Other women your age can have children and you can't. Other women your age aren't faced with the consequences of having a reproductive system that has essentially stopped working. They don't have to come to grips with concerns about aging, debates about HRT, and thoughts of osteoporosis and heart disease. "It's just not fair!" you want to scream sometimes. And, honestly, it *isn't* fair. Some people may tell you to get past that feeling by remembering others who are less fortunate than you but while that may help a bit, you still have that deep-down feeling of having been cheated.

To make matters worse, many of the physical symptoms of menopause, such as hot flashes, insomnia, and night sweats, help feed the fire of your anger. You're often exhausted, which makes you more jumpy, which, in turn, makes it easier for you to get angry and stressed out.

Oddly enough, though, the anger you may be feeling is a very positive force—a healing force for you. Often you'll find that the anger, the feeling of being cheated or shortchanged, happens after you've gone through a period of grieving. Instead of sinking into a mire of depression, you find yourself lashing out instead. This is common and very healthy. It's a natural step on the road to acceptance of your premature menopause.

The problem is that you may sometimes turn that anger you feel about premature menopause against other people or other situations that have nothing to do with menopause. Many women find themselves yelling at their children or starting fights with their husbands, and end up feeling even worse once the anger has passed. Instead of the rage they felt, they're consumed with guilt and consider themselves bad mothers or wives.

While it is understandable to feel guilty about taking your anger out on someone who has nothing to do with it, do recognize that the emotional upheaval you are going through is the cause. You're not "bad" for reacting badly, you're just stressed out.

Some women turn their anger about premature menopause into anger at themselves: "I should have had a child earlier,"

"I should have been healthier," "I should have guessed what was happening." There are hundreds of ways you can blame yourself. I know how tempting it can be to do this, but dwelling on these "should-haves" can only make you feel worse. Premature menopause isn't your fault. It's something that happened to you, something you couldn't prevent.

If you notice that the anger you feel is getting the upper hand in your life, you can work through it in a number of different ways:

- *Take time out when you feel the anger building*—If you know that you're ready to blow up, stop and cool off. Try deep breathing, just sitting quietly, or anything else that helps you cycle down the rage.
- *As with depression, if there is a certain person or situation that makes you get stressed or angry, try to distance yourself*—Give yourself a break, literally, by getting away from the person or situation that is setting you off, even if it's just for a little while. If you find that you're blowing up more at your children, see if someone else can watch them for a while.
- *Channel your anger into other activities*—When you find yourself overwhelmed with anger, use that energy to do something else: exercise, garden, read . . . do anything to defuse that hot feeling into calmness.
- *Destress yourself as much as possible*—Stress often leads to tension, which leads to frayed nerves and anger. Try some of the stress-busters mentioned later in this chapter, such as yoga, meditation, or exercise. Or again, take time for yourself by doing an activity you enjoy.
- *If you fly off the handle at your husband, children, or friends for no real reason, explain that your anger was misdirected*— Honesty to yourself and others can heal the hurts caused by your anger. Be as frank as possible. Explain that you were wrong and that you need them to understand that you are going through a difficult time.
- *Finally, don't beat up on yourself for blowing up*—Adding

guilt or self-loathing to everything you're dealing with won't help you cope. Remember that your anger is a natural reaction to a bad situation and that with time it will pass.

Feeling Powerless: How to Regain Control

> I felt like I was going insane. I had hundreds of hot flashes each day, so bad that my clothes would be drenched. I would cry for no reason at all. Sometimes I'd be furious for no reason—I'd find myself yelling at my daughter and then I'd feel so bad for yelling. It was a nightmare. I didn't feel like myself. And I didn't like the person I had become.
>
> —Celia, age 26

One of the most disconcerting aspects of premature menopause is the feeling of being out of control. Your body is going bonkers, and you're stuck going along for the ride whether you want to or not. And, worse, you can't do a thing about it.

Well, actually, you *can*. While you can't reverse premature menopause, you can fight back against that "out of control" feeling by taking charge of your body and your mind. It is a way of being active, of seizing power when you feel the most powerless.

Regaining control of your body and mind allows you to regain control of your life. It is a way of making premature menopause only one aspect of your life, not the be-all and end-all that it often seems to be, especially at the beginning.

* *Learn as much as you can about your condition, so you can take an active role in treating it*—This, to me, is one of the most positive and empowering acts a woman in premature menopause can do for herself. The more you know about what is happening to your body, the more you can be involved in the whole treatment process, both with your doctor and by yourself. In addition, when you know the whys and hows of premature menopause, you can better understand

why you feel the way you do, and figure out how to cope better. Fear of the unknown is one of the most potent fears. By making premature menopause a known quantity, you can reduce the fear and powerlessness it may create in you.

- *Take positive actions about your lifestyle*—Often, dealing with premature menopause can be the jump-start you need to push you into a new, healthier lifestyle: begin eating better, follow a good exercise program, quit smoking, start taking vitamins. There are a number of positive moves you can make that will not only help your body in handling menopausal symptoms and consequences, but also help your psyche. By doing something positive—actually, just by doing *something*—you are taking charge of the situation and turning it into an opportunity for you to improve yourself and take charge of your health as you may not have before.

- *Give yourself the chance for small victories*—Feeling in control is often a matter of feeling victorious, feeling that you've conquered something, no matter how small. Set small goals for yourself so you can be sure you'll meet them. For example, if you've put on weight since premature menopause, decide that through diet and exercise you want to lose a pound in a week or two. Or if you are starting an exercise program, you can decide to begin with 15 minutes of exercise a day four days a week. By setting small, workable goals, you can ensure yourself small victories and enjoy the feeling of having made a positive, take-charge move.

- *Rid yourself of stress*—Premature menopause in and of itself is a stressful condition to deal with, physically and emotionally. So the more you eliminate stress from your life, the better able you are to take charge of your situation. Listen to your body and begin to pick up on the signs it sends you about stress. If you notice that you're having problems sleeping or are suffering from indigestion or fatigue, chances are your body is telling you that it's stressing out and you need to take time to relax.

- *Try relaxation techniques for both your body and mind*—Yoga, deep breathing, muscle relaxation, tai chi, and the like are great ways of calming your mind and relaxing (sometimes even toning) your body. (For some simple techniques that work see page 55.)

Get the Support You Need

Getting support from others, whether it's your husband, your family or friends, or a more formal support group of other women in the same situation, is probably the most helpful thing you can do for yourself.

Because premature menopause wreaks such havoc on you physically and emotionally, it's important to vent sometimes, to find people you trust who you can talk to, unload on, and just draw comfort from.

> **My friends are all going through so much negative stuff, we all are a welcome understanding ear to each other. Spouse problems, teenage children problems, our own premenopause problems, etc. My mom is the only person who understands everything I've been through, including the premenopausal things, and has been my ultimate support system.**
> **—Bryana, age 38**

Virtually all the women I have spoken with who are going through premature menopause said that talking out their concerns, worries, and fears was a great help in adjusting to this change in their lives.

Possibly one of the best ways of coping with the emotional fallout of premature menopause and maintaining a sense of calm once you've passed through the worst of the transition is to join a support group of women who are experiencing the same things and can truly understand what exactly you are going through.

> **Finding women who have "been there/done that" has been of help. It always makes you feel better when some-**

one says "I know what you mean" and you know that they mean it.

—Steph, age 28

As I said before, I think the one thing that helped me most was finding a group of women on America Online who were also going through premature menopause. For the first time since I was diagnosed, I felt like I wasn't alone. I could ask questions, share experiences, and discuss my feelings with other women like me. In many ways, I was more able to be completely open and honest about many issues because I knew I would be understood.

Support groups are a very special form of community because you can share in a special way. While you may confide in friends and family, other women in premature menopause are in tune with you; they're going through the same ups and downs you are. They have many of the same fears and are fighting the same battles with their bodies and emotions. Most important, you realize that you aren't alone. There are other women out there like you.

How can you find a support group? If you have a computer, you can explore a number of them online. For example, America Online has a message board I participate in called "Early Menopause" for women in premature menopause whether naturally, through surgery, or due to cancer treatments, as well as a weekly support chat group meeting. I can't begin to express how helpful this group has been for me. Talking on line with other women who were going through premature menopause kept me going when I was still reeling from the diagnosis. And now, two years later, I still find the group a wonderful source of much-needed support, information, and camaraderie. (The "Early Menopause" message board is at Keyword: Women Talk. Go to the message boards; click on "Wellness," then on "Health Central," and you'll see it.) There's also a support group for women with POF reachable at http://pofsupport.org. Infertility sites are often a good place to find other women in premature menopause, such as INCIID (the International Council on Infertility Information Database) at www.inciid.org. If you're in premature menopause due to surgery, there are numerous support groups for women who've had oophorectomies or hysterectomies. In addition, you can often find young women who've gone through menopause on general menopause sites. See the Appendix (page 367) for a complete listing of different Web sites and support groups available to you.

You don't necessarily need to find a support group that's already established. The computer is also a great means of setting up your own support group. As I mentioned before, the early menopause group that I belong to began informally. A few of us met through posts on a general menopause message board on America Online, we all began corresponding by e-mail and eventually we set up a group that meets for weekly chats and even has its own message board now. I've also met dozens of other women via the Internet by posting on other general Web menopause boards, and exchange regular correspondence with them. As one woman from England recently wrote to me, it is wonderful to be able to share concerns and advice with someone across an ocean who can truly understand what you're going through. So you may want ot reach out on your own— check out menopause message boards on the Web, see if there are other women who have posted about premature menopause, and e-mail them directly. Also check infertility sites (See the Appendix for some of the major ones). You would be surprised at how many women are out there going through premature menopause, and how many would be grateful to establish contact with others like them.

But, of course, you don't need a computer to find or set up a support group. You can check with associations dealing with your situation to help you find a local support group. For example, if you have gone through premature menopause due to cancer, check with your local branch of the American Cancer Society. National infertility associations often have local offices and maintain programs and support groups for women. One of the largest of these is RESOLVE, which has both a national headquarters and local branches across the country. Contact them at:

RESOLVE
1310 Broadway
Somerville, MA 02144-1731
617/623-1156
617/623-0252
www.resolve.org

You can also talk to local reproductive centers to see if they have any special groups or programs for women like you. Finally, you may want to speak to your doctor to see if she is treating other women going through your situation who would want to join an informal support group of your own.

Also keep in mind that support groups can be extremely informal. If you don't know women your own age going through menopause, then you can recruit family members or older friends who are going through menopause. While they may not completely empathize with the difficulty in adjusting to this transition at a young age, they'll certainly understand the symptoms you're going through and can often give you great advice or at least an understanding ear.

PREMATURE MENOPAUSE AND YOUR PARTNER: WORKING TOGETHER THROUGH YOUR CHANGE

I think it is hard on my husband and I'm not sure if he really understands what actually is going on. There is a lot to know about and I'm not sure he realizes what I am going through. It has affected my daughter also as she is asking why she cannot have a baby brother and sister. How do you explain that to a six-year-old?
—Stacey, age 33

Going through premature menopause isn't only an individual process. It also affects those around you, especially your partner. And in turn, his reaction may have an enormous effect on you.

Dealing with your partner (and his dealing with you) is a very special, sometimes very helpful, sometimes very difficult, element in coping with premature menopause. Even if your husband is extremely supportive, you may find that premature menopause puts new stresses on your relationship. You may feel guilty because of your condition or angry because he can't fathom how you're feeling. You may worry that he won't love you any more. He might not understand why you're crying so much, or where the anger and feeling of loss is coming from. You both may feel confused, concerned, and crazed by the change in your life.

In many ways, premature menopause becomes another partner in your relationship, a new factor that you and he aren't used to dealing with. When you go through such a major transition, by necessity your partner goes through it too, even though it's not happening to him personally. So it is important to understand what you may confront in your relationship and how to deal with the changes that *your* change is causing.

"He Doesn't Understand": How to Communicate What You're Going Through

> I've been extremely lucky in that my husband has always been 110 percent supportive. When he proposed to me, I told him that I would not marry him if having his own children was important to him. Deep down I knew then. He somehow kept his sanity amidst me losing mine, he remained caring, loving, and understanding through my search for my lost libido. He's been wonderful for me!
> —Steph, age 28

Many women find that their husbands are their best source of support—everything they hoped for and more. But sometimes, at a time when you can least handle it, you'll find that you aren't getting the support you need from your husband.

You are going through hormone hell, your emotions are all over the map, you are depressed and upset, and your husband isn't giving you what you need.

> **I was an emotional basket case when I first learned I had POF. I wasn't on HRT, so my hormones were seesawing, plus I was trying to get used to the idea that I wouldn't have a kid, and that I was actually in menopause. My husband tried to be supportive, but I don't think he completely understood how much this whole thing hit me. He kept saying that it could be worse, that I wasn't sick or anything. But I think I really wanted him to feel as bad as I did about the whole thing, and to understand that my entire life felt like it had been turned upside down.**
> **—Diana, age 31**

Maybe he looks confused when you start crying in the morning. He can't figure out why you are obsessing about looking older or feeling older. He comments that you seem edgier and he can't figure out why. He argues back when you fly off the handle, which escalates what could have been a minor argument into a major one. To put it simply, he just doesn't get it.

Even women whose partners are as sympathetic as possible say that their husbands often don't seem wholly to grasp what a wrenching change premature menopause is.

It's no wonder, really. Words can't adequately convey what a hot flash feels like or how your self-image has been rocked. But words are your best tool. Open, honest communication is always important in a relationship, and it's especially important when you are going through something that affects your moods and body so much.

Going through premature menopause is a difficult transition, and you need all the support you can get—especially from the person closest to you. Give him the tools to help support you by communicating your feelings.

• *When in doubt, talk it out! Then talk some more!*—Don't assume your partner understands what you are going through.

Tell him in clear language. This is without a doubt the most important thing to do with your partner. Let him know what you are going through. Explain how you feel, both physically and emotionally. Tell him to ask questions about your condition, and answer them for him.

- *Teach him about premature menopause*—If your partner doesn't know what your body is going through and how it is affecting your moods and psyche, he won't be able to give you the support and understanding you vitally need in this time. Give him books to read so he can truly understand what premature menopause is and how it affects your body and emotions.

- *Give your partner concrete suggestions for helping you cope*—You know better than he what you need. Tell him. If you are having terrible night sweats and need to have a window open at night, explain that this will help you get at least a little sleep. If you need a hug, need to be reassured that you are still a sexy woman, be honest and let him know. Often your husband wants to do the right thing to help you out, but doesn't know what it is that he should do. Be explicit and you'll both be happier for it.

- *Be sure he doesn't feel that he is being lost in the shuffle*— Sometimes when you are going through premature menopause, you are so wrapped up in yourself and your sense of loss or traumatic change that you forget that your partner has needs and feelings too. You're just not as emotionally available as you used to be, and this can cause stresses in your relationship. So it's important to reassure him and let him know that you still care. In any relationship, there comes a time when one person is more needy than the other, and when you're going through premature menopause, you're that person. But don't forget that your husband has needs and emotions as well, and he may be feeling somewhat rocked by the change in you, as you are. Again, talk to him and be sure that he doesn't feel neglected.

- *Keep him aware of your mood changes or physical symptoms so they don't surprise him*—If you feel yourself beginning to spin out of control into a teary episode or a temperamental rage, let him know when you first get the signal. This will enable him to know what to do and, more importantly, what *not* to do. For example, if you feel your nerves getting shot and your stress levels rise, give him a warning. This way you won't wind up in an argument that starts for no real reason other than your premature menopause symptoms.

Guilt and Your Partner: When You (or He) Feel You've Let Him Down

> My husband was an only child and always missed having brothers and sisters, so he wanted us to have a big family. We have one son, but I know he is disappointed that, as it turns out, I can't have the family he had dreamed about. He doesn't talk a lot about it, but I know he is upset about the situation. Sometimes I wonder if he blames me for not having children sooner. Sometimes I blame myself too. I worry that this will drive us apart.
> —Lynda, age 34

Guilt and blame—both, unfortunately, can play a role in a relationship affected by premature menopause.

Sometimes it's you: you feel as though you've let your husband down. He married a woman who could give him children, and now you can't. And sometimes he consciously or unconsciously believes that you're at fault.

Of course, there should be no guilt or no blame involved in the situation. Premature menopause isn't something you cause, and if you did delay having children, you did so with no idea that you would wind up in this situation. Nevertheless, often you or your partner find yourself caught in the blame game.

• *Again, talking this out is critical to your relationship*—If you blame yourself or if your husband blames you for your infertility, you run the risk of causing real damage to your relationship. Confront the issue head-on. Set up a time to talk with your partner when you are feeling emotionally able to handle this conversation, and openly communicate your fears about his reaction to your inability to have children.

• *Work as a team in exploring alternative methods of having a child*—If you want to pursue the options open to you in having a family, go over them with your partner. For example, if you are considering donor eggs, be sure that he too understands what is involved and make an appointment for both of you to go to a fertility clinic to explore this. If adoption seems the right thing for you, you can both go to agency open houses.

• *If you feel that your relationship is suffering a great deal, consider couples counseling*—Often a time of change rocks even the most stable relationship. If you think that your premature menopause is causing a problem you can't work through on your own, it may make sense to see a family therapist to give you the means to handle it.

Your Romantic Life: Sex and Premature Menopause

As far as my libido goes, it is way down. This is the one thing that my hubby has a problem with, but he is still understanding about it.

—Karen, age 39

My husband thinks this is all very bizarre; aside from his concerns for my future health, he is disheartened by my loss of libido.

—Cathy, age 37

First, the good news: no matter how you feel right now, there *is* sex after premature menopause. Good sex. Satisfying sex. Sex like you used to have.

But often, especially in the beginning stages of premature menopause, sex is a problem. It may be painful for you. Your libido might be lagging, or virtually nonexistent. Or it might just be that you aren't in the mood because you feel so depressed.

As you can imagine, this definitely has repercussions in your relationship. Your partner often can't figure out what is happening, and may feel angry, upset, or both.

Again, the best thing to do is to explain. This is no time to be shy. If you are having problems with sex, the worst thing to do is say nothing. Going along with sex when you're not enjoying it can breed resentment and lead to bigger problems. By the same token, not having sex but not explaining can cause problems as well.

Before I went on HRT, I found sex uncomfortable. Added to the discomfort was the fact that premature menopause had made me feel distinctly undesirable. I felt old, fat, and generally unsexy. So I found that I wasn't interested in sex. I'd try to avoid it or hope to get it over with quickly. Eventually I realized that by saying nothing, I was hurting both myself and my husband. So I told him about my discomfort and about my terrible self-image. And I explained that it wasn't that I had lost interest in him—it was me. Through my opening up to him and explaining what I felt, physically and emotionally, we were able to work through the sexual problem and strengthen our relationship.

Sex is an important part of a relationship, so it is important to let your partner know how you feel, what you need, and what you want. By the same token, talking openly with him will enable you to know the same about him, which can help you enrich your sex life in the long run.

- *Be explicit*—If you find that you need more foreplay to be adequately lubricated, say so. If certain positions are more comfortable than others, explain which ones you'd rather try. Even if you're not used to talking about this or taking charge, remember that you're the only one who knows what feels good and what doesn't.
- *If you are feeling undesirable and unsexy, let him know*— Your partner doesn't necessarily know what's going on in your head. In fact, the chances are that from his perspective you're the same woman you've always been. But often this physical change has caused your self-image to founder, and

you may need reassurance about your sexuality and desirability. Instead of feeling this way, explain to your husband that now, more than ever, you need to know that you are loved and attractive. A little love goes a long way to erasing the self-doubts that may have arisen since you entered premature menopause.

* *Encourage your partner to talk about his feelings about sex as well*—Communication is, of course, a two-way street. And often your partner may be feeling a bit neglected or upset if you aren't as interested in sex as you used to be.

COPING WITH THE OUTSIDE WORLD

"When are you going to finally have a baby?" I don't know how many times I've heard that. I want to scream, "I *can't* have a baby! Don't you get it! Don't you think I would if I could?"
                                        —Marianne, age 32

I haven't told anyone but my family that I am in premature menopause. I don't think it's anyone else's business and I don't want people treating me differently. I'm scared that, if they know I'm in menopause, they'll act like I'm old or sick or something.
                                        —Sarah, age 28

Being 21 when diagnosed, I have found that people treat you a little differently. They pity you. So, I don't bring it up unless I feel it would be of some help or comfort to them. I told my family. They don't really treat me any differently, although at times I think they should. At least be more considerate—meaning my younger (by six years) sister is one of the most fertile women in the world. That is very hard at times and they don't always understand that.
                                        —Steph, age 28

Dealing with the outside world—friends, relatives, coworkers, and the like—can be another emotionally sticky area for the woman in premature menopause.

People who don't know your condition can make you feel very uncomfortable by asking when you plan to have children, or by talking on and on about their own children or pregnancies. Often, even if you tell people, you run into awkward situations. I remember telling one older friend that I was in menopause, only to have her explain to me that it was impossible, I was too young, and clearly I had made some sort of ridiculous mistake.

The problem is that, as I've stated before, premature menopause is something that isn't apparent to the outside world and few people know about it or can wholly understand.

It is a strange situation having to explain something so private to others. You worry if it will change how they act toward you. You may be concerned that people will begin acting as if you are older, especially since menopause is something that usually happens to older women. Or you worry that people will be walking on eggshells around you, scared that they may say something that will make you feel bad.

There is a plus, however, in talking with others about your condition. Many women going through premature menopause find it a useful tool in coping. By talking about what they're going through, they find it easier to work through their emotions and often get a built-in support group.

> I told my women friends, sisters, and my mother, partly to get used to the idea myself. I find people are curious and want to know what it's all like. Some people (my mother for one) are uncomfortable with the whole idea of someone so young experiencing old ladies' problems. What's funny is that my older sister (by eleven years) is menopausal, and we are enjoying having each other to talk to.
>
> —Cathy, age 37

The bottom line, then, is that there is no right or wrong way to handle this situation. Whether or not you tell other people about your condition is, of course, entirely up to you. Some women feel more comfortable letting people know about it. Others, though, feel that their premature menopause is a personal issue and one that is best left unmentioned. It is a personal decision and one only you can make.

- *Just because you have told some people, don't feel obligated to tell everyone*—You don't owe anyone anything but you owe yourself a lot, especially during this tough change in your life. If you don't want to tell your coworkers, if you are concerned it will affect their opinion of you or simply don't want their sympathy, there's no need to say a thing. You know your own comfort level.
- *Be honest with those people you do tell*—Let them know if something bothers you: if their talking about their children or their plans to get pregnant upset you. By the same token, explain that you may be more emotional than usual or more prone to irritation. This is a difficult transition for you, and you don't need any more stress in your life caused by misunderstandings between you and your friends or family.
- *Let your friends know how they can support you*—Some women might prefer to be left alone for a while; others may prefer open sympathy. If you don't let your friends know how to treat you, you may end up causing problems for yourself. A friend of mine wanted to be helpful, so she kept getting information for me about adoption. I knew she meant well, but at that time I was so overwhelmed by my premature menopause that I couldn't think straight about adoption or anything. Worried that she might think I was ungrateful, I finally came out with the truth and explained that, while I understood she was trying to help, it was actually making me feel more pressured and more upset. It cleared the air a great deal because she had been feeling hurt that I wasn't responding to her suggestions.
- *Don't take things too personally*—This is one of those "easier said than done" bits of advice. It is very difficult not to get upset when someone wonders why you waited to have

children, or makes inappropriate comments. But keep in mind that this is often simply ignorance or thoughtlessness. These words aren't intended to hurt you. Again, if you are upset by something, either speak up and let the person know or try to avoid that person for a while, if possible.

When You're Single: Premature Menopause and Meeting Potential Partners

Dealing with the outside world at large is one thing, but it's often more difficult when you're single and dealing with the idea of meeting prospective partners. In this case, premature menopause often becomes an unwelcome companion in your dating game.

> **The fact of not being able to have my own biological child is the major problem for me. This is what is tearing me apart greatly. I am only 28, not married and no boyfriend currently. My fear is having to explain this to my signifi-cant other-to-be and having him accept that we will never have our own child.**
>
> **—Iris, age 28**

This is a common fear for women in premature menopause who don't have a partner: How will I find someone who will understand that I probably can't have my own biological child? How will someone understand that, at this early age, I'm al-ready menopausal? Will I ever find someone who can handle this?

Dealing with premature menopause is not easy for anyone. But it can seem harder for a woman who isn't already in a relationship. Again, a great deal of this difficulty is in the link we often feel exists between fertility and femininity. Many women who are prematurely menopausal and single worry that they're no longer sexually desirable and will never find a part-ner with whom to share their life.

This can greatly affect your romantic life. In effect, premature menopause can become an obstacle to establishing intimate ties.

You may worry about how to explain this to someone, how that person will react, and if your condition will ruin what could have been a promising relationship.

> **When I meet someone, I keep wondering how—and when—should I tell him about my condition. Will it scare him off? It's always at the back of my mind . . . and makes starting a relationship really tough for me.**
> **—Jamie, age 31**

It isn't easy. It's difficult enough to start and maintain a relationship. And having the knowledge that you're prematurely menopausal can definitely complicate matters. Most women in this situation, though, have said that if the relationship is meant to be, the premature menopause becomes much less of a factor than they initially thought it would be.

Think about it—a person with whom you can fall in love can and should accept you as you are. Premature menopause hasn't changed the essential "you," the person you are inside. Yes, it has changed your body and your options for having a child. But you are the same person you always were.

It's important, then, to focus on the positives about yourself, and not think of yourself as less of a woman just because of a quirk of biology. It may sound simplistic, but a person who can't accept what you're going through is probably not the right person for you. Yes, premature menopause is unpleasant. Yes, it means that you are facing the prospect of not having your own biological child. And, yes, it means that you're coping with physical and emotional symptoms that most women wouldn't dream about facing until they're much older. But this doesn't mean that you're not going to find a partner who can cope with this.

As I said much earlier in this book, you're much more than simply functioning ovaries. The trick to meeting someone with whom you can get involved is to accept your premature menopause yourself first.

Keep the following thoughts in mind:

- *If your infertility is a key factor in your concerns about meeting a partner, remember that you can have a child through such options as donor eggs or adoption*—It's absolutely vital to keep this in mind. If you worry that you will have problems finding a partner because you can't have a child, remember that you *can*. And through donor eggs, your partner will be able to have *his* biological child if this is vital to him. This and other options open to you are explored in Chapter 8. Having premature menopause doesn't mean you can't have a family—which is something you can and should tell prospective partners when the issue arises.

- *Don't worry too much about the "when will I tell my prospective partner" timing syndrome*—This may sound easier said than done, but many of the single women I've spoken with who have gone through premature menopause said that they were able to tell when the time was right. Opening up to a person in a relationship is always a slightly frightening prospect. And it can seem even more daunting when you know you have to explain about your condition. But there is no right or wrong time. Only you will know when it seems natural to talk about your premature menopause. Going by your "gut" feel is usually the best way to proceed.

- *Don't feel compelled to go into a confessional mode when you've just met someone*—Think about it: when you first meet someone, you don't automatically start telling him everything and anything about yourself. You're not being deceptive if you don't explain about your premature menopause from the very beginning. Give yourself time to get to know the person; see how comfortable you feel, where the relationship is going, and so forth. Again, you'll know when the time is right to discuss it.

- *As with women in relationships when they're diagnosed, remember that open communication is crucial*—As I said before, most misunderstandings arise with lack of communication. Once you feel comfortable with someone, don't let fear keep you from being open and honest about what you're going through. Often this will help strengthen a relationship, and will enable your prospective partner to feel closer to you.

LIVING WITH PREMATURE MENOPAUSE: ACCEPTANCE, COPING, AND MOVING ONWARD

I used to dwell on how I felt and how it seemed unfair at my age to not feel great or as good as I did 10 years ago, but feeling sorry for yourself never does any good, only serves to make things worse, so I don't waste my time with negative thoughts and moods.
—Bryana, age 38

I am really not the kind of person to ask "why me?" I just figure this is something to deal with.
—Cathy, age 37

I went through a time of confusion, pain and uncertainty. Now, I'm taking control of my life once again.
—Steph, age 28

Premature menopause won't go away. It is a condition you will live with for the rest of your life. But once you have accepted it—once you are past the initial shock and grief and depression—you will be able to move ahead. You can expect your period of mourning, depression, and anger to last at least six months. But there will come a time when you will discover that you are getting past the initial emotional fallout. You may still be depressed periodically or still feel a pang when you see a baby with its mother, but these moments will be fewer. You are beginning to feel like you again—perhaps a new you, but you all the same.

The most crucial step on the way to accepting premature menopause is finally realizing that your ovaries aren't you. Your ovaries have failed, but you haven't. Yes, the "change in life" coming so early does require readjustment of your life plans, your lifestyle, and your outlook. But you are still *you*. Just because you have gone through a transition usually gone through in middle age doesn't mean you are suddenly middle-aged.

No transition is easy, and premature menopause is a particularly difficult one because it comes unexpectedly, and years before you ever dreamed it would happen. Yet it is within your power to handle this transition and emerge stronger.

In some ways, the negative change of premature menopause can be a positive force in your life. You are going through a change you didn't want and didn't expect, but you can turn this change into something beneficial. Recognize that this can be a milestone marking a new beginning. Some women find going through premature menopause has actually helped them because they made it through a difficult transition and they are more self-confident, more directed, and better able to accept the things they can't change.

Perhaps this is because by going through such a major change in life so early, you grow up in ways you never expected to. You have had to cope with a body that is going through major physical changes, emotions that careen all over the place, and the reality that you have moved past your normal reproductive life. Some women say it's like going through puberty again, only this time they're adults and can handle the raging hormones a little better. Others simply feel that they've weathered a tremendous shift in their lives and emerged into a calm after a storm. And others feel as though they've moved to a different place in their lives and in their selves.

> Going through premature menopause was in a funny way a growing experience for me. It wasn't easy, and I definitely would have rather not had to go through it. But it has changed me in some positive ways. I'm more self-confident now. I figure if I could deal with all that, I can deal with almost anything.
> —Marianne, age 32

Sometimes, though, being in premature menopause will get to you. You'll think you've got the whole thing licked, and bam! That familiar mood will hit you, or the questions will reemerge in your mind. When the going gets tough, remind yourself:

- *You're not older just because your body is acting as if it's older*—Menopause doesn't confer instant age, no matter how it may seem sometimes. You are still a young woman—just one who happens to be going through a transition that usually doesn't happen for years.
- *You are still feminine, sexy, desirable, and everything else!*— A change in reproductive ability doesn't make you less female. You are a woman who can't have a biological child, perhaps, but you *are* a woman!

Finally, remember that this too shall pass.

When you're having your seventy-eighth hot flash of the day or when you're feeling as though you're going to explode, remember that you will get through it. When you see a baby and you're ready to cry because you won't be able to have one of your own, or when you're looking at yourself in the mirror and wondering how this could have happened to you, remember that you are strong enough to handle this. With time, it will get easier.

I speak from experience on this one. A year ago I would never have dreamed that I could sit down and write about the emotional fallout of premature menopause without breaking down myself. Yet I have gotten to a place where I can cope. And yes, I realize I have accepted it. Premature menopause has become just one reality in my life. It isn't the focal point it once was when it seemed that everything was related to premature menopause. Now premature menopause is something I live with every day. It's an unfortunate reality, to be sure, but it is something I can deal with. There are days when I don't think about it at all; and other days, when I do get a little down about it and wish that somehow it had never happened. But it has happened. And I am in premature menopause. However, it no longer affects my every thought.

I now realize that I'm still the same person—if anything, a little better of a person. Premature menopause forced me to come to terms with many personal issues. It made me think long and hard about who I really was, how I defined myself, what mattered in life. It pushed me to open up to other people, to speak out and to communicate what I felt and thought. It has made me *grow*. I'm not going to pretend that I wouldn't have preferred never having gone through menopause at such an early age. But I have discovered that the worst times do pass and the good things in life do endure.

Chapter 5

Hormone Replacement Therapy

The Pros and Cons

Hormone replacement—this was one of the most confusing aspects of premature menopause for me. I'd read so many articles about the negatives and the positives, too. The problem was, all the articles I read assumed that I was in my fifties. And I wasn't. What did HRT mean for a woman in her thirties? What were the consequences if I went on HRT—or, for that matter, if I didn't? I realized that I couldn't base my decision on the arguments put forth for the older woman. I had to keep digging and try to understand what hormone replacement meant for a younger woman.

Hormone replacement therapy (or HRT, as it's commonly called) is based on a very simple principle: you replace the hormones that drop during menopause, and by so doing, you can alleviate the uncomfortable symptoms (like hot flashes) and can help prevent long-term consequences like osteoporosis and heart disease.

If you are like me, you may have heard a lot of discussion about the risks and benefits of HRT as they apply to an older woman—the "average" woman in menopause—and very little, if anything, about what HRT means to a younger woman in premature menopause. However, while there is some debate about the use of HRT for menopausal women in general, there has been little debate among doctors about its use for women in premature menopause.

The consensus is that HRT may be the one best thing you can do for yourself if you're in premature menopause, whether your menopause is natural or surgical.

Perhaps the most convincing argument of all is this: Even most doctors who are generally against HRT and who advocate natural alternatives for the average (that is, older) woman in menopause believe HRT is important for women in premature menopause.

You may be surprised to learn this. I know I was. When I was first diagnosed with premature menopause, I read articles about HRT that questioned whether it was necessary for a woman in menopause. So for a year, I threw away the prescription my doctor gave me, stayed off HRT, and figured I'd handle my menopause naturally. But I also kept on researching about premature menopause. And the more I read specifically about my condition, the more I became aware that I had jumped to my conclusion too quickly. I realized that I hadn't made a decision based on the facts as they related to *me*—a 38-year-old woman, not a 48-year-old woman or a 58-year-old woman. Instead, I had automatically assumed that HRT was wrong, without really understanding the repercussions for a woman of my age.

Put simply, you're faced with many different needs and consequences from those of an older woman because you're dealing with lower hormone levels at a much earlier age. So, to make a truly educated decision about HRT, you need to know about HRT as it applies to a woman in premature menopause, not the average woman in menopause. It's actually a very different situation.

The many articles and books you may have read debating the HRT issue don't necessarily apply to women in premature menopause. Yes, there are risks associated with HRT, which are explained in this chapter. But the consensus in the medical community seems to be quite straightforward: when you are in premature menopause, the benefits of HRT usually strongly outweigh the risks.

This chapter, then, addresses the HRT issue in terms of *premature* menopause, not menopause in general. It will enable you to understand how HRT works for the younger woman and examines the very real positives and negatives of HRT so you can make an informed decision about your body based on your particular situation, not on the generalities you might have read or heard. This chapter examines what HRT is, the benefits and risks as they apply to a younger woman in menopause, the different types of HRT available to you and how they work, as well as giving you a framework to make your decision making easier.

HRT BASICS: WHAT IT IS AND WHAT IT IS REPLACING

Okay, let's start at the beginning of this all: What exactly *is* HRT?

Not surprisingly, hormone replacement therapy is exactly what is says it is: you take hormones to replace those that your body has stopped producing.

Usually HRT involves replacing both estrogen and progesterone, the two main female hormones. In the past, ERT (estrogen replacement therapy) was the norm, but research showed that unopposed estrogen (that is, estrogen taken without progesterone) increased chances of uterine cancer. So doctors began replacing progesterone as well to protect the uterus. Plain ERT is still prescribed, but usually only to women who have undergone surgical menopause and who don't necessarily need the protective benefits of progesterone. Even this is becoming less common, however, as more doctors believe that progesterone has important benefits whether or not you have a uterus. In addition to traditional estrogen/progesterone replacement, HRT may sometimes involve replacing testosterone as well, since your ovaries produce a small amount of this too.

To make things a little clearer, here's a quick breakdown of the hormones involved in HRT.

Estrogen

Estrogen is the hormone most commonly prescribed in HRT, and it's the one that attracts so much of both the negative and positive claims. On one hand, replacing estrogen is what helps fight symptoms and long-term risks; on the other hand, it may also increase chances of cancer. It's also a little misunderstood, for lack of a better term.

Estrogen, as you know, is one of the major sex hormones but it also appears to do more in your body than work with your reproductive system. Your body has estrogen receptors in the brain, heart, liver, and other organs, as well as throughout the body. Researchers are still trying to determine the many roles of estrogen in addition to its reproductive role.

Many people assume that estrogen is just one single hormone, but actually it's a family of hormones. In fact, researchers have identified two dozen different estrogens produced in a woman's body. But virtually all doctors agree that there are three principal estrogens.

Estradiol (also known as E2) is the primary estrogen produced by your ovaries. It's the strongest estrogen and the one that you have the most of during your reproductive years. Because it is the strongest, it has the most effect on your tissues, which is why, if you take too much of it for a long period of time, you can suffer from a range of negative side effects, including breast tenderness, bloating, headaches, heavy bleeding, and, at the worst, breast or uterine cancer. Your body can convert estradiol to the weaker estrogens, estrone and estriol.

Estrone (E1) is an end product of estradiol produced when your liver converts estradiol to estrone, and it is also produced by your adrenal glands. This is the estrogen you have the most of in your postmenopause years. While it is weaker than estradiol, it too is associated with many of the same negative side effects if taken to excess for a prolonged period of time. Most commonly, if you have excessively high levels of estrone, you may get fluid retention and blood sugar fluctuations, but like estradiol, estrone appears to be associated with endometrial and breast cancers. While estrone can be made from estradiol, it can also convert into estradiol.

Estriol (E3) is the weakest estrogen of the three. Your liver can convert both estradiol and estrone into estriol, and during pregnancy, your body (more specifically, the placenta) produces very high amounts of estriol to protect the fetus. Overall, estriol is the "protective" estrogen. Unlike the other, stronger ones, it doesn't overstimulate your breast and uterine tissues, so it doesn't cause cancer as the other ones may, and it may protect against cancer as well as minimizing other menopausal symptoms.

When you go through menopause, your estrogen levels drop. In addition, the balance between them changes: before menopause, you produce higher amounts of estradiol, the strongest estrogen, than estrone, but after menopause, even though both estrone and estradiol drop, the ratio changes, reversing the balance so that you have more estrone than estradiol. While the estrogen prescribed in HRT is designed to boost your low estrogen levels, it doesn't necessarily provide your body with the same balance of estrogens you had prior to menopause. Instead, you will often be getting one form of estrogen only—for example, Premarin, a commonly prescribed estrogen made from pregnant mares' urine, consists primarily of estrone and equilin (a horse estrogen), and Estrace, a commonly prescribed estrogen made from plants, is 100 percent estradiol. (See page 190 for a more thorough explanation of the different prescription estrogens available).

Progesterone

This is the next most commonly replaced hormone in HRT, prescribed to balance the effects of estrogen and to protect the uterus. Before menopause, progesterone is essentially the "pregnancy hormone." It aids ovulation and builds up your uterine lining in preparation for a fertilized egg. Recent studies have determined that it also appears to help build bone. However, in HRT, you often take not natural progesterone but a synthetic progesterone, called a *progestin* or *progestogen*. Progestin is similar but not identical to the progesterone naturally produced in your body. It is associated with a higher rate of side effects and doesn't appear to have the same bone-building ability. We'll take a look at this later in this chapter, as well as the differences between natural and synthetic progesterone.

Testosterone and DHEA

These are the other hormones sometimes prescribed in HRT. Until recently, little attention was paid to them, but many researchers now believe that they may play more of an important role in HRT than previously thought.

Testosterone is an *androgen*—a hormone produced in both men and (to a lesser extent) women that promotes masculine characteristics such as hair growth, among other things. Most importantly, it keeps your libido strong, boosts energy, builds bone and maintains muscle. In addition, the right level of testosterone in relation to estrogen and progesterone helps to minimize the body changes that often arise in midlife such as body fat shifting from your hips to your middle in more of a male pattern of fat distribution. It's prescribed most often to women who have gone through surgical menopause because the ovaries produce testosterone in women. In general, however, it's not uncommon for a woman's testosterone levels to drop as much as 50 percent after menopause, which is one of the reasons doctors are beginning to look into testosterone replacement especially for those women for whom regular HRT doesn't seem to help enough.

As for DHEA, this is the new kid on the block in hormone replacement, and is still the subject of a great deal of scrutiny. It's a building-block hormone, one from which the other sex hormones are made. According to recent studies, it appears to help prevent osteoporosis, heart disease, and Alzheimer's disease. However it is not commonly prescribed in HRT at this point, and further studies need to be done to determine its benefits and possible negatives. One apparent problem: A recent study found that post-menopausal women with the highest levels of DHEA were more likely to develop breast cancer. Clearly more research is needed before DHEA becomes part of HRT.

THE HRT CONTROVERSY: OR, WHAT'S ALL THE NOISE ABOUT?

By replacing all or some of the above hormones, you can alleviate menopausal symptoms and help fight the long-term consequences. But the questions persist: How effective is it? And do the risks outweigh the benefits? Most important, does HRT actually increase the risks of breast and uterine cancer, and, if so, to what degree?

The medical community has been conducting clinical trials on HRT for years, and unfortunately, there is no clear-cut answer to any of these questions. Some studies point to estrogen as causing an increased cancer risk; others point to progestin (the synthetic progesterone often prescribed); still others have found that the risk is minimal. To make matters even more confusing, many studies have indicated that estrogen replacement is a definite plus in the fight against cardiovascular disease. For most American women, cardiovascular disease is more of a threat than breast cancer. So many doctors believe that the benefits of preventing heart disease outweigh the risk of breast cancer. But to complicate matters even more, some studies have shown that adding progestins to estrogen may actually minimize the positive cardiac benefits. Finally, many researchers and doctors point to the so-called "healthy woman" bias in positive claims about HRT. In other words, the women who are on HRT are often healthier to begin with—they usually are nonsmokers, eat a healthy diet, exercise, and so on—and thus may show a reduced rate of heart disease not due to estrogen, but due to a healthier lifestyle.

It's extremely complicated, to say the least, which makes it difficult to wade through all the claims and counterclaims to get to the heart of the matter. Basically, though, most studies conducted so far have concluded that:

• HRT does reverse most menopausal symptoms such as hot flashes, vaginal dryness, and so forth.
• HRT appears to help combat osteoporosis.
• HRT helps lower the levels of bad cholesterol and so may reduce incidence of cardiovascular disease.
• Unopposed usage of estrogen increases the risk of endometrial (uterine) cancer. This is why most doctors prescribe progesterone or progestin, a synthetic form of progesterone, instead of just estrogen.
• HRT, and specifically long-term usage of estrogen, that is, the use of estrogen for 10 or more years, *may* increase the incidence of breast cancer according to some studies; other studies have found no increase in breast cancer. The long-term effects of estrogen usage are still under study.
• HRT can increase the chances of gall bladder disease and liver disease.

There are still a lot of unanswered questions. In most cases, no one is sure what the very long-term risks of HRT are, since the studies have tracked women for up to 10 years only. Moreover, the majority of the studies have been based on women taking a standard dosage of estrogen (0.625 mg of conjugated estrogen—specifically, Premarin), so there are still questions about the effects of different forms of estrogen, different dosages, and the role that progesterone plays. An ongoing study by the Women's Health Initiative will be completed in 2008, at which point the medical community hopes to have more of the questions about HRT answered. Until then, you can expect to see more studies, more articles, and more debate about the benefits versus the risks of HRT.

Why Is HRT Different When You're in Premature Menopause?

> I feel that the issues surrounding HRT are different for young(er) women, and these issues are absent from most of the literature I have found. I am concerned about hormones and breast cancer (mother and sister had it) and I have not found studies related to women my age. This is upsetting.
>
> —Cathy, age 37

So that's the HRT debate in a nutshell. But it's important to realize that this debate doesn't necessarily apply to you.

Most of the negatives about HRT are due to a simple fact: older women are in effect *adding* hormones to their bodies, not really replacing them. Their bodies have low hormone levels because they have reached a certain age at which point it is natural to have this happen. So when they go on HRT, they're adding hormones beyond that point.

A woman in premature menopause, however, is *replacing* hormones that she normally would have had until she reached age 50 or thereabout. In other words, HRT is giving the prematurely menopausal woman the hormones her body "expects" to have.

Yet many of us in premature menopause don't think about that aspect of HRT. Instead we read about the health risks of hormone replacement and automatically put ourselves in the same risk groups as older women in menopause. And this is a mistake. Yes, there is some overlap. Many of the benefits and risks do apply to a younger woman as well as an older one. However, there is also a decisive difference because of the longer time frame. When normal menopausal women go on HRT, they're exposing their bodies to hormones for a longer time than naturally designed. And it is this prolonged exposure to estrogen that seems to increase the risk of breast or uterine cancer.

But—and here again is the key difference for women in premature menopause—when you are prematurely menopausal and take HRT, you're not prolonging your exposure to estrogen, you're taking estrogen in those years when your body would normally have maintained higher levels of estrogen on its own; you're literally replacing it. I can't say it enough times. So your cancer risks aren't necessarily increased to the levels that appear in the studies because as a younger woman, you start out with a much lower risk of breast cancer than that of the older women involved in the studies. (To make a rough comparison of odds, the average 35-year-old woman has a one in 622 chance of developing breast cancer, while a 55-year-old woman has a one in 33 risk—quite a large difference.)

On the other hand, because you've entered menopause earlier than normal and are facing a prolonged period of time with low levels of estrogen and progesterone, your risk factors for osteoporosis and heart disease are much higher than both other women your age and the normal woman in menopause.

This is why, according to most research and doctors, the benefits appear to outweigh the risks where women in premature menopause are concerned—and why you should strongly consider HRT.

There are exceptions: if you have certain risk factors (such as a past breast cancer, which will be covered on page 184–85), then HRT may not be right for you. But most women in premature menopause are likely to benefit from HRT in terms of preventing osteoporosis, heart disease, and simply preserving quality of life.

Once you reach the age of 50 or so, the normal arguments against HRT apply. This is when you should rethink your position about HRT, based on the benefits and risks that apply to the older woman in menopause and the impact of long-term exposure to hormone replacement. But until that point, HRT can make a huge difference in your current and long-term health.

Of course, this is a personal decision and one that you shouldn't undertake lightly. Read through the following benefits and risks so that you can be sure you understand what HRT can do for you and, for that matter, what it *won't* do for you.

WHAT HRT CAN DO FOR YOU: THE BENEFITS OF REPLACING HORMONES

For all of the debate about HRT, there is definite good news: it does have a number of proven benefits, both in the short-term and in the long-term. This is why so many doctors are quick to prescribe HRT to women in premature menopause and why so many of these women decide to go on HRT. Here's a quick breakdown of the positive side of HRT—the immediate benefits you'll notice and the benefits over the long term, as well as the claims that researchers are still trying to prove.

Short-Term Benefits of HRT

RELIEVING MENOPAUSAL SYMPTOMS (HOT FLASHES, MOOD SWINGS, BRAIN FOG, AND ALL THE OTHER NOT-SO-FUN REMINDERS OF MENOPAUSE)

> I decided to go on HRT because my doctor prescribed it. I really didn't do any research. I just wanted the symptoms to end!
> —Steph, age 28

> I was flashing more than a strobe light! But when I finally went on HRT, I actually felt normal again—no more red face, no more sweating, no more hot flashes at all! It was a minor miracle!
> —Barbara, age 31

Hot flashes, night sweats, brain fog, and general weepiness may not be life-or-death issues, but they definitely affect your quality of life. And HRT does help alleviate these symptoms—there's no debate about this benefit whatsoever.

Because most of these annoying menopausal symptoms are caused by low estrogen levels, replacing estrogen—boosting it back up to "normal" levels—relieves the unpleasant symptoms of estrogen deprivation. Your body also goes through changes due to low progesterone and testosterone levels, which the appropriate HRT can help. In fact, relieving symptoms is one of the main reasons a lot of women decide to go on HRT in the first place. You'll often notice an improvement very quickly. In fact, some women say that the first day they took HRT, they felt a difference. In all fairness, they're probably exaggerating— it usually takes at least a few days for your symptoms to disappear. But they do normally disappear or at the least become less intense and frequent within a few weeks of beginning HRT. If you still do have symptoms after a month of going on HRT, you may need a higher dosage or a different form of HRT, so should speak to your doctor.

One final point: remember that these menopausal symptoms are natural signs that your hormone levels are dropping. If you don't go on HRT, your body often adjusts to the new lower levels and the symptoms slowly stop. However, some unlucky women can have hot flashes and the battery of other symptoms for years after menopause—some for the rest of their life. This means that if and when you decide to stop HRT, these symptoms will probably return as your body goes back through the process of adjusting to lower levels of estrogen.

REVERSING VAGINAL DRYNESS AND ATROPHY

This is another undebatable benefit of hormone replacement therapy, and one I can definitely swear to. With low levels of estrogen, your vagina becomes dryer and, over time, actually thins and becomes less elastic. Taking HRT replenishes the moisture in your vaginal tissues and prevents the thinning of vaginal walls; in effect, it rejuvenates your vagina—and, very possibly, your sex life! It also helps restore the natural pH balance in your vagina, which helps fight infections.

Usually, you'll see this benefit within a few weeks of starting HRT. If you've already begun to suffer from vaginal atrophy, it will probably take longer because your vagina needs more time to regain its elasticity. However, after few months of HRT, your vaginal walls and tissues will improve.

PREVENTING URINARY STRESS INCONTINENCE

Just as estrogen helps your vaginal lining and muscles, it also helps other muscles in your pelvic area—most notably, your urethra muscles, which push urine out of your bladder. When your estrogen levels are low, you may experience urinary stress incontinence: leakage of urine. Taking estrogen helps reverse this by strengthening the muscle and rebuilding the mucous membranes of your urethra. It works in 40 to 70 percent of the women who use it. Again, you'll usually see results within a few weeks of starting HRT.

Long-Term Benefits of HRT

Relief of symptoms is great for quality of life, but HRT is also linked to much more. Call it *extension* of life. No, I'm not talking about a fountain of youth here. You don't suddenly get to live hale and hearty until age 100 because you're on HRT. But HRT does appear to help prevent major diseases, most notably osteoporosis, which cripples thousands of older women, and heart disease, the number-one killer of American women.

These long-term benefits of HRT are the key reason so many doctors recommend it to women in premature menopause. Remember, because your hormones have dropped at an earlier age than other women, you are exposed to low hormone levels for a longer period of time, which can lead to a much higher risk of both osteoporosis and heart disease. If you boost your hormone levels, though, through HRT, you can decrease this risk.

FIGHTING OSTEOPOROSIS

> I guess I was lucky because I really didn't have very bad symptoms. But I went on HRT because I was very worried about osteoporosis. The more I read, the more I realized that osteo was a very worrisome threat, so even though I wasn't sure about taking HRT, I decided it was a good idea.
>
> —Cindy, age 31

Fighting osteoporosis is one of the most compelling reasons for a woman in premature menopause to strongly consider taking HRT—and for good reason. As I mentioned in Chapter 3, when you are in premature menopause you are at a much higher risk for debilitating osteoporosis than the average woman your age—or than the average woman in menopause, for that matter. This is because your bones are exposed to lower levels of estrogen than normal for a longer period of time than an older woman in menopause. Added to this is the fact that you typically reach peak bone mass at age 35. So if you go into premature menopause before the age of 35, you might have less bone than an average woman to begin with, which makes the effects of bone loss even more dramatic.

Studies have consistently shown that HRT will help you prevent osteoporosis and may in fact help you build more bone. In the past, most researchers and doctors believed that you couldn't restore your bones to their premenopausal density by taking hormones. But more studies are showing that this might not be the case. The key is to replace not only estrogen, but also progesterone, *not* progestin. Natural progesterone seems actually to build bone, not just halt bone loss. Similarly, researchers have found that testosterone replacement appears to build bone as well. So HRT including one or both of these hormones not only may stop osteoporosis, it may be able to reverse it.

Unfortunately, there have been no large-scale controlled studies to prove these theories yet, but this is an exciting and interesting area of research. It's a good idea to keep abreast of any developments in this area, since premature menopause puts you at such a high risk for bone loss. As I mentioned in Chapter 3, the National Institutes of Health are currently working on an estrogen/testosterone patch specifically for women in premature menopause, in the hopes that this will help stop the rapid bone loss observed in women with premature ovarian failure.

In the meantime, however, estrogen itself has been proven to prevent osteoporosis in 75 to 80 percent of the women taking it and to greatly reduce the risk of fractures. Calcium and exercise alone just won't help your bones the way HRT will.

According to most research, to prevent osteoporosis, you need to raise your estradiol levels in your blood to above 50 picograms per milliliter. Typically you can reach this level by taking 0.625 mg of conjugated estrogen (Premarin) or the equivalent dosage of another form of estrogen. If you're also taking 1,500 mg of calcium daily, you can take about half the dosage of estrogen. However, if you have a high risk for osteoporosis (family history, etc.), you may need a higher dosage than usual of estrogen.

One important point: to fight osteoporosis, it is best to start HRT early—preferably within a year of being diagnosed with premature menopause. According to several studies, you begin losing a substantial amount of bone in the first six to 18 months of premature menopause, so the earlier you begin replacing your hormones, the less bone density you lose and the quicker you begin fighting back against the effects of hormone deprivation.

Now for the downside: when you stop using HRT, you begin losing bone again—which is why many doctors recommend staying on HRT for a very long time, sometimes for the rest of your life. This has led doctors who are against the use of HRT to question if it's really necessary to prevent osteoporosis by staying on a medication for your entire life and possibly exposing yourself to the risks of this prolonged exposure to hormones. Again, though, this argument against HRT doesn't necessarily apply if you're in premature menopause. Because premature menopause leads to such a rapid loss of bone at such an early age, you are taking HRT to prevent this early and immediate risk. Once you reach age 50, you should reconsider HRT—and the negatives associated with it. Remember: going on HRT now doesn't have to mean a lifelong commitment, but a way of fighting rapid bone loss until the time when you would normally have gone through menopause.

FIGHTING CARDIOVASCULAR DISEASE

Heart disease is serious business, and unfortunately, an increased risk of both stroke and heart disease has been linked to menopause. For a woman in premature menopause, the increase is even higher. As I mentioned in Chapter 3, if you go through natural menopause before the age of 35, your risk of heart disease increases two to three times. If you go through it between the ages of 35 and 40, your risk is about double. If you go through surgical menopause before the age of 35, your risk of heart disease increases *seven* times.

These are frightening figures, which is why so many doctors recommend HRT for a younger woman—at least until she reaches age 50.

Cardiovascular disease is tied to your arteries—more precisely, to *atherosclerosis,* a narrowing of the arteries that lead to your heart. When this happens, not enough blood goes to your heart, causing heart disease, or to your brain, causing stroke. In addition, you may get high blood pressure, which increases your chances of heart attack or stroke.

In the past, many people thought that HRT, or more specifically estrogen, actually increased your risk of heart disease or stroke. But the opposite may be the truth: according to several recent studies, postmenopausal women taking estrogen for 10 years or longer have about half the risk of heart disease compared with women who don't, and a 50 percent reduction in death from stroke. (One important note: Recent data released from the HERS study *did* find an increased risk of heart disease in women on estrogen who already had heart disease—but the risk appeared to diminish after several years.)

The studies done examining HRT's role in preventing cardiovascular disease have focused on older women. Nevertheless, the findings do apply to those of us in premature menopause, especially since one of the key consequences of premature menopause where cardiovascular disease is concerned is a rise in cholesterol.

I speak from experience: with no change in my lifestyle whatsoever, my cholesterol went from 126 to over 200 when I entered premature menopause. After only a few months on natural HRT (plant-derived estrogen and progesterone), my cholesterol levels dropped back to normal.

My situation isn't uncommon. According to the studies done on older women in menopause, HRT does help to lower cholesterol, and it can do the same for a younger woman in menopause. But HRT doesn't just help with cholesterol.

More specifically:

- On average, estrogen lowers LDL (bad cholesterol) by 8 percent and raises HDL by 15 percent.
- HRT lowers *fibrinogen,* a blood coagulant that increases the chances of heart attacks and strokes.
- Estrogen helps improve blood flow, helps the elasticity of blood vessel walls and the aorta, and appears to help fight—and reverse—plaque formation in arteries and blood vessels.
- Estrogen also appears to lower your levels of a specific type of LDL cholesterol, *small-molecule LDL cholesterol,* and *lipoprotein(a),* both of which cause your arteries to clog.
- While many people had thought that estrogen caused blood pressure to rise, recent studies show that not only is this not the case, but it may actually help lower blood pressure.
- Natural progesterone (available as a prescription HRT in a micronized pill or in a vaginal gel) also appears to help reduce blood pressure. In addition, according to the PEPI study (Postmenopausal Estrogen/Progestin Intervention, a three-year trial sponsored by the NIH to study HRT), when taken with estrogen, blood cholesterol levels were better than with estrogen taken with a progestin.

This is pretty compelling evidence in favor of HRT.

But, in the interest of fairness, let's take a look at the flip side. There are doctors and researchers who don't believe this evidence is as good as it sounds. First, as I mentioned before, some believe that most of these studies fall prey to the "well woman" bias—that is, the women taking HRT on the whole appear to live healthier lifestyles than those who don't, so perhaps their lessened risk of cardiovascular disease is a function of their lifestyle, not the HRT. Secondly, there are those who say that lowering cholesterol can't necessarily be equated with preventing heart disease. Finally, many doctors rightly point out that there are other things you can do to help prevent cardiovascular disease, such as exercise, eating right, and taking certain vitamins and other supplements. Their conclusion? Since the cardiovascular benefits of HRT aren't proven, perhaps you shouldn't needlessly expose yourself to the risks.

However, it's important to remember yet again that they are talking about older women who aren't facing as many years of estrogen deprivation as a woman in premature menopause and who may not be facing the same risks of heart disease and osteoporosis. This is why even some of these doctors and researchers have said that HRT might be a logical choice for a younger woman in menopause.

The bottom line, then: Don't discount the good news about cardiovascular disease prevention. Yes, the studies aren't as conclusive as one might want, but there is evidence that HRT might be a big help to your heart. As a woman in premature menopause, your risk of cardiovascular disease is dramatically increased, so it's important for you to consider these possible benefits and weigh them against the possible risks as they apply to you.

PREVENTING WRINKLES

Okay, okay, I know wrinkles are far from a major health risk. But increased wrinkles and loss of skin tone are side effects of low estrogen levels, and HRT can help prevent them.

When you go through premature menopause, the change in your skin is often more noticeable than it is in women who go through normal menopause simply because you're younger. You don't expect to have thinner, less elastic skin in your thirties like you might in your fifties. Granted, some of the wrinkles you'll start noticing in your thirties are probably due to sun damage or other causes. But low estrogen does contribute to collagen loss, and the results are evident on your face. Taking estrogen helps prevent collagen loss and, according to some studies, may even increase the amount of collagen in your skin by about 3 to 5 percent. On a personal note, before I started HRT, my skin was showing definite signs of age, and many people thought I was older than I was. Only a few months after I began taking it, I noticed a definite difference. I actually looked my age again.

ALZHEIMER'S DISEASE

This is a relatively new area of research where HRT is concerned, but one that is again pointing to a possible benefit from estrogen replacement. It appears that estrogen loss may be linked to an increased risk of Alzheimer's disease, and that using estrogen may help reduce that risk. While low estrogen levels don't cause Alzheimer's themselves, they do appear to increase susceptibility to other factors that cause Alzheimer's. In other words, low estrogen may increase your chances of developing an Alzheimer's risk factor—which, in turn, could result in Alzheimer's.

A study by the National Institute on Aging found that women who used estrogen reduced their risk of Alzheimer's disease by 54 percent. Other studies have indicated that estrogen may help improve memory function and memory loss in women who already have mild to moderate forms of Alzheimer's. And research released in 1999 found that estrogen appeared to affect the brain—but didn't appear to increase memory.

So the evidence isn't conclusive yet. First, the tests that have been conducted so far have been on older women who were already, by virtue of their age, at an increased risk for Alzheimer's or already suffering from it. It isn't clear if taking estrogen replacement at an earlier age has any effect on your brain and the prevention of Alzheimer's. Second, as with so many other areas about HRT, there have been other studies that showed no link between Alzheimer's and the use of estrogen. All in all, then, this is a positive claim for which the jury is still out.

RECTAL AND COLON CANCER

This is a benefit of HRT that isn't well known, but it looks promising. Rectal and colon cancer is the third most common malignancy in women over 50. One reason for the increased risk of this form of cancer may be low estrogen and progesterone levels. When they drop, you secrete more irritating bowel bile acids, which may lead to a higher chance of rectal and colon cancer. HRT appears to help fight this. A recent University of Wisconsin study that included over 600 women with cancer and 1,600 without found that rectal and colon cancer was reduced by 46 percent in women who were using (or recently had used) HRT, and by 30 percent in women who had once used it. Again, this is a long-term benefit that hasn't been studied much and isn't directly tied to younger women, but it's yet another example of how replacing estrogen may help fight diseases that are ordinarily associated with older women but that you may be at a greater risk for because of your premature menopause.

OSTEOARTHRITIS

Here's another possible long-term benefit of HRT that looks promising. About 16 million Americans suffer from this form of arthritis, the majority of whom are women aged 45 and over. So while preventing osteoarthritis may not be much of an issue for you now, preventing it in the future should be, and replacing estrogen may help. A recent study of women over the age of 65 found that those taking estrogen had the lowest incidence of the disease. Further studies clearly need to be done to substantiate this finding, but so far this appears to be yet another potential benefit from HRT.

THE NEGATIVE SIDE OF HRT: WHAT YOU NEED TO BE AWARE OF

You've read about the positive side of HRT, now what about the negatives?

Obviously there wouldn't be a debate about HRT if the whole picture was a rosy one. And frankly, it isn't. There are, as mentioned earlier, certain negatives about HRT that you should know about to make the best possible decision for yourself. Some of these negatives are minor, but others are definitely worrisome.

However, to repeat the point I keep making over and over again: it is important to remember that virtually all of the studies that are cited in articles and books, the bulk of the publicized research and the news stories, are about the average woman in menopause, a woman in her fifties who is taking hormones after her body expected to have lost these hormones. This is why the increased risks discussed below don't always apply to the younger woman who is in premature menopause. Even so, you should know about these potential risks. The risks that don't apply to you now will probably apply to you eventually and should be taken into consideration when you decide if and how long to take HRT.

Side Effects of HRT

Let's start with the not-so-pleasant but not life-threatening negatives from HRT: the annoying side effects like bloating, breast tenderness, nausea, headaches, and a general "blah" PMS feeling.

The bad news is that these side effects are fairly common. Most of the women I've talked to who are on HRT have had complaints at some point or another. Some of these side effects are from estrogen, but most are associated with progestin, as you'll see when you read through the following lists. You may experience many or few of these side effects. It depends on the dosage of your HRT, the type of HRT you're using, the length of time you've been using it, and your body chemistry in general.

The good news is that side effects often go away after a few weeks of HRT, once your body gets accustomed to the new hormone levels. In addition, many side effects can be diminished or even completely eliminated by changing the dosage or form of the HRT you're taking. For example, if you're on cyclical therapy (you take estrogen and/or progesterone part of the month, then stop), your hormone levels change throughout the cycle, which can cause some of these side effects. But if you take a continuous dose of HRT, the side effects may disappear after a while because your hormone levels remain level. Similarly, switching from a pill to a patch often helps with side effects. Finally, where the progestin side effects are concerned, switching from a progestin to a natural progesterone often makes a big difference.

This is why, if you go on HRT and find you have unpleasant side effects, it makes sense not to give up immediately and go off HRT. Many women test different dosages or forms of HRT until they find the right one for them. Just be patient, talk to your doctor, and keep trying to find the right combination of hormones that can give you the benefits you want without the annoying side effects.

ESTROGEN SIDE EFFECTS

Most women don't report a high number of side effects from estrogen itself, and find it's the synthetic progesterone that really does them in. But there are some side effects reported with estrogen replacement. You might have all, some, or none of these:

- migraine headaches (especially if you already suffer from them)
- breast tenderness and enlargement

- increase in the number and size of uterine fibroids (benign tumors in your uterus)
- dark spots or blotches on your skin
- heavy menstrual bleeding
- varicose veins

PROGESTIN SIDE EFFECTS

> I'm happy on HRT when it's just the estrogen part of the month. But I dread the days when I take Provera. It's like going through PMS without the chance of ever getting pregnant.
> —Sarah, age 28

> Bloating? I don't just bloat, I become like a water balloon! When I go on the Provera, I feel like my body is going to explode, like water would gush out of me if you stuck a pin in me. It's really uncomfortable.
> —Julia, age 36

With progestin you may run into more side effects, many of which are a great deal like PMS. But remember, if you use a natural progesterone instead of a progestin as part of your HRT or if you're only on estrogen replacement, you will probably avoid some, if not most, of these unpleasant side effects:

- bloating; water retention
- breast tenderness
- irritability and mood swings
- breakthrough bleeding (bleeding or spotting at times other than the end of your monthly cycle)
- nausea and stomach upset
- pressure or discomfort in your lower abdomen
- constipation
- acne

TESTOSTERONE SIDE EFFECTS

As with the others, these are the most commonly reported side effects—but that doesn't mean you'll necessarily have them:

- hair loss
- acne
- hirsutism (excessive hair growth, facial hair, etc.)

Long-Term Risks of HRT

Side effects are one thing. But the most important negative side to HRT is long-term health risks—very real and scary health risks, to be blunt.

The main risk, and the one that most women are frightened of, is cancer. Studies have shown that HRT can increase your risk of endometrial cancer and may also do the same for breast cancer, although this still isn't certain. In addition, it has been linked to stroke, high blood pressure, gall bladder disease, and kidney disease.

Not a great list of possible consequences. . . . You can see why there is a debate about HRT, and why many women are leery of it.

But, as you'll note when you read about the different risks, some of these risks haven't been proven, but are speculative; others are controllable, and still others have been proven not to be linked to HRT after all. In addition, many of these dangerous risks are the result of replacing hormones in women who are 50, 60, or older. Our bodies aren't designed to keep producing hormones at a later age. But when you're in premature menopause, you're replacing hormones a woman your age normally has. In some cases, then, the risks don't apply, and in others, the increase in risk isn't as dramatic as is appears in the studies because you start out with a much lower risk than the women studied. Finally, you have to keep in mind the positive side of HRT and the potential to fight the very real threats of osteoporosis and heart disease, both of which are unfortunately connected to premature menopause.

In any case, you shouldn't completely discount the risks of HRT. Even if you feel they don't really apply to you, you need to know about these downsides to make an educated decision. Only when you weigh these possible risks against the benefits and factor in your own lifestyle and health history can you come up with the right answer for you.

INCREASED RISK OF ENDOMETRIAL CANCER

An increased risk of endometrial cancer is unequivocally linked with estrogen but fortunately is not something most women need to worry about. This is because it is *unopposed* estrogen (taken without progesterone or progestin) that causes the problem. Estrogen stimulates your uterine lining. If there is no progesterone to cause this lining to slough off, the estrogen causes the lining to keep growing, resulting in *hyperplasia* (overgrowth) and eventually endometrial cancer.

If you still have a uterus, your doctor will prescribe a progestin or progesterone in addition to estrogen. Even relatively small doses of progesterone oppose the estrogen's effect on your uterine lining and prevent endometrial cancer. In fact, using progesterone with estrogen appears actually to reduce your chances of endometrial cancer, to less than that of women taking no hormones at all.

The bottom line, then—while endometrial cancer has been linked to estrogen replacement therapy, it's not a major concern any longer, because nowadays women with uteruses aren't prescribed estrogen alone, but estrogen and progesterone. And, when you're on this combined HRT, you are actually reducing your risk of endometrial cancer as compared with a woman who isn't on HRT.

INCREASED RISK OF BREAST CANCER

I worry at times about taking such a high dose of estrogen. I have a family history of breast cancer, but it's all

paternal. My current gyn/oc states that because the family history isn't maternal, I don't have anything to worry about. I'm unsure, I guess. Or just concerned.
—Steph, age 28

One reason I have avoided HRT so far is because of my maternal aunt's death from breast cancer. She had a hysterectomy, started HRT, and five years later she died. Did it have anything to do with the HRT? I don't know for sure, but I am afraid to find out. The endocrinologist said that several years ago they used stronger estrogen in a shot form. She says that today's HRT is much safer, but still??
—Karen, age 35

Many of the women I've spoken with who aren't on HRT immediately say that one of their reasons is their fear of breast cancer.

This is understandable, since breast cancer is the most common cancer affecting Western women. By the age of 75, about one in every 13 women will get breast cancer, and it will affect one in every eight women with a family history of this disease.

The concerns about estrogen replacement being linked to increased breast cancer risk began because certain cancerous tumors have *estrogen-receptor proteins*. Scientists have hypothesized that this type of tumor may grow more rapidly if you are taking estrogen. So the focus of much of the concern about ERT and breast cancer isn't so much that estrogen will cause normal cells to become cancerous, but that it may cause cancer cells already in your breasts to grow much more aggressively.

But is this the case? Is the risk as bad as it seems to be?

The answer is that no one is completely sure. As you might expect, many of the studies are inconsistent, inconclusive, and often completely contradictory.

- Some studies have found an increase in the risk of breast cancer in women who used hormones for over five years. More specifically, the Nurses' Health Study found a total 28 to 32 percent increase in the risk for breast cancer in women who were currently on HRT and had been taking it for at least five years. Other studies have reported that the risk for breast cancer increases only after 15 years of HRT.

- On the flip side, a University of Washington study showed *no* increase in breast cancer in women who had been using HRT for up to 20 years. And a smaller study, a California population control study, found that women who used both estrogen and progesterone for eight or more years had, if anything, a reduced risk of breast cancer. Finally, recent analyses of 23 different studies concluded that there was no change in risk of breast cancer at all in HRT users. In addition, statistics show that 90 percent of post-menopausal women who get breast cancer never have taken HRT.

- Finally, many of the studies that do show an increase in the risk of breast cancer indicate that the risk doesn't increase during the first five years of HRT. (But of course, if you're in premature menopause, even if you intend to be on HRT only until you reach 50, you're looking at well over five years of HRT.) Yet a 1998 analysis of 51 different studies published in the Journal of the National Cancer Institute found that each year of HRT increased the risk of breast cancer by 2.3 percent—a risk the report said is ''comparable to that associated with delaying menopause by a year.''

Obviously the jury is still out. As I mentioned earlier, the results of the long-term study by the Women's Health Initiative, due in 2008, should help draw more definitive conclusions.

In the meantime, though, who or what do you believe?

Let's try to make sense of this complicated issue. It seems safe to say that there could be a link between long-term use of HRT (specifically estrogen) and an increased risk in breast cancer, although this hasn't been conclusively proven. But it's important to understand that this increased risk sounds more threatening than it actually is. Put simply, if the studies that show an increase in breast cancer after five or more years of HRT are correct, this means that instead of one woman in 500 getting breast cancer, the risk rises to 1.3 or 2. On an individual level, this means that one woman's chances of cancer increase by about 0.3 to 0.5.

Second, and probably most important, the studies that have been done deal with women aged 50 and over. But what does this increased risk mean to you, not a woman in her fifties or sixties, but one in her twenties and thirties? What are you increasing your risk from, in other words?

You may have heard the frightening statistic that one in eight women is expected to develop breast cancer in her lifetime. But that's actually one in eight women up to the age of 85. The actual risk of breast cancer for a woman age 20 to 40—that is, the usual age of someone in premature menopause—is much lower. A woman of 25 has a one in 19,608 chance of getting breast cancer. At 35, the risk increases a great deal, but it's still not as high as you'd think—one in 622. By 45, the risk has increased even more, to one in 93, and by 55, to one in 33. It's a very large jump from one in 19,608 or one in 622 to 1 in 33. As a younger woman, on average you are at a much lower risk of breast cancer than the women who have been studied.

But will taking estrogen, then, increase your risk dramatically from this relatively low number? Again, it's difficult to be sure. If we are to believe the studies, yes, the risk will be increased, but still not to the level of older women. In addition, to be as safe as you can, you have to factor in the risks you already have.

The main risk is for women who have a family history of breast cancer, especially if relatives on your mother's side got breast cancer befor menopause. To get a little technical, there are two major breast cancer genes that have been identified (among others): BRCA-1 and BRCA-2. If you have a mutated BRCA-1 gene *and* have a strong family history of breast cancer, you have an 80 to 85 percent risk of developing breast cancer and a 50 percent risk of ovarian cancer over your lifetime. If breast cancer doesn't run in your family but you have the mutated BRCA-1 gene, you may have inherited a ''blocking'' gene as well that prevents the mutation from causing the cancer. About one in 200 to 400 American women probably carry a mutated BRCA-1 gene. If you have a mutated BRCA-2 gene, you also run an 80 percent risk of breast cancer, but not ovarian cancer. Overall, your risk increases two times if your mother had breast cancer before the age of 60, and about one and a half times if she got breast cancer after 60.

You're also at a higher risk if you've been exposed to estrogen for a long period of time—your own estrogen, not HRT. This is one instance where premature menopause is actually a positive thing: the older you are when you start menopause, the higher your chances of getting breast cancer. It's a similar effect if you start your period at a very young age—before you reach 12. If you have your first child after the age of 30 or if you never had a child, you also increase your risks. The key here is exposure to estrogen without the protective benefits of your natural progesterone. A prolonged exposure to unopposed estrogen is associated with an increase in breast cancer. Other risk factors for breast cancer include obesity, smoking, high-fat/low-fiber diet, alcohol consumption, and a history of breast cysts.

These other risk factors—genetic predisposition, exposure to estrogen, and so on—are the ones that you have to take into account when weighing how much of a risk it is for you to go on HRT. Is your risk of breast cancer so high already that adding to your odds of getting it outweighs the very high risk of osteoporosis and heart disease that premature menopause causes? Or do your risk factors of osteoporosis or heart disease outweigh the possible increase in breast cancer?

Next, take into account that, according to several research studies, a woman has a much greater risk of dying from heart disease because she isn't on HRT than she has of dying from breast cancer if she does take it. And when you're in premature menopause, your risk of heart disease is much higher than the average woman.

Finally, many studies have determined that the breast cancer caused by HRT, *hormonally promoted cancer* or *estrogen-related cancer*, seems to be more contained, less invasive, slower growing, and more easily treatable than cancers in women who aren't on HRT. (There is debate on this issue, but so far most studies have borne this out.) Obviously, this still isn't great news—no one wants breast cancer, no matter how much more easily controlled it may be. However, according to these studies, if you get estrogen-related breast cancer, your tumors will respond well to therapy and you'll face a much lower death rate than a woman who isn't on HRT and gets breast cancer.

So does HRT cause breast cancer, and should this possible risk be enough to keep you off it? Unfortunately, this is a situation where there is no definite black and white, and where your individual risk factors must be taken into account. All in all, as with so many of the other aspects of HRT, the risks probably aren't high enough to counterbalance the positives in most cases. Again, the key would be taking HRT until you

---

BREAST CANCER RISK FACTORS

Certain women are at a higher risk for breast cancer to begin with. Risk factors include:

- family history of breast cancer

- never having given birth or having your first child after age 30

- being overweight

- early puberty (before the age of 11) or late menopause (after the age of 54)—a risk factor that clearly doesn't apply to us

- high-fat/low-fiber diet

- smoking

- alcohol—as little as one drink a day can increase your risk by 11 percent

- history of breast cysts

reach the age of 50, then reconsidering the positives and negatives. If, however, you have a family history of breast cancer,
you will need to think even more carefully, study the facts, go
through all the possible negatives, and discuss the issue with
your doctor.

OVARIAN CANCER

This is another frightening cancer, and another one that may be
linked to estrogen. Yet again, no one is sure. The problem is
that this hasn't been studied much as yet, and the few studies
that have been done are inconclusive.

Briefly, according to some studies, estrogen increases the risk
of ovarian cancer. One study found a higher death rate from
ovarian cancer in women on estrogen replacement and a higher
incidence of the disease. There need to be more studies done
before any hard-and-fast conclusions can be drawn. However,
it's important to realize that ovarian cancer is relatively rare. A
35-year-old woman with no family history of ovarian cancer
has only a 1.5 to 1.6 percent chance of developing it in her
lifetime. If she has a mother, sister, or daughter with it, she has
a 5 percent risk. But here's a case where going through premature menopause actually has a positive benefit: the more you
ovulate, the higher your risk of ovarian cancer. So the earlier
you enter menopause—that is, stop ovulating—the lower your
risk.

Moreover, the studies that have suggested that estrogen replacement may increase your risk of ovarian cancer looked at
women taking estrogen alone, not with the progesterone or progestin that is now commonly prescribed as part of HRT. Since
adding a progesterone or progestin can decrease the risk of
endometrial cancer, there is a chance that it would do the same
with ovarian cancer. Again, however, more studies are needed
to determine if this is the case.

All in all, then, this is an area that needs further research to
determine whether or not ovarian cancer is linked to estrogen
and if so, whether there is a way to diminish the risk.

GALLBLADDER DISEASE

Gallbladder disease isn't usually fatal, but it's not something most of us would welcome. And unfortunately, taking estrogen, with or without progesterone or progestin, does increase your risk. According to most studies, you have about two times the risk of gallbladder disease requiring surgery when you're on estrogen replacement.

This happens because estrogen raises the amount of cholesterol in your bile. For example, a 1.25 mg dose of Premarin raises the bile's cholesterol level by 18 percent. The more cholesterol in your bile, the higher the chance of gallstones, which cause intense pain and usually lead to surgery.

There are other risk factors for gallbladder disease as well: being female (which, obviously, you can't control!), a family history of the disease, a high-fat diet, being overweight, multiple pregnancies, and age. In fact, doctors used to sum up the risks for gallbladder disease as the four "F's"—forty, fat, female, and fertile.

If you decide to go on HRT, it's a good idea to reduce your other risks as best you can through proper diet and exercise. In addition, some studies indicate that using a patch instead of a pill form of estrogen helps, since estrogen then isn't broken down in the liver.

What You *Don't* Have to Worry About, Even if You've Heard Otherwise

WEIGHT GAIN

I'll be completely honest: this was one of the main side effects about HRT that I'd heard about, and the one that made me very hesitant about trying HRT even after I realized that the health benefits outweighed the risks in my case. I've always been extremely weight-conscious—the legacy of having been a fat child—and didn't want to see my hard work go down the drain or maybe more accurately, on my hips! So when I read books and articles that talked about weight gain as pretty much a given if I went on HRT, I was upset. I didn't want to be a 38-year-old with the body of a much older, middle-aged woman.

But, happily, recent studies have indicated that this isn't the case. The PEPI trial and other smaller studies found that while women on HRT did often put on a few pounds, those women who weren't on HRT gained more weight. In fact, some studies have shown that many women actually lose weight on HRT.

One possible reason is that when you're in premature menopause, your estrogen levels drop, so your body may try to increase its fat content to store and produce as much estrogen as possible. When you go on HRT, you're getting the estrogen your body expected to have, so it doesn't need that extra fat any more. In addition, when your estrogen levels are low, you tend to put on weight around your middle—more like a man. This accounts for the "disappearing waistline" that so many women in premature menopause experience. When you replace estrogen, your body reverts to its normal weight distribution, which for most women means putting weight on in their hips, thighs, and lower abdomen instead of the middle.

To some degree, though, whether or not you gain weight on HRT may depend on the type you're taking. Progestins tend to make you retain water and bloat more. So even if you haven't actually gained weight, you may feel (and look) as though you have, especially if you're on cyclical progesterone—that is, taking it for only part of the month. Natural progesterone doesn't seem to have this side effect as much, and it often works as a diuretic instead, helping you lose water weight. Other women have found that lowering their dosage of estrogen or progesterone helps keep bloating down. Finally, others report good luck with patches instead of pills. You can read more about this in the discussion about the different forms of HRT.

But, all in all, weight gain isn't something you should worry about when you consider going on HRT. Yes, you may gain weight when you go through premature menopause, but this could just be a function of growing older or of poor diet or exercise habits. If you eat right and exercise enough, you won't put on weight just because you're taking HRT.

Blood Clots

In the past, women were warned that estrogen caused blood clots, so anyone with a history of abnormal blood clots was automatically told to steer clear of HRT. But now more doctors are shifting position on this.

The reason? The studies that alarmed people about a possible link between clotting and estrogen were based on birth control pills, which have a much higher dose of estrogen than the amount you get in HRT. Some recent studies done haven't shown any clear evidence linking ERT or HRT with an increased risk of blood clots, thrombophlebitis, or pulmonary embolism. (In fact, many studies have shown that HRT reduces the amount of fibrinogen, a blood coagulant associated with artery blockages.)

So blood clotting doesn't appear to rule out HRT. In fact, some doctors now believe that if you've had no sign of thrombosis for two to four years, HRT may be safe. That said, you should be sure to have your doctor monitor you closely. Moreover, you may be better off using estrogen in a patch form, which, because it bypasses the liver, appears to have less of an effect on clotting.

Stroke

This is yet another case in which something that people think is caused by HRT may actually be helped by HRT. Many studies have shown that replacing estrogen reduces the risk of death from stroke by 30 to 50 percent. Again, this appears to be due to estrogen's effect on your cardiovascular system, including lowering cholesterol, blood pressure, and fibrinogen, and maintaining the tone of the arterial walls. According to these studies, adding a progesterone or progestin didn't appear to detract from these positive effects. In general, then, most doctors believe that if you are a candidate for a stroke (due to family history, diabetes, high blood pressure, or atherosclerosis), HRT may help you prevent it.

HYPERTENSION

As with stroke, hypertension, or high blood pressure, is another example of a disease that is probably helped, not hurt, by HRT. Many women and doctors have believed that HRT raises your blood pressure, which made it appear to be a bad choice for women who either already have high blood pressure or have risk factors for high blood pressure. But recent studies have indicated that the opposite is the truth: as mentioned in the section on HRT's cardiovascular benefits, studies have shown that HRT may actually help lower blood pressure.

DIABETES

In the past, many doctors believed that estrogen replacement would raise blood sugar levels, making it a no-no for diabetics. This isn't the case, though. Studies have shown that taking oral forms of estrogen actually helps lower blood sugar levels and improves the metabolism of blood glucose. In addition, HRT is usually a good choice if you have both premature menopause and diabetes, because you are at a double risk for heart disease: not only is your risk increased due to premature menopause, but heart disease is also two to four times more common in people with diabetes.

On the negative side, estrogen can raise blood triglycerides, which are often associated with diabetes: In this case, you should talk to your doctor about using a patch form of estrogen, which doesn't raise triglycerides as a pill form does, or about taking testosterone in addition to estrogen, which appears to help offset the rise in triglycerides.

SMOKING

No, HRT won't make smoking good for you, but the old myth that you can't go on HRT if you smoke is just that, a myth.

To a great degree, this myth arose from studies about birth

control pills. Birth control pills can increase clotting factors, which are promoted by smoking. If a clot lodges in a coronary artery, you'll get a heart attack, if in your brain, you'll get a stroke. So smoking and birth control pills are not a good mix. But birth control pills contain a much higher dosage of estrogen than that which is usually prescribed in HRT. HRT, then, doesn't cause the same problems as birth control pills. In fact, if you're a smoker, you're at a much greater risk for heart disease and osteoporosis, which means you may need the probable benefits of HRT even more than a nonsmoker. HRT won't reverse the effects of smoking, but it may cut your risk somewhat.

But there is a negative aspect to smoking and HRT: when you smoke, you have lower levels of estrogen, even when you are on estrogen replacement. This may be due to an increase in liver breakdown of estrogen or an increase in hormones that oppose estrogen. But whatever the specific cause, usually a smoker needs higher dosages of estrogen to get the amount necessary to prevent osteoporosis and heart disease, as well as to eliminate symptoms. If you smoke, be completely honest with your doctor about your habit so you can be sure you're getting the estrogen you need. Often you'll need to have your estrogen levels tracked and retested to double-check how much estrogen you're actually getting from your prescribed dosage.

WHO SHOULDN'T BE ON HRT— AND WHO SHOULD BE CAREFUL?

Most women in premature menopause are able to take HRT safely. But there are some women who may be told by their doctors to steer clear of HRT, and others who should be very careful while on it and have a doctor track them closely. This isn't an exact science because studies are still being done. However, in general, the following applies.

You shouldn't be on HRT if you have:

- *unexplained vaginal bleeding*
- *estrogen-related breast cancer*
- *had a recent heart attack*
- *severe liver disease, such as cirrhosis*

This is common sense. If you have unexplained vaginal bleeding, you could have endometrial cancer, which is promoted by estrogen. It's a similar case with breast cancer. The first step in either of these cases is to treat your problem. HRT may be something you can take later on, but taking it now is risky business. As for severe liver disease, this is a problem because oral forms of estrogen are broken down and metabolized by your liver. Taking estrogen may cause your liver to work even harder, which could cause its function to worsen. Using an estrogen patch, however, may be possible for you—but, of course, you would need to discuss this with your doctor.

You may be able to take HRT, but need to discuss it carefully with your doctor, if you have had:

- *endometrial cancer*
- *breast cancer or a family history of breast cancer*

This sounds surprising, but it's true. A number of women in premature menopause have entered it because of treatment for these cancers, and until recently, their doctors probably would have told them to stay away from HRT. But recent studies are beginning to question this. A 1997 study found that HRT didn't have a significant effect on a recurrence of cancer. As with so many other areas in HRT research, there still needs to be a full-scale randomized trial to draw more precise conclusions. In the meantime, though, in many cases having had cancer or a family history of cancer doesn't necessarily rule out HRT. In these cases, it is wise to discuss HRT with a cancer specialist as well as with your gynecologist.

Where endometrial cancer is concerned, the issue is usually time. Many doctors prescribe estrogen and progesterone within three to five years of surgery, which will eliminate symptoms, help fight osteoporosis and heart disease, and (because of the progesterone) prevent any cells from becoming cancerous due to unopposed estrogen.

As for breast cancer, most doctors still hesitate to prescribe HRT to women who have been treated for breast cancer since there is a chance that the cancer could be restimulated by the estrogen. Often, you'll be prescribed an alternative to estrogen, such as tamoxifen, to help fight osteoporosis and cardiovascular disease. However, these alternatives don't eliminate symptoms, which are often quite intense for women with premature menopause. In addition, they don't seem to have the same level of benefits as HRT. This is one of the reasons doctors are beginning to rethink prescribing HRT to women who have had breast cancer or have a family history of it. Their belief is that the benefits may outweigh the risks when you're in premature menopause. Moreover, no studies have shown that HRT will cause a recurrence of breast cancer.

Given this, if you had breast cancer treatment five to 10 years ago and no recurrence of symptoms, or if you had non-estrogen-related breast cancer, and you have bad symptoms or a high risk of cardiovascular disease, osteopenia, or osteoporosis, you and your doctor may want to consider HRT or tamoxifen plus estrogen. This is a difficult situation and one that you'll have to consider very carefully. If you do choose to go on HRT, you need to have regular breast examinations and see a cancer specialist or gynecologist who is well versed in breast cancer.

You can take HRT but need to be tracked closely while on it if you have:

- *seizures*
- *diabetes*
- *hypertension*
- *mild liver disease*
- *lupus*
- *gallbladder disease*

- *benign breast disease such as fibrocystic breast disease, mastopathy, chronic cystic mastitis*
- *endometriosis or fibroids*

These conditions may be worsened by HRT. If you have any of these, talk to your doctor. In some cases, different forms of estrogen (such as a patch) or dosage adjustments may help you avoid aggravating these conditions.

DIFFERENT FORMS OF HRT: SYNTHETICS, NATURALS, PILLS, AND PATCHES

HRT in general is confusing enough, but it can get even more so when you're faced with an array of different products—natural estrogen, equine estrogen, progestin, natural progesterone gel, patches, pills, and so on—all with different names, claims, positives and negatives.

Yet you may not even know about all the choices you have. All too often, your doctor will simply come out with the pat recommendation that you need HRT, hand you a prescription for the HRT "biggies," Premarin and Provera, and tell you to fill it—end of story.

But it *isn't* the end of the story where you're concerned.

Even if you agree that you should be on HRT, you need more information than just a quick "you need to be on this." Remember, you're the one who is considering taking the hormones. You deserve to know exactly what you're taking, why, and if there is a better choice for you. Yes, some women do automatically fill the prescription, start taking Premarin or Prempro, or one of the other widely prescribed HRT drugs, and hope things will work out. But just as taking HRT itself shouldn't be a knee-jerk action, taking a specific kind of HRT shouldn't be either.

To make an informed, educated choice about the type of HRT you should take, you need to know about the different options available to you, the pros and cons of each, and how they can fit into your health picture and lifestyle.

The Synthetics Versus the "Naturals": A Broad Difference Between Forms of HRT

Before I run through the commonly prescribed forms of HRT, let's take a quick look at one of the main issues regarding HRT in general: Should you take synthetic or natural forms of HRT?

This is yet another area of debate in the whole HRT arena. Some researchers claim that synthetic forms of HRT aren't as effective as natural; others disagree. But to understand your options better, you have to understand the terms. To begin with, what is "natural"? It is a bit confusing (as with so much concerning HRT), but I'll try to make it as simple as possible.

As used in this book, as well as by most people discussing HRT, "natural" refers to estrogens and progesterone that are actually man-made, but from *natural* sources. Most important, they are *naturally occurring* and *bioidentical to the hormones your body makes.* In other words, they don't just approximate your hormones; they have the same exact chemical structure as the hormones made by your ovaries. This is one of the reasons many women and researchers believe natural hormones are preferable. Because they are the same as what we make, our bodies can work better with them. We can more easily metabolize them and break them down so our livers and kidneys can excrete them once they've done their work, and so they don't accumulate in the body and cause side effects.

"Synthetic" refers to man-made hormones, as you'd expect, made from synthetic sources but also to Premarin (and its offshoots) which, although made from a natural source (horse urine), *isn't* exactly the same as the estrogen that is made in your body. The "synthetics" aren't bioidentical. The synthetic versus natural issue is most clear-cut when it comes to progesterone. Until very recently, the only easily available choice was synthetic progesterone (or progestin). Progestin isn't exactly like progesterone, but has many of the same attributes and opposes estrogen in your body as natural progesterone does. But now natural prescription progesterones have become widely available, both in vaginal gel form and in micronized pill form. These natural progesterones are very different from the synthetics in that they are, again, bioidentical to your own progesterone. They have fewer side effects and—the best news of all—may help grow bone in addition to just preventing bone loss.

In general, then, where the synthetic versus natural debate is concerned, it may make more sense to opt for a natural progesterone than a synthetic because of its effect on bones. Beyond that, however, it really boils down to a personal decision. While many doctors claim that naturally occurring forms of estrogen are a better choice because they are exactly the same as the hormones your ovaries produce, others feel more comfortable prescribing Premarin because it has been studied more extensively.

Ask yourself the following: What argument do you agree with? What do you feel comfortable taking? What works for you? There are many ethical, political, and practical opinions floating around about HRT and its different forms, but I'm a believer in taking whatever works for you as an individual. Some women feel uncomfortable taking hormones made of horse urine and talk about the mistreatment of the horses used in the preparation. This is a legitimate concern on their part, and I agree that they shouldn't take Premarin since the concept bothers them. Others, however, don't feel this is a problem, and feel comfortable taking Premarin because it has been so widely studied. This too seems to be a legitimate decision. In honesty, I think the different views are all valid. When it comes to health risks, you'll note that some forms of hormones do appear to be associated with a higher risk than others, but, in fairness, nothing has been unequivocally established.

The bottom line, then: HRT is such a personal decision, you shouldn't allow yourself to be bullied into anything. Remember that everyone is different, and what doesn't work for one person may work well for another. For example, I opted against Premarin and Provera, having read about the possible side effects and having a personal preference for taking natural HRT. Moreover, my risk of osteoporosis is high since I have a family history of it, so natural progesterone seemed to be a better choice for me than synthetic. So I chose to take a natural estrogen and progesterone (in my case, Estrace and Crinone) based on my attitudes and health concerns. However, I know several women who are taking Premarin and Provera and are very happy with the results. Many have no side effects at all; others have side effects, but don't feel that they're a major issue. They are as pleased with their choice as I am with mine.

Estrogens

Estrogen is the major component of HRT, and the one for which there is the widest range of choices. Different types of estrogen are available—conjugated estrogen, estradiol, estropipate, and so on—and different forms of estrogen are available as well—pills, patches, and creams. Following is a quick explanation of these different forms, including the commonly prescribed brands.

ORAL ESTROGENS

This is probably the most common form of estrogen used in HRT—estrogen tablets or capsules. But as you'd expect, there are several different forms of oral estrogen.

Conjugated Estrogen (Premarin)

Premarin is the biggest brand name of estrogen—in fact, it's the number one selling drug overall in the country—and is the one that doctors often automatically prescribe when you say you're ready to go on HRT. On the market since the 1950s, Premarin is currently the only form of conjugated estrogen available. It's also the form of estrogen used in the bulk of the research studies on HRT, which means that most things you read about estrogen are actually specifically about Premarin.

Premarin is a mixture of over ten different estrogens, including estrone (which we make in our own bodies), and equilin and equilenin (both horse estrogens, which, of course, we *don't* make in our own bodies). In fact, the name Premarin comes from "pregnant mare's urine," which is its source. Because it comes from horse urine, the pharmaceutical company that makes Premarin (Wyeth-Ayerst Laboratories) considers it a natural estrogen. They are technically right; after all, horse urine is definitely natural! But by most standard definitions of "natural" as it applies to HRT, Premarin isn't considered one of the "naturals" since it isn't identical to the estrogen we produce in our own bodies.

When you take conjugated estrogens, your body converts them into active estrogens and uses them as it would estrogen your ovaries have produced. About 10 to 15 percent of the estrogens, however, can't be used.

Some people have a bias against Premarin because of its source, but, in all fairness, because conjugated estrogen is similar to our own estrogen, Premarin has been shown to eliminate the symptoms of menopause and prevent bone loss, and appears to protect against cardiovascular disease. In addition, studies conducted by the pharmaceutical company indicate that the horse estrogen may be more effective than human estrogen in improving blood cholesterol levels and may actually help prevent the increased risk of breast cancer. These findings, however, haven't been corroborated by an outside study, so it's difficult to be sure about these claims. In fact, other studies hold that Premarin, because it isn't natural to your body, may cause cancer, while natural estrogens won't. It's yet another facet of the ongoing HRT debate.

On the downside, it appears that you get a higher amount of estrogen in your blood with Premarin than you do with other estrogens. The culprit here is the equilin. The amount of equilin you get from Premarin is much higher than your normal level of the human estrogens, estradiol and estrone. Because it is so strong, it appears to tax your liver more than other nonequine estrogens do, which can be a problem especially if you have a history of liver disease in your family or have had liver disease yourself, or if you smoke, are obese, or have high blood pressure.

In most cases, however, the issue as to whether or not Premarin is the right choice for you boils down to whether you want a natural (that is, bioidentical) estrogen or one that only approximates the estrogen you naturally make. Studies have shown that Premarin will work to combat osteoporosis and heart disease and eliminate symptoms as well as do other forms of estrogen. Moreover, because it has been studied so widely, doctors often feel most comfortable prescribing this.

One final note: as of this writing, a pharmaceutical company (Duramed) was awaiting approval from the Food and Drug Administration (FDA) for Cenestin, a conjugated estrogen made from plants instead of horse urine.

Form:	Tablet.
Standard dosage:	0.625 mg—this is the amount most studied and has been shown to be the lowest amount required to protect against osteoporosis and heart disease, although recent studies also indicated that 0.3 milligram will also eliminate symptoms and prevent osteoporosis. The lower dosages' effect on heart disease isn't known yet. Also available in 0.9, 1.25, and 2.5 mg.
Pros:	Widely studied; most commonly prescribed estrogen; appears effective in relieving symptoms and maintaining bone density.
Cons:	Not identical to the estrogen your body makes; some women feel uncomfortable taking an estrogen made from horses' urine; stronger than many other estrogens, so may cause changes in your liver.

Estradiol (Estrace)

Estradiol is the estrogen our ovaries produce the most of during our reproductive years, so when you take estradiol in

HRT, you are to some degree replacing the estrogen you used to make with its identical twin.

The most commonly prescribed estradiol is Estrace; however, you also can get generic estradiol. In either case, it is a natural, bioidentical estrogen, made from plant sources, that is *micronized*—broken down into little pieces—so it is easily absorbed and used by your body. When you take estradiol orally, it enters your gastrointestinal tract, is metabolized by your liver, and is converted into estrone, the estrogen your body has the most of after menopause.

According to studies, micronized estrogen helps prevent bone loss and so fights against osteoporosis, helps lower cholesterol, and appears to prevent the risk of cardiovascular disease. Another plus is that estradiol is the form of estrogen that appears to be involved with memory, learning, and other mental functions that often decline with age.

While most studies have been conducted using a standard dose of 1 mg of Estrace (which is comparable to the 0.625 mg of Premarin), recent studies have also shown that a half-dosage of 0.5 mg also helps fight osteoporosis if taken with a calcium supplement. One other often unreported plus is that micronized estradiol increases sex-hormone-binding globulin, so women with high levels of androgens that cause such side effects as excessive facial hair growth may see improvement with this estrogen.

But there has been some concern about taking micronized estradiol because estradiol is the strongest form of estrogen and the one that is most carcinogenic. According to a Scandinavian study of over 23,000 women, there was an increased risk of breast cancer over time—up to 1.7 times the risk after nine years. However, the study looked at women taking 2 mg of estradiol, which is double the most commonly prescribed dose of 1 mg. Moreover the study has been criticized because only one in every 30 women participating in the study was sent questionnaires. Yet again, then, this is a case where it's difficult to say whether the findings of a study should concern you.

On the whole, most doctors believe that micronized estradiol is a good choice of estrogen for women wanting to prevent osteoporosis and heart disease and to minimize menopausal symptoms. And, since it is naturally occurring and identical to the estrogen the ovaries produce, it's a good choice for women who prefer a natural estrogen to a conjugated one.

Form: Tablet.

Standard dosage: 1 mg; also available in 2 mg tablets, which may be prescribed if the initial 1 mg dose fails to help eliminate symptoms, and 0.5 mg, which, combined with calcium, has been shown to prevent osteoporosis.

Pros: Plant-derived; identical to the estrogen your body makes; easily absorbed; helps fight osteoporosis and heart disease and eliminates symptoms.

Cons: Higher-than-usual doses were shown to increase the risk of breast cancer in one study (however, the findings of this study have been criticized); easily excreted from your system, so if you take it in the morning, you may have symptoms at nighttime. You can easily get around this, though, by taking a half dose in the morning and another half-dose before bedtime.

Estropipate (Ogen, Ortho-Est)

Another natural estrogen that is bioidentical, estropipate is made from purified crystalline estrone. In effect, then, when you take estropipate, you're getting the final by-product of estradiol and conjugated estrogens, since the liver converts the estrogens in them to estrone.

Estropipate is weaker than the other estrogens, so you need to take a higher dosage to get the same levels of estradiol and estrone in your blood system that you get from taking a standard dose of either conjugated estrogens or micronized estradiol.

You get the same benefits from estropipate, however, in terms of eliminating symptoms and fighting osteoporosis and heart disease. In addition, because it is the weaker end product of estradiol, estropipate is often prescribed to women who have side effects from the other estrogens, such as breast tenderness and bloating.

Form:	Tablet.
Standard dosage:	0.75 mg estropipate in 0.625 mg; Ogen: 0.625, 1.25, 2.5, and 5 mg tablets. Ortho-Est: 0.625 mg; 1.25 mg.
Pros:	Natural; bioidentical to the estrone in your body. Like the other estrogens, fights osteoporosis and heart disease. Often tolerated better by women who suffer from estrogen side effects such as breast tenderness, bloating, migraines.
Cons:	Weaker than the other estrogens, so you may need to adjust your dosage to eliminate symptoms such as hot flashes. In addition, you may need a higher dosage than you would of Premarin or micronized estradiol.

Esterified Estrogen (Estratab, Menest)

Esterified estrogen is a plant-based product made from yams and soy. It was introduced in 1998, so is relatively new. Its big claim to fame is that you can take a much lower dosage than other forms of estrogen but still get the same benefits in terms of eliminating symptoms, preventing osteoporosis, and helping to fight heart disease.

According to studies, esterified estrogen prevents osteoporosis at half the dose of conjugated estrogens (Premarin), and apparently has fewer side effects. One study conducted by researchers at the University of California-San Francisco found that esterified estrogen didn't cause the increase in vaginal bleeding or buildup of the uterine walls—the precursor to endometrial cancer—that conjugated estrogens do. In fact, some researchers believe that you may not need to take a progestin or progesterone with this form of estrogen (since these are usually prescribed to fight against the possibility of endometrial cancer) or may be able to take a lower dose. This looks promising because the side effects many women report from HRT are caused by progestin. However, more studies will be done to determine whether this theory is correct. In addition, perhaps because of the lower dose than that of Premarin or micronized estradiol, esterified estrogen doesn't seem to cause as great an increase in breast tenderness, headaches, or nausea as Premarin.

Form: Tablet.
Standard dosage: 0.3 mg.
Pros: Natural; low dosage appears to prevent os-
                     teoporosis and heart disease as well as
                     minimize menopausal symptoms, but with
                     fewer side effects than other higher-dose
                     forms of estrogen.
Cons: Because it's relatively new, no long-term
                     studies have been conducted, so it's un-
                     clear how effective it is in preventing os-
                     teoporosis, etc. over a prolonged period.

Tri-estrogen: Estrone, Estradiol, and Estriol

This is a form of estrogen replacement that has been get-ting a lot of attention lately, although it's still not widely prescribed. There is no major pharmaceutical company put-ting out tri-est, but you can get it with a doctor's prescription from a compounding pharmacy.

Tri-estrogen is, not so surprisingly, a combination of the three major estrogens your body makes—estrone, estradiol, and es-triol. Usually it is produced in the proportion of 10 percent estrone, 10 percent estradiol, and 80 percent estriol, but this ratio can be adjusted depending upon your specific needs.

The theory behind tri-estrogen is a simple one: by taking it, you get the benefits from three different estrogens, and they are in a ratio similar to that which your body produces. The bulk of tri-est is estriol, which is the weakest form of estrogen pro-duced in our bodies, and, as mentioned before, not only is it the least likely to cause breast cancer, but some studies have shown that it actually helps prevent it. So by taking all three estrogens—very small doses of the stronger ones and a higher one of the weakest one—you can eliminate menopausal symptoms, fight osteoporosis and heart disease, and help prevent the increased risk of breast cancer.

It's a great theory, and one that bears watching. The only problem is that, as with other newer forms of estrogen, there haven't been any long-term studies done on this.

Form:	Capsule.
Standard dosage:	1.25 mg twice a day to treat mild to moderate symptoms; 2.5 mg twice a day for moderate to severe estrogen deficiency; also available in 5 mg dosage.
Pros:	Natural; appears to have fewer health risks than other estrogens, while preventing osteoporosis and heart disease and eliminating symptoms.
Cons:	May be too weak for some women, particularly those who have just had surgical menopause; no long-term studies have yet been conducted on this form of estrogen replacement.

Estriol

As mentioned earlier in this chapter, estriol is the weakest of the three major estrogens in your body. It appears to give a lower risk of breast cancer, and may possibly have a protective effect on the breasts. Unlike conjugated estrogens or estradiol, when you take estriol, it isn't converted into estrone, which means you aren't exposing yourself to the estrogens that have been linked to cancer.

This is one of the main reasons more researchers are looking into the use of estriol alone as an estrogen replacement in place of the commonly prescribed conjugated estrogens or estradiol.

The key plus of estriol is its weakness: it appears to offer the benefits of the stronger estrogens with fewer of the risks. Tests have indicated that it relieves menopausal symptoms, and protects against heart disease and osteoporosis, as the other estrogens do, but appears not to increase the risk of breast cancer or endometrial cancer. In fact, many studies indicate that it has an anticancer effect and may actually work better than tamoxifen for women with breast cancer. In addition, studies conducted in the United States found that estriol seemed to be a good choice for women who had trouble tolerating the stronger estrogens.

But the weakness of estriol is also a negative factor. Because it is so weak, you need a much higher dosage to get the results you do from the standard dosages of conjugated estrogens or estradiol. For example, 4 mg of estriol equals 1.25 mg of conjugated estrogens. In some studies, many women needed as much as 8 mg a day to get relief from menopausal symptoms, but a high dose of estriol can cause nausea. Remember, estriol is the estrogen that rises when you're pregnant—and suffering from morning sickness. One way to get the benefits of estriol without the high dosage is to opt for tri-est (see page 196).

Estriol has been widely used for years in Europe and China with great success, but is currently rarely prescribed in the United States. It's not a patented drug, so there is no major pharmaceutical company putting out a brand-name estriol. But doctors can have it formulated by compounding pharmacies, and the use of it seems to be growing. Because of its unique properties, estriol seems to be a good and safe choice for estrogen replacement. It's well worth talking to your doctor about this.

Form:	Capsule.
Standard dosage:	Ranges from 2 to 8 mg.
Pros:	Natural; appears to have low risks compared to other estrogens; may help prevent breast cancer.
Cons:	You may need a very high dose to eliminate symptoms, which can cause nausea.

ESTROGEN PATCHES

Estrogen is also available in a patch form, which is often recommended for women who have problems absorbing estrogen through their digestive tract, women with liver problems, diabetes, history of blood clots and high blood pressure, and for women who just seem to have trouble with oral estrogens.

When you use a patch estrogen, the estrogen is absorbed through your skin and directly into your bloodstream. Because it doesn't go through your digestive tract, it isn't broken down by your liver, which keeps side effects caused by changes in the liver to a minimum. In addition, the estrogen is released continuously into your system, which is like your natural estrogen production and helps prevent the hormone highs and lows you may get when you take a pill and get all of your estrogen at once. Because it mimics your natural estrogen production, some doctors believe this is the best form of estrogen for women in premature menopause.

But there are downsides: not only do the patches often cost quite a bit more than pills, they also often cause skin irritation and can fall off if you sweat. In addition, the amount of estrogen you actually get through your skin varies from woman to woman, depending on skin thickness, pore size, and amount of perspiration. This is why it makes sense to have your doctor double-check your estradiol levels once you're on the patch—you need to make sure you're getting what you need (at least 50 picograms per milliliter). Finally, there haven't been any long-term studies of the patch yet, so it's unclear if it helps prevent heart disease. It does lower blood cholesterol levels, though—a little slower than oral forms of estrogen, but ultimately to the same levels. All in all, depending upon your specific situation, the patch may be a good choice for you.

Transdermal Patch (Estraderm)

The Estraderm patch was the first widely available estrogen patch and is still one of the most widely used. It comes in two different sizes—the 0.05 mg patch, which continuously delivers

PILLS VERSUS PATCHES:
HOW TO CHOOSE BETWEEN THEM

Consider a patch if:

• you experienced uncomfortable symptoms with oral forms of estrogen, such as nausea;

• you've noticed highs and lows when you take oral estrogens—you feel great for part of the day, then start getting hot flashes, etc. about 12 to 18 hours after taking your estrogen pill;

• you suffer from migraines or have noticed an increase in migraines with estrogen tablets;

• you are at risk for gallbladder disease or have already had it;

• you have a history of blood-clotting problems;

• you have had liver disease or have a high risk of it;

• you have diabetes;

• your blood pressure has risen since you've been on oral estrogen;

• you have very high triglycerides;

• you smoke.

On the other hand, the patch may not be your best choice if:

• you perspire a lot because you live in a hot climate or you often exercise strenuously, or if you swim a great deal (in these cases, you may have problems keeping the patch sticking to you);

• you have sensitive skin and are prone to skin allergies and irritations such as contact dermatitis;

• you are having problems absorbing enough estrogen from the patch to raise your estradiol levels to at least 50 picograms to help prevent osteoporosis and/or heart disease;

• you are uncomfortable about the idea of wearing a visible sign of your menopause (this is something many single women with premature menopause may feel particularly self-conscious about).

50 micrograms (mcg) of estradiol to your system each day, and the 0.10 mg patch, which delivers 100 mcg of estradiol. Both are transparent ovals with adhesive like a Band-Aid and a fluid reservoir like a bubble in the middle. This bubble contains the estrogen that is transmitted through your skin. You apply the patch to unexposed skin—your buttocks, thighs, or lower abdomen—and forget about it until it's time to change it, which you do every three-and-a-half to four days. It usually takes less than four hours to reach the therapeutic level of estrogen in your system, and the estrogen is delivered continuously to your body.

It's a nice and easy way to get estrogen, plus you get the benefits of bypassing your liver and getting a steady, continuous dosage of estrogen into your system. But, unfortunately, it's not always as great as it sounds. First, there's something about the adhesive in the Estraderm patch that apparently causes skin irritation, especially if you use it in more sensitive areas, such as your lower abdomen. About 15 to 20 percent of the women using the Estraderm patch develop blotches and welts under and around the patch. You may be able to get around this, though, by moving the patch to less sensitive skin areas, such as the buttocks or thighs. In addition, using vitamin E or cortisone cream may help soothe the irritated skin. But according to Ciba Pharmaceuticals, the manufacturer, at least 2 percent of Estraderm users stop using the patch because of skin irritation. The second problem that a number of Estraderm users have reported is that the edges often get rolled, less sticky, and generally messy. This isn't a huge problem, but it can get annoying—and sometimes embarrassing if the patch suddenly stops sticking at an inopportune moment.

Form:	Patch.
Standard dosage:	0.1 mg; 0.05 mg (usually prescribed to eliminate symptoms; possibly not strong enough to prevent osteoporosis).
Pros:	Easy to use.
Cons:	Skin irritation under and around the patch is common; studies haven't been done to show how effective the patch is against heart disease.

Matrix (Climara, Vivelle, FemPatch, Alora)

This is the newer, improved estrogen patch. Like the transdermal, it continuously releases estrogen into your system, but it causes less skin irritation. According to one manufacturer, only about 9 percent of users developed significant skin irritation, about half that of Estraderm users.

The Matrix patch was first introduced in 1995, when the Climara patch came out. A year later, the makers of the Estraderm patch came out with their version of a matrix patch, Vivelle. Next came FemPatch, a lower-dose estrogen patch, and Alora. Finally, in January 1999, the FDA approved yet another patch by Noven Pharmaceuticals, the makers of Vivelle. This patch is the smallest yet—only a little larger than a nickel, but delivers as much as .10 mg. of estradiol. In all cases, the patch doesn't have the bubble that the Estraderm does. Instead, it's a flat, translucent patch that lies flat under your clothes and sticks better than the Estraderm patch, even when you shower or swim. In addition, the matrix delivery system appears to deliver estrogen more steadily, maintaining more stable blood levels of estrogen. But you get a slightly lower level of estrogen in your blood from the Climara or Vivelle than you do with the Estraderm—about 70 picograms of estradiol from the 0.1 mg matrix patch, as compared with 100 picograms from the corresponding Estraderm patch.

Form: Patch.

Standard dosage: Climara: 0.1 mg; 0.05 mg (usually prescribed to eliminate symptoms; possibly not strong enough to prevent osteoporosis). Vivelle: 0.1 mg (also available in 0.0375, 0.05, 0.075 mg dosages). Fempatch: 0.025 mg. Alora: 0.1 mg; 0.05 mg; 0.075 mg.

Pros: Easy to use; source of continuous estrogen, less obvious and better adhesion than the Estraderm patch; Vivelle's wide range of available dosages allows for more flexibility than other patches.

Cons: Can cause irritation.

ESTROGEN CREAMS

The three common forms of estrogen (conjugated estrogen, estradiol, and estrone) are also available in vaginal creams. Premarin, Estrace, and Estratrab, among other major brands, all make vaginal creams. The problem? It's difficult to measure absorbability of the cream, and you may get much less estrogen than you actually need. For example, while 1 gram of Premarin cream contains 0.625 mg of estrogen, just like the standard tablet dosage, you usually absorb enough to bring your blood levels of estrogen to only about 25 to 50 percent of the levels you would get from taking the tablet. And you get even less with Estrace cream. This is why most doctors don't prescribe estrogen creams to women in premature menopause. All in all, vaginal creams are usually recommended only for preventing vaginal dryness, not for the overall effect on osteoporosis and heart disease prevention as provided by other forms of estrogen.

Estrogen skin creams appear to be even weaker than the vaginal ones. Again, the problem is one of measuring absorption. If your skin is thicker or less permeable than average, you may get much less estrogen than you need. However, many women have reported great results from a combination tri-estrogen-progesterone cream. The problem? This product hasn't been widely tested, so results are anecdotal at this point. This is something that you may want to look into in the future and discuss with your doctor, but until more studies have been done, you may want to steer clear, since you might be feeling relief from symptoms but still not be getting the estrogen your body needs to fight osteoporosis and heart disease.

Finally, there is estrogen gel, which is used in other countries but not yet in the United States. Sold under the brand name Estrogel, it was approved for sale in Canada in early 1999, has been used in Europe for over 20 years, and is the most widely prescribed form of estrogen in France. Estrogen gel seems to work well: like the patch forms of estrogen, you are delivering estradiol continuously into your system while bypassing your liver, but unlike the patch, you don't have to worry about skin irritation since there is no adhesive involved. The gel has been proven to help prevent bone loss but has less of an effect on your blood cholesterol levels. Another downside is that it's difficult to be sure of the exact dosage you're getting, so a doctor would have to track your estrogen levels. While the gel isn't available yet from a major pharmaceutical company in the United States, it may be introduced in the future because of its success in Europe and because more women are interested in exploring alternative forms of HRT. Currently, though, alternative hormone-formulating companies do put out similar alcohol-based estrogen gels. Again, though, it's important to discuss this with your doctor.

Progesterones

Progesterones are the number two in HRT—the hormone most of us take in addition to estrogen. As mentioned before, progesterone is usually prescribed if you have a uterus, to balance out the estrogen and protect against endometrial cancer. In addition, even women who have had their uteruses removed are often prescribed progesterone.

But all progesterones are not created equal. As with estrogen, you do have choices. Actually, until recently you *didn't* have much of a choice—the synthetic progesterones were the only ones widely prescribed. This was because plain, natural progesterone isn't that easily absorbed in oral form, yet women need to take a progesterone to counteract the endometrial-building effects of estrogen. So scientists came up with synthetic progesterones, or progestins, to enable women on HRT to balance out the estrogen.

The problem? While progestin does help prevent endometrial cancer, it has several unpleasant side effects which are extremely common in women taking it. Most are like PMS symptoms: bloating, fluid retention, breast tenderness, cramping, headaches, depression, mood swings, irritability. In addition, progestins seem to interfere with some of the heart-healthy benefits of estrogen. More specifically, they block the increase in HDL and the positive effects on the coronary blood vessels.

Recently, however, researchers developed ways of making natural progesterone more absorbable. They developed a micronizing process that breaks the progesterone down into small particles, allowing it be more easily absorbed and delivered in a stable amount. In addition, a vaginal gel form of natural progesterone was developed that delivers the progesterone to your uterus in a bioadhesive gel with a consistent amount of progesterone. These developments have led to a wider use of prescription natural progesterone, especially as major pharmaceutical companies have begun introducing products of their own. In addition, natural progesterone is available from compounding pharmacies—pharmacies that formulate hormones based on a doctor's prescription. Natural progesterone is bioidentical to the progesterone your body makes, causes fewer side effects than progestin, and may help build bone in addition to preventing bone loss.

Even so, some women prefer the synthetic progestins because they have been more widely prescribed and closely studied, or they simply take them because it's what most doctors automatically prescribe. Others prefer a natural progesterone because it is identical to their body's progesterone and because of the lower risk of side effects. In addition, some scientists speculate that natural progesterone may work better in preventing the increased risk of cancer caused by estrogen. Again, the choice is yours. Here's a quick rundown of the different options open to you to help you make your decision.

PROGESTINS

Medroxyprogesterone acetate or MPA (Provera, Cycrin)
MPA is, in effect, the conjugated estrogen of the progesterone world. In other words, it is the oldest form of progestrone used in HRT, the most commonly prescribed, and the type of progesterone that has been used in most HRT studies.

This synthetic form of progesterone is called a C21 progestin and is made by adding chemical groups to progesterone, which makes the progesterone more stable and more easily available for use by the body. But MPA causes PMS-like side effects in many women, sometimes to such a degree that women want to stop HRT completely. In addition, MPA may detract from some of the heart-healthy aspects of estrogen. So it's recommended that you take the smallest amount that will protect against endometrial buildup.

Form:	Tablet.
Standard dosage:	2.5 mg daily (on continuous therapy); 5 mg daily for two weeks of your cycle (on cyclical therapy); also available in 10 mg dosage.
Pros:	Widely studied.
Cons:	Linked to a number of side effects ranging from breast tenderness to bloating to depression; blocks some of estrogen's effects on cholesterol.

Norethindrone Acetate (Aygestin)

Another synthetic progesterone, norethindrone acetate (NTA) is a C19 progestin, made from testosterone. Different chemical groups are added and subtracted, eliminating the male properties from the hormone and forming an absorbable, stable progestin.

It is stronger than MPA, so you need smaller dosages. It's commonly prescribed to women who have had problems dealing with side effects from Provera or Cycrin, and is said to help reduce the breast tenderness and bloating that are often caused by MPA. In addition, it lowers triglycerides, which is a plus because estrogen tends to raise them. The downside? Because it's made from testosterone, some studies have indicated that it has androgenic effects—in other words, it may cause masculinizing side effects such as acne, hair growth, and excessive oil production. But there is one plus to its androgenic roots: one recent study conducted in Denmark found that women on estradiol and norethrindrone acetate showed a decrease in fat, especially in the abdominal area, and an increase in muscle mass. The doctor in charge of the study pointed out that it wasn't conclusive, but this could be due to the androgenic source of the progestin.

Form:	Tablet.
Standard dosage:	Comes in 5 mg tablets, but dosage can range from 2.5 to 10 mg, taken five to 10 days of the month.
Pros:	Often causes fewer side effects than Provera or Cycrin; may reduce breast tenderness and bloating, lowers triglycerides; may help decrease fat and increase muscle mass.
Cons:	May cause weight gain (but primarily lean mass, not fat), increased cholesterol levels, acne, excessive oil production, other masculine characteristics.

Norethindrone (Micronor)

Also known as the "minipill," norethindrone is another synthetic progesterone that is similar to Aygestin, but has another chemical group attached to it. It's widely used as a progesterone-only birth control pill, one that has fewer risks because it doesn't contain estrogen. But it's also used in HRT as a progesterone replacement. It's a very low-dose progestin—only 0.35 mg. Because it's such a low dose, it's most commonly prescribed in continuous HRT—you take both estrogen and Micronor every day. In addition, its low dose is a plus because it causes fewer side effects than other progestins. The other big plus? It stops breakthrough bleeding (bleeding while on continuous HRT) quickly, usually within nine months.

Form:	Tablet.
Standard dosage:	0.35 mg taken daily.
Pros:	Low dose, so causes fewer side effects; swiftly reduces breakthrough bleeding.

Cons: Low dose may require closer tracking to be sure to avoid endometrial problems; may cause increase in cholesterol levels and weight gain as well as other androgenic effects.

NATURAL PROGESTERONE

Micronized Progesterone (Prometrium, Generic)

Micronized progesterone is natural progesterone that has been broken down, or micronized, to enable your body to metabolize it more easily. Before this process was discovered, women couldn't take natural progesterone orally because it was absorbed badly and became inactive when swallowed. But now it's easily available, allowing you to get the benefits of natural progesterone in the ease of a pill.

Most often, you get micronized progesterone at a compounding pharmacy that formulates its own drugs according to a doctor's prescription. But in 1998, a micronized natural progesterone called Prometrium became available from the large pharmaceutical company Schering, which is good news for women who couldn't find a compounding pharmacy in their area.

Briefly, the big plus about natural micronized progesterone is, as I said before, the lack of side effects. It's often prescribed to women who have had bad luck with progestins. In addition, it doesn't inhibit estrogen's raising of good cholesterol and may help build bone. All of this, plus the normal protective benefits of adding progesterone to your HRT, makes natural micronized progesterone a good choice.

The only real downside is cost: natural micronized progesterone is usually much more expensive than Provera or the other progestins. In addition, micronized progesterones from compounding pharmacies may come in different bases, which may affect absorption. However, with the introduction of Prometrium from a large pharmaceutical company, both costs and standardization may improve.

Form: Tablet.

Standard dosage: 100 mg twice daily (cyclical therapy taken five to ten days each month); 100 to 200 mg daily (continuous therapy taken every day); 100 mg in the AM; 200 mg in the PM.

Pros: Minimal side effects; may help build bone in addition to preventing bone loss; doesn't interfere with estrogen's raising of HDL.

Cons: More expensive than progestins; absorption rate may vary depending upon the formulation; can cause drowsiness and sleepiness. Prometrium is in a peanut-oil base, so can't be used by women with peanut allergies.

Natural Progesterone Vaginal Gel (Crinone)

Another natural form of progesterone, the vaginal gel has one major benefit: because it is applied through your vagina and goes to your uterus, the progesterone is absorbed right where you need it most.

Crinone, currently the only natural progesterone gel on the market, was introduced in 1998. It comes in two different formulations: 8 percent, which is used for infertility treatments, and 4 percent, which is used for HRT. The 4 percent gel delivers 45 mg of progesterone into your system in a sustained release. The major plus of this method is that because the progesterone goes directly from the vagina to the target organ, the uterus, you don't get high blood levels of progesterone, which means that you get the benefits of progesterone without the side effects. Furthermore, when you take progesterone in pill form, about 95 percent of it is metabolized and eliminated from your system, which is why you often need a high dosage. The vaginal gel form, on the other hand, is more bioavailable—that is, it is able to be used by your system more easily and isn't metabolized—so you don't need as high a dosage, cutting back on side effects. Studies conducted by the pharmaceutical company showed that the majority of women studied who used the vaginal gel didn't have the side effects normally associated with progestins, and even had fewer side effects than women taking natural micronized progesterone.

Now for the negatives: since it is a vaginal gel, it's not nearly as neat or simple as swallowing a pill. But it's not as messy as many women assume it must be. Yes, you sometimes get a pelletlike discharge, sort of like Styrofoam, but it's minimal and can often be completely avoided if you stay seated or lie down for a few minutes after first inserting the gel. This allows the gel to be absorbed better. The second downside to Crinone is that it is more expensive than progestins or even oral micronized progesterone. However, these are very minor drawbacks when compared with the many positives. All in all, this is another good choice when it comes to replacing progesterone in your system.

Form:	Vaginal gel.
Standard dosage:	4% gel (containing 45 mg progesterone) used every other day for 12 days of the month.
Pros:	Delivered directly to your uterus; very few side effects; may help build bone in addition to helping prevent bone loss.
Cons:	May cause limited discharge; more costly.

Natural Progesterone Cream

Natural progesterone cream has attracted a lot of attention, with books, articles, Web sites, and so forth devoted to it. It is a nonprescription form of natural progesterone available at health food stores and through mail order.

The problem is that on the whole, it isn't a great answer to progesterone supplementation for women in premature menopause. The reason? As with estrogen creams, progesterone cream doesn't necessarily supply you enough progesterone to counterbalance estrogen. The amount you get can vary greatly, depending upon how well your skin absorbs it. You may get enough for reduction of symptoms, but there is a good chance you won't get enough to help fight osteporosis and, most importantly, to balance estrogen that you are taking (or even still producing). This is why, if you're taking prescription estrogen, natural progesterone cream probably doesn't fit well into an HRT scenario.

Combination HRT

These were designed to make HRT as easy as possible by combining both estrogen and a progestin in one tablet or patch. The big plus with combination HRT is the simplicity. You don't have to remember to take two pills, or to put on a patch and take a pill. Instead, you get everything you need in one product.

Conjugated estrogen plus medroxyprogesterone acetate (Prempro, Premphase)

These are the most commonly prescribed forms of combination HRT. Both Prempro and Premphase contain the standard dosages of both conjugated estrogen and progestin that you would get if you took them individually.

With Prempro, you take both estrogen and progestin every day, which emulates continuous therapy. With Premphase, you take the estrogen daily, and the progestin for the first two weeks of every month, which is cyclical therapy.

There's really no difference between taking one of these combination pills or taking two separate estrogen and progestin tablets. The only difference is the simplicity. You take one tablet every day and don't have to think about what day of your cycle it is (if you're on cyclical HRT) or don't have to worry about getting two prescriptions filled. That's the upside, of course. The downside is the same as if you were taking Premarin and a progestin separately. Again, there's a good chance of PMS-like side effects from the progestin; and you face the negatives of Premarin as well.

Form: Tablet.
Standard dosage: 0.625 mg conjugated estrogen/2.5 mg
                     MPA.
Pros: Very easy to use.
Cons: Because these contain progestins, you may
                     have a number of side effects.

Estradiol/Norethindrone Acetate Tablet (Activelle)

Approved by the FDA in late 1998, Activelle is the newest
oral form of combination HRT. It combines estradiol, the estrogen that is identical to that which your body makes, and norethindrone acetate (NTA), the progestin that has been associated
with fewer side effects than MPA, making this a great alternative to Prempro and Premphase. It's continous-combined HRT,
meaning that you get both estrogen and progestin continously—
a schedule that should eventually cause you to stop having
periods.

Form: Tablet.
Standard dosage: 1 mg estradiol; 0.5 mg norethindrone
                     acetate.
Pros: Easy to use; contains estradiol, which is
                     bioidentical to human estradiol; the pro-
                     gestin NTA may cause fewer side effects
                     than the other common progestin, MPA.
Cons: Low amount of progestin.

Estradiol/Norethindrone Acetate Patch (CombiPatch)

Introduced in late 1998, CombiPatch is notable because it is
the first patch that delivers both estrogen and progesterone—more
specifically, estradiol and norethindrone acetetate. Like the
estrogen-only matrix patches, the CombiPatch is a thin, unobtru-
sive patch that delivers hormones through your skin. But because
you get both estrogen and progestin from the patch, you don't
have to take any pills in addition to using the patch; all you
have to do is stick the patch on and change it twice a week. It's
that simple.

The clinical trials conducted before CombiPatch was approved found the most common side effects to be breast tenderness and breakthrough bleeding. But because the progestin in the patch is NTA, it will probably cause fewer side effects than other progestins. All in all, this looks like an excellent choice for a woman who prefers a patch to a pill and likes the idea of getting everything in one simple step.

Form:	Patch.
Standard dosage:	0.05 mg estradiol; 0.04 mg norethindrone acetate.
Pros:	Very easy to use—one patch gives you everything you need; supplies steady dosage of both estrogen and progestin.
Cons:	As with other patches, may cause allergic skin reactions.

Testosterone

Although adding testosterone to HRT isn't a necessity, it is becoming more common and may be particularly useful for women in premature menopause. As I mentioned before, more researchers are beginning to explore the relationship between testosterone and bone growth. The National Institutes of Health (NIH) is studying a combination estrogen/testosterone patch specifically for women in natural premature menopause to see if this will help offset the rapid bone loss that many women experience. But there's more to testosterone than bones. In fact, one of the most common reasons you'll go on testosterone is to help boost your libido.

A 1998 study concluded that adding small amounts of testosterone to HRT can restore a lagging libido and fight against hot flashes, in addition to increasing bone density. Most research finds that testosterone is especially important for a woman who has undergone surgical menopause. When you have your ovaries removed, you aren't producing the tiny amount of testosterone that a woman with ovaries does even after menopause. So there is a good chance that you may suffer from more intense hot flashes, more rapid bone loss, and a loss of interest in sex. By replacing the testosterone in addition to estrogen, you can usually reverse these symptoms.

The bad news? Some studies have shown that testosterone may raise blood pressure. The important factor is the ratio of testosterone to estrogen, so if you do take Estratest or another testosterone in HRT, you should be sure to have your testosterone levels as well as your estrogen levels checked initially and tracked while you're on the HRT. There are other side effects with testosterone as well, including acne, facial hair, weight gain, increased anger, and liver disease. In addition, some studies indicate that it may increase your risk of breast cancer. Finally, perhaps the biggest problem of all is that testosterone still hasn't been studied closely, so it's difficult to be sure what the long-term side effects may be. That said, though, it still may fit into your HRT picture, especially if you've been through surgical menopause. As with everything else, it's wise to discuss this carefully with your doctor.

You may be prescribed either natural testosterone or methyl-testosterone (a variation)—usually the latter, because testoster-

---

WHEN TO CONSIDER TAKING TESTOSTERONE

You may want to take testosterone or discuss it with your doctor if:

- You've undergone surgical menopause.

- Your menopausal symptoms such as hot flashes, night sweats, insomnia, depression, and mood swings haven't improved on regular HRT.

- Your libido is extremely low and hasn't improved on regular HRT.

- You are suffering from extreme breast tenderness on HRT.

- You already have significant osteoporosis, especially in your vertebrae.

one is quickly converted to estrogen in your body and so has less of an effect, while methyltestosterone isn't as rapidly metabolized. Both are available from compounding pharmacies in pill and cream forms, and an oral form of methyltestosterone is also available from a major pharmaceutical company. In all cases, you'll be adding testosterone to your HRT regimen. You'll still have to take an estrogen and a progesterone or progestin, since testosterone doesn't protect your uterus. Because this may mean you're juggling three different hormones at the same time, you may want to consider taking a combination pill, as listed below, which combines estrogen and testosterone.

Methyltestosterone (Android-10, Generic)

This variant of testosterone is less easily converted into estrogen than plain testosterone, which is why it's more widely prescribed. To avoid the possible side effects listed above, many doctors recommend starting with a low dosage of methyltestosterone; take a quarter or a half of a tablet and put it under your tongue (the sublingual method of taking oral hormones). By taking it sublingually, you avoid your digestive tract, minimizing its effect on your blood cholesterol and lipid levels. And by beginning with such a low dose, you cut down on your chances of acne, facial hair, and other side effects. If this mini-dose doesn't work, your doctor may slowly up your dosage, trying to keep it as low as possible while still gaining the benefits you're after.

Form:	Tablet.
Standard dosage:	10 mg (although you'll usually only take a half a tablet).
Pros:	Boosts libido; may help prevent bone loss; can help eliminate menopausal symptoms that regular HRT couldn't.
Cons:	May cause secondary sexual characteristics like hair growth, acne, and so on.

Estrogen and Testosterone (Estratest, Premarin with Methyltestosterone)

This is a form of HRT that was recently FDA-approved—a combination of estrogen and testosterone. The most commonly prescribed brand is Estratest, which contains esterified estrogens (Estratab) plus testosterone; however, Premarin is also available in a testosterone-included form.

In general, the pros and cons are the same as you'd face taking testosterone and estrogen individually. The major decision in this case is whether you'd prefer taking the natural estrogen in Estratest or the conjugated estrogen in Premarin with methyltestosterone. The Premarin plus testosterone has a much higher dosage of testosterone in it than Estratest does— over double the amount. Since many doctors advocate starting on a low dose with hormones, then building up if there's no effect, you may be better off opting for the Estratest.

Form:	Tablet.
Standard dosage:	Estratest H.S.: 0.625 mg esterified estrogen/1.25 mg methyltestosterone
	Estratest: 0.625 mg esterified estrogen/2.5 mg methyltestosterone
	Premarin with methyltestosterone: 0.625 mg conjugated estrogen/5 mg methyltestosterone
	Premarin with methyltestosterone: 0.625 mg conjugated estrogen/10 mg methyltestosterone.
Pros:	Need to take only two hormone pills, including a progesterone, instead of three; can help libido, bone loss, and so on.
Cons:	May cause side effects; Premarin testosterone dosage is very high.

ORAL ESTROGENS

Name	Drug Company	Type	Dosages
Premarin	Wyeth-Ayerst	conjugated estrogens (equine); 45% estrone sulfate, 55% equine estrogens	0.3, 0.625 (standard), 0.9, 1.25, and 2.5 mg
Estrace	Mead Johnson	micronized estradiol (from plant sources)	0.5, 1, 2 mg
Ogen	Abbott	Estropipate (piperazine estrone sulfate)	0.625, 1.25, 2.5, 5 mg
Ortho-Est	Ortho	Estropipate	0.625, 1.25 mg
Estratab	Solvay	Esterified estrogens (from plant sources)	0.625, 1.25, 2.5 mg
Menest	SmithKline Beecham	Esterified estrogens (from plant sources)	0.625, 1.25, 2.5 mg
Tri-Est	compounding pharmacy	estradiol, estrone, and estriol (usually in a 10%, 10%, 80% ratio)	1.25, 2.5, 5 mg
Estriol	compounding pharmacy	estriol	2 to 8 mg

ESTROGEN PATCHES

Name	Drug Company	Type	Dosage
Estraderm	Ciba Pharmaceuticals	transdermal patch, estradiol	0.05, 1 mg
Climara	Berlex	matrix patch, estradiol	0.05, 0.1 mg
Vivelle	Ciba Pharmaceuticals	matrix patch, estradiol	0.0375, 0.05, 0.075, 0.1 mg
Fempatch	Parke-Davis	matrix patch, estradiol	0.025 mg
Alora	TheraTech	matrix patch, estradiol	0.075, 0.05, 0.1 mg

PROGESTERONE/PROGESTINS

Name	Drug Company	Type	Dosage
Provera	Upjohn	medroxyprogesterone acetate	2.5, 5, 10 mg
Cycrin	Wyeth-Ayerst	medroxyprogesterone acetate	2.5, 5, 10 mg
Generic MPA	varies	medroxyprogesterone acetate	2.5, 5, 10 mg
Aygestin	Wyeth-Ayerst	norethindrone acetate	2.5, 5 mg
Micronor	Ortho	norethindrone	0.35 mg
Prometrium	Schering	natural micronized progesterone	100, 200 mg
Generic Progesterone	compounding pharmacy	natural micronized progesterone	100, 200 mg
Crinone	Columbia Labs	natural progesterone vaginal gel	4% gel (delivering 45 mg of progesterone; used every other day)

COMBINATION ESTROGEN/PROGESTIN

Name	Drug Company	Type	Dosage
Prempro	Wyeth-Ayerst	oral: conjugated estrogens (Premarin), medroxyprogesterone acetate (Cycrin)	0.625 mg estrogen; 2.5 mg progestin
Premphase	Wyeth-Ayerst	oral: conjugated estrogens (Premarin), medroxyprogesterone acetate	0.625 mg estrogen; 2.5 mg progestin (progestin included in first 2 weeks only)
Activelle	Novo Nordisk A/S	oral: estradiol, norethindrone acetate	1 mg estrogen; 0.5 mg progestin
CombiPatch	Rhone-Polenc-Rorer	patch: estradiol, norethindrone acetate	0.05 mg estradiol; 0.04 mg NTA

TESTOSTERONE AND COMBINATION ESTROGEN/TESTOSTERONE

Name	Drug Company	Type	Dosage
Android-10	ICN	methyltestosterone	10 mg
Methyltestosterone	generic	methyltestosterone	10 mg
Estratest	Solvay	esterified estrogens, methyltestosterone	0.625 mg estrogen; 2.5 mg testosterone
Estratest H.S.	Solvay	esterified estrogens; methyltestosterone	0.625 mg estrogen; 1.25 mg testosterone
Premarin with methyltestosterone	Wyeth-Ayerst	conjugated estrogens, methyltestosterone	.0625 mg estrogen; 5 or 10 mg testosterone

COMMON HRT SCHEDULES: CONTINUOUS VERSUS CYCLICAL

Here's yet another decision about HRT that you or your doctor will be making if you're taking both estrogen and progesterone: What kind of schedule will you follow?

There are three common ways of taking HRT: *cyclical therapy,* which means you take both estrogen and progesterone only part of the month; *continuous estrogen and cyclical progesterone,* which means you take estrogen every day and progesterone only part of the month; and *continuous therapy*, which means you take both estrogen and progesterone, well, continuously. If you're in premature menopause due to surgery and taking estrogen only, you have two choices: cyclical estrogen or continuous estrogen.

As you'd expect, the different therapies have different results. No one method is better than the other, however; there are pros and cons to each method of taking HRT. You have to think about which you would feel most comfortable with, which you can live with most easily, and, of course, which works best for your specific situation.

Cyclical HRT

When you take HRT cyclically, you're trying to mimic your natural menstrual cycle as it was before you entered premature menopause. Before menopause, your body produced estrogen for about two weeks; then you ovulated and produced progesterone in addition to the estrogen for another two weeks. Your endometrial lining built up in reponse to these hormone surges, preparing for a fertilized egg. But if the egg wasn't fertilized, both estrogen and progesterone levels plunged, and your uterine lining was sloughed off. In other words, you got your period.

Cyclical HRT follows this natural game plan: you take estrogen alone for days 1 through 25 of your cycle. You add progesterone for the last 10 to 14 days (begining on either day 12, 14, or 16, depending on how many days you'll be taking the progesterone). Then you stop both hormones for five days.

This regimen is often recommended for women when they first start HRT because it's what your body still "expects"— the surge of hormones, then the dropping off. So what can you expect if you go on this regimen?

- *Usually you'll get a period on those days off, which can be good or bad, depending upon your perspective*—On the plus side, many women like having their "regular" cycle again. Since premature menopause is such a shock, having normal periods can make you feel like your old self again; you're not ovulating any more, but you feel as though everything is relatively normal. But if you felt that one of the only positives about premature menopause was not getting a period any more, then you're out of luck. With the cyclical regimen, you'll probably keep getting a period each month like clock-work. Furthermore, if you're having problems with progesterone, you may get mega-PMS symptoms for the 10 to 14 days you're on it.

- *On the other hand, if you're having side effects from proges-terone, taking the time off may make you feel better*—Since you're only taking progesterone for a few days each month, you're limiting your exposure to it, so you'll experience the side effects only for those days, not for a complete month as you might with continuous therapy.

- *During your five days off, you may notice a resurgence of menopausal symptoms such as hot flashes and insomnia*—It makes sense: your hormone levels are low, so you may feel the effects of these low levels.

- *Cycling hormones may increase headaches and migraines if you're already prone to them*—Again, it's a function of low hormone levels.

You will probably adjust fairly quickly to this regimen, but it sometimes takes three or four months for your bleeding to occur on schedule. Your body has to adjust to the HRT, so at first you might not automatically get your period exactly when it's expected and instead may notice bleeding at different times of your cycle. This is normal, but if three or so months have passed and you're still bleeding when you're on estrogen only or when you're only a day or two into your progesterone, then you should check with your doctor. Usually, this regimen causes less breakthrough or abnormal bleeding than other forms of HRT therapy. After several years on cyclical HRT, your periods will usually get lighter and lighter, and may even disappear completely.

Continuous Estrogen with Cyclical Progesterone

This is a variation on the cyclical theme: you take estrogen every day of the month, with no time off at all. But you still take the progesterone for 10 to 14 days to protect your uterus. You're mimicking your natural cycle, but with a twist: by main-taining the estrogen throughout your cycle, you don't have the recurrence of menopausal symptoms you do with straight cyclical HRT. And although you're taking a continuous dosage of estrogen, 10 to 14 days of progesterone are enough to protect against endometrial buildup or, worse, cancer.

What to expect with this method?

- *Again, you will probably get a period when you cycle off the progesterone*—As with cylical HRT, it may take three to four months before you bleed when you cycle off the progesterone. If you bleed at other times, you should speak with your doctor.
- *Often, your periods will get lighter and disappear with this regimen*—It will take time, but this is a common occurrence.
- *Unlike cyclical HRT, you shouldn't experience a return of hot flashes and other symptoms*—This is the big plus of this method; because your estrogen levels remain constant, you don't go through the minimenopause you may have with cyclical HRT.

Continuous HRT

On a continuous cycle, you take estrogen and progesterone every day. That's it, plain and simple. This is based on a very simple theory: since unopposed estrogen can cause endometrial cancer, why not balance it by taking progesterone every day with the estrogen? By doing this, you get constant protection while receiving steady levels of both hormones.

Here's what to expect:

- *Because you're taking the progesterone every day, you are given a lower dosage*—Generally, you'll be prescribed half the dosage of progesterone that you would get in cyclical HRT. This is good news for women who are sensitive to progesterone and get bad side effects from it. Since you're getting a lower dosage, you'll probably have fewer side effects.

- *With constant hormone levels, you experience few (if any) PMS-like symptoms*—Another big plus: with no hormonal changes caused by cycling off either estrogen or progesterone, you don't have side effects like bloating, mood swings, and so on.
- *You may have periods initially, but over time, your endometrial lining gets thinner and inactive, and your bleeding stops*—This is a big plus for many women: no more periods. Yes, sometimes bleeding also stops with the other regimens, but it also may continue. But on continuous HRT, you usually stop bleeding completely.
- *On the downside, it's very common to have breakthrough bleeding, especially at the beginning of continuous HRT*— Although continuous HRT is supposed to stop your bleeding eventually, the chances are that you'll have breakthough bleeding for the first three or four months, if not longer. About 40 percent of all women have this problem, especially if they're in the first year or so of menopause, and it's an annoying one. You can't tell when your bleeding will start, or for that matter, when it will stop. The good news is that this becomes much less common the longer you're on continuous HRT.

Because breakthrough bleeding is common with continuous HRT, many doctors prefer to start women on cyclical therapy, then, a year or so later, switch over to continuous.

TO HRT OR NOT TO HRT: MAKING AN INFORMED DECISION

You've learned the facts and the hypotheses. Now comes the hard part—determining not only if you should go on HRT, but also what type to choose.

It's a tough decision. There are so many variables, so many forms of HRT, so many brand names, so many pros and cons and so forth to make sense of. But it's a decision you have to

make, and one that can make a huge difference in both your
quality of life now and your long-term health.

> **I will have to take hormones for close to twenty years.
> Most hormone replacements are deemed safe for the short
> term, not too clear on long-term results. Great. As I stand,
> without HRT, I have no hormones whatsoever. So I do,
> in my opinion, need replacement for long-term bone
> health as well as heart benefits. I am still unsettled as to
> what meds I will end up with. I started with birth control
> pills, which provided the hormone levels of a normal 35-
> year-old. These caused weight gain and puffiness. I
> switched to Premphase. Then I wanted to add some testos-
> terone since my own levels came back "negligible." Now
> I have been on Estratest for about five months. Now I've
> been hearing bad things about Estratest so I plan to
> switch to either a natural estrogen/progesterone or go
> back to Premphase. I'm going to make a consultation ap-
> pointment with my gyno next week. The problem is that
> she lumps me in with other postmenopausal women who
> are in their fifties. This is really not accurate; I am a
> special case. So the HRT issue is still changing, month by
> month, until I find something that my body and my mind
> can both agree on.**
>
> **—Susan, age 35**

As I mentioned before, the real problem is that so many of the
studies and articles you may have read about HRT assume
you're a women in her fifties. So it does get a little difficult
reading between the lines, trying to determine what the story is
for a woman your age. It would be wonderful if there were
several (or even one!) clear, conclusive studies that unequivocally laid it all out in black and white.

All in all, though, it seems that most doctors agree that, as
a woman with premature menopause, you probably are better
off taking HRT now; consider dropping it later, when you reach
age 50.

Again, the key in deciding about HRT is *relative risk*. In

other words, you have to balance the potential problems with the potential benefits; factor in your own risks for certain diseases, including family history; and carefully determine what HRT can do for you, both on the positive and negative side.

Chapter 6

Nature's Way:
Taking the Other Road to
Managing Your Hormones

Vitamins, Herbs, Minerals, and
Other Natural Sources

I've always been a vitamin taker and someone who is interested in natural methods of staying healthy. So before I went on natural HRT, I first tried natural everything *else* to cope with my premature menopause. I read everything I could get my hands on about natural supplements that were supposed to help with menopause and tried black cohosh, extra vitamin E, and citrus bioflavanoids. I tried ginseng and chaste berry and dong quai—anything I had read about that seemed like it could help. Some things I tried worked well; others didn't seem to do anything for me. And it seemed to be the same with other women I spoke with. Yet again, I realized that it was as important to research the natural way just as closely as I had researched premature menopause in general. Now I'm on HRT, but I'm still taking certain vitamins and other supplements, and I feel like I've found the best of both worlds.

For some, nature's way is an *alternative* to HRT for coping with the miseries of premature menopause and the long-term health risks; for others, it's an *additional* way of maintaining health.

If you can't go on HRT due to health risks, you can use natural alternatives—vitamins, herbs, and food sources—to replace the hormones in your body that are at low levels. These alternatives can minimize uncomfortable symptoms such as hot flashes and vaginal dryness, and can even help prevent the risk of long-term health problems such as heart disease and osteoporosis. You won't get the same level of protection as you can from HRT, but you will get some important benefits, certainly more than you would if you opt for no therapy at all.

But there's more to taking natural supplements than simply replacing HRT. If you're on HRT, natural supplements also can have an important role in your menopause management. You can use vitamins, herbs and other therapies to complement your HRT—to assist in the fight against premature menopause's potential negative effects on your heart and bones, and to provide a natural way of coping with quality-of-life problems such as depression and anxiety.

Both methods of managing menopause through natural supplements are getting more attention these days. Many women find the natural way of approaching health to be an appealing one, and for good reason. Often natural supplements have fewer side effects than other drugs. And many people feel more comfortable taking something natural than taking traditional, often synthetic drugs.

You may have heard about many of these natural menopause managers such as black cohosh, dong quai, and evening primrose oil. Magazines, Web sites, books, and news stories have been focusing on natural menopause management, especially as more baby boomers enter menopause. There are dozens of different theories about what works and what doesn't, but, unfortunately, not all that many studies to back up claims. In fact, many women find that their doctors are leery of natural supplements, and these women aren't sure if they should try natural supplements or not.

The problem is that until recently, most doctors and researchers have followed the traditional Western style of medicine and have paid little attention to alternative methods. So there haven't been a large number of studies done testing the claims and effects of different herbs, vitamins, and other alternative forms of medicine, especially as they apply to menopause. Luckily, this is changing. More researchers have begun focusing on alternative medicine and more studies are being conducted to assess scientifically different natural forms of menopause management. In the meantime, however, the jury is still out on many of these natural alternatives.

This is one reason it's often difficult to be sure what natural supplements work for menopausal symptoms. It's even more difficult when it comes to premature menopause specifically. Many of the articles and books praising the natural way are (here we go again) written for an older woman, one who is in menopause at the typical age and who isn't facing the same risks as a younger woman.

Again, most doctors, even those who advocate alternative approaches to menopause, tend to believe that you are probably best off opting for HRT if you can while supplementing this with certain vitamins and herbs. As I've said before, the key issue here is your age: since you're younger than the average woman in menopause, you face higher risks from low levels of estrogen and other hormones. And while natural alternatives can help boost hormone levels to some degree, it's difficult to be sure you're getting enough of an effect to ward off long-term health risks. Moreover, because of the lack of studies, we don't know all of the long-term effects or possible risks.

That said, you definitely shouldn't discount natural supplements, whether you're on HRT or not. Natural supplements can be an important part of your overall health plan when you're in premature menopause. They may help you fight against some of the long-term consequences of premature menopause and help with the immediate issues you're dealing with. This chapter covers the natural supplements you should consider, from phytoestrogens to vitamins to herbs, and explains what they can do for you. Whenever possible, I've mentioned studies that back up claims, but unfortunately, in many cases, no scientific study has been conducted yet.

One final and very important point: always research any vitamin, herb, or other natural supplement you are thinking of taking before you plunge in and try it. Remember, just because they're natural, this doesn't mean they're risk-free. Be sure you know about any possible side effects or potentially dangerous interactions with other drugs. And, most importantly, always discuss what you are taking or plan to take with your doctor. If you are interested in trying herbs, you may also want to consult with a licensed herbal practitioner. The bottom line is that, as with any form of medication, natural or otherwise, you should be safe, careful, and sure about what you are taking.

> **"Alternative" to me means natural—building the immune system naturally and helping it out naturally when worn down; Licensed and qualified *always*. As with any type of doctor, you want an educated, qualified, legitimate, licensed professional. Healing comes many ways. You have to find the method that works for you.**
> **—Bryana, age 38**

PHYTOESTROGENS: THE NEW (OLD) KID ON THE BLOCK

Phytoestrogens are nature's way of increasing flagging estrogen levels in your body, and best of all, they seem to have few side effects. This is why they are heralded as a wonderful new option for menopausal women. But, actually, they're not new at all. Phytoestrogens have been used for years in Asia and other areas as a way for women to ease menopausal symptoms. In fact, Asian women tend to have very few hot flashes, apparently because they get most of their protein from soy and other phytoestrogen-rich foods.

The word "phytoestrogen" sounds superscientific, but phytoestrogens are simply plants (herbs and other foods, including soy, flaxseed, red clover, alfalfa, even beer!) that have either plant-based estrogen or precursors to estrogen in them. These estrogens are weaker than the estrogen your body produces—

at the most, they're only about 2 percent of the strength of estradiol. Nevertheless, they produce an estrogenic reaction in your body. When you consume a phytoestrogen, it binds with estrogen receptors in your body. Sometimes it actually blocks the stronger estrogen in your body (either your natural estrogen or the estrogen you're getting from HRT) by taking its place at an estrogen receptor site. So phytoestrogens can both *raise* your level of estrogen if it's low by binding to receptor sites, and *lower* it if it's high by blocking the stronger estrogens.

All the hubbub about phytoestrogens, then, boils down to some simple facts: they act as a balancing agent where your estrogen is concerned; they can protect you against stronger estrogens, which may help reduce cancer risks and other side effects; and they also can boost your estrogen levels if you need it, which can relieve menopausal symptoms.

The Different Types of Phytoestrogens

Just as there are different forms of estrogen, there are different forms of phytoestrogen. The main types are:

- *Lignans*—Found in sources including cereals and vegetables, flaxseed (also called linseed), and other oil seeds.
- *Isoflavones (genistein, daidzein, biochanin, and formono-netin)*—Found in legumes and are especially high in soybeans.
- *Coumestans*—Found in red clover and alfalfa sprouts; this is the most potent phytoestrogen, although it is still about 200 times weaker than human estrogen.

As you'd expect, these phytoestrogens are found in a wide range of foods and herbs in addition to the major sources listed above (see the table on page 233 for a list of phytoestrogen-rich foods). You'll also notice that some of the herbs and other natural menopause therapies covered later in this chapter have phytoestrogenic components.

What Can Phytoestrogens Do for You?

Until recently, there hadn't been many scientific studies concerning phytoestrogens and, more specifically, their role in managing menopause. But with the interest in natural therapies rising, more researchers are focusing on this area. As more studies are being conducted on specific phytoestrogens or phytoestrogen sources, we are beginning to see more evidence about how phytoestrogens can help a woman going through menopause. However, keep in mind that this is an area that still hasn't been studied in depth, and researchers are especially unclear about long-term effects.

So far, the studies have shown that:

- *Phytoestrogens appear to help fight high blood cholesterol.*
- *Phytoestrogens appear to help alleviate menopausal symptoms, such as hot flashes and vaginal dryness.* However, many studies show that these effects are much more minimal than those of estrogen.
- *Some phytoestrogens, such as genistein (an isoflavone), have antitumor effects and can help fight against cancer.* In addition, because phytoestrogens compete with estrogen and can bind with the breast's estrogen receptors in place of the more carcinogenic estrogens, they can help cut the risk of breast cancer. Several studies have shown that women with a diet high in phytoestrogens, particularly legumes and soy, had a lower rate of uterine cancer. (One important note, though: other estrogenic supplements, such as ginseng, have a reverse effect.)
- *Phytoestrogens may help fight osteoporosis, although not to the degree of HRT.* More specifically, one study found that isoflavones, particularly genistein and daidzein, modestly improve bone mass. However, they also found a negative impact on bone when very high doses were taken.
- *Phytoestrogens may have beneficial effects on cardiovascular risk factors.* One animal study found that they reduced blood sugar levels, produced smaller LDL particles, and lowered

cholesterol. Most interestingly, the combination of soy plus estrogen produced the lowest cholesterol, which shows how phytoestrogens may work well for you even if you're on HRT.

Overall, then, phytoestrogens can help provide some of estrogen's benefits when you're in premature menopause. Because they are weaker than estrogen replacement, you won't get all the benefits from phytoestrogens that you would get from HRT. In addition, the effects of phytoestrogens depend upon how well your body absorbs them, and studies have shown that different women have different absorption rates.

The different phytoestrogens also have different potencies and effects. There can even be differences in effect with the same type of phytoestrogen or the same food source. For example, one study showed that the amount of isoflavones found in tofu varied from brand to brand. Another study found that the amount of phytoestrogenic power in flaxseed varied according to time of harvest. Not only is this one of the reasons it has been difficult for researchers definitively to assess claims about phytoestrogens in general, it's also an example of how difficult it is to be sure you're getting enough estrogenic activity to prevent such long-term problems as osteoporosis and heart disease.

However, if you can't or won't go on HRT, they can help you deal with symptoms and even fight some of the long-term negative consequences of premature menopause. If you are on HRT but would like to bolster it by taking phytoestrogens, you should speak to your doctor. In some cases, they may interfere with your HRT, which is the last thing you need. Sometimes you may block the estrogen you're taking and supplant it with the weaker estrogen, which can result in a recurrence in symptoms or worse. But in other cases, phytoestrogens can actually work well with your HRT, complementing and balancing it.

PHYTOESTROGEN-RICH FOODS

If you want to add phytoestrogens to your diet, the following foods are great choices. They're all rich in the different phytoestrogens, and they're also packed with vitamins, minerals, fiber, and fatty acids, and are low in saturated fat.

Alfalfa	Corn and corn oil	Peas	Soybeans
Anise seed	Cucumbers	Plums	Split peas
Apples	Fennel	Potatoes	Squash
Baker's yeast	Flaxseeds	Pumpkins	Sunflower
Barley	Garlic	Red beans	seeds
Beets	Green beans	Red clover	Tempeh
Black-eyed peas	Hops	Rhubarb	Tofu
Cabbage	Licorice	Rice	Wheat
Carrots	Oats	Rye	Yams
Cherries	Olive oil and olives	Sage	
Chickpeas	Papaya	Sesame seeds	
Clover	Parsley	Soybean sprouts	

Some Specific Phytoestrogen-Rich Supplements That Can Help

SOY

In cultures where soy is the main source of protein, people tend to have lower rates of heart attacks, cancer, and osteoporosis, not to mention hot flashes, which is why more people are beginning to think that soy may well be the miracle food where menopause is concerned. It's rich in phytoestrogens, specifically isoflavones, it's cholesterol-free, and it contains protein, omega-3 fatty acids, calcium, folic acid, iron, and other vitamins and minerals. And here's a big plus: it has been studied more closely than many other natural supplements for menopause.

These studies have so far been promising. It appears that soy may help prevent heart disease, stroke, cancer, hot flashes, and osteoporosis. Among some specific recent findings:

- *Soy may help cut your risk of developing endometrial cancer*—A University of Hawaii study found that women who ate the highest amount of soy had a 54 percent reduction in the risk of endometrial cancer compared with those who consumed the least.
- *Soy also appears to help fight against a range of other cancers, including breast cancer*—Even one serving of soy food a day appears to help lower your risk of a number of cancers. This is because soy isoflavones block tyrosine kinase, a key enzyme involved in the growth of cancer cells. In addition, several studies have shown a much lower incidence of breast cancer in Asian women, who consume very high amounts of soy. More specifically, one study showed that women who ate 55 or more grams of soy a day had a 50-percent or lower risk of breast cancer. But the key here may well be the amount of soy you consume or how you get your soy. According to a laboratory study on isoflavones, low levels of genistein and daidzein (the soy isoflavones) actually caused a growth in estrogen-sensitive cancer cells, while high levels reduced the growth of both estrogen-sensitive and non-estrogen-sensitive cancer cells. This wasn't tested on humans, however. Moreover, since most other studies indicate that soy inhibits breast cancer growth, it could mean that isoflavones alone cause this effect, not dietary soy. This is one argument in favor of getting your soy through your diet, not by taking soy isoflavones.
- *Soy may help reduce menopausal symptoms, such as hot flashes*—It's difficult to state this completely conclusively because different studies disagree. In some studies, the reduction of hot flashes was minimal and could have been attributed to placebo effects. However, several recent studies have found that soy helped decrease hot flashes. Two different studies followed women eating at least 60 grams of soy a day for three months,

and in both studies, the women reported a 45-percent reduction in hot flashes. One important factor to keep in mind though is that if you're using soy to handle symptoms such as hot flashes, you may need to take it more than once a day. One study showed that daidzein and genistein, the soy isoflavones, may be broken down by your body in as little as seven and a half hours, so if you start your day with soy milk or with a soy isoflavone capsule, you might experience hot flashes or night sweats by the end of the day.

- *Soy may help reduce your risk of heart disease*—Like estrogen, soy appears to help lower cholesterol and help your coronary blood vessels dilate, both of which are important in fighting heart disease. A University of Kentucky study found that people who ate at least 30 grams of soy protein a day reduced their risk of heart disease by up to 28 percent. More specifically, one study found that eating about 47 grams of soy a day lowered overall cholesterol by over 9 percent, LDL (the bad cholesterol) by nearly 13 percent, and triglycerides (which often rise when you take estrogen) by over 10 percent.

- *Soy may help prevent osteoporosis*—Soy isoflavones appear to help inhibit bone resorption and keep calcium from being excreted from your body. More specifically, two recent studies showed that postmenopausal women who consumed soy had healthier bones. More specifically, these studies have found that not only does soy increase bone density (by about 3 percent, according to one study), but it also increases bone mineral content, which means that bone quality is better and less prone to osteoporosis. In particular, it appears that *ipriflavone*, a phytoestrogen in soy, is responsible for this increase in bone mineral density. In Japan, Italy, and Hungary, ipriflavone has already been approved as an osteoporosis treatment, so expect to see more research done to follow up on this promising therapy. Soy is also high in vitamin K—an important vitamin for healthy bones.

The bottom line, then? Taking soy appears to be a health-conscious choice. By doing so, you can help fight heart disease, osteoporosis, and cancer, as well as alleviate uncomfortable symptoms. True, some claims touting soy as a menopausal miracle food haven't been scientifically proven, but there have been enough studies done that point to conclusive benefits, and as of yet, there don't appear to be any negative side effects.

The good news is that if you want to add soy to your diet, it's not that difficult even if you don't like soy. Remember, soy isn't just tofu. There is a wide range of soy products available, some traditional, others newer variations that are great for those who are not soy lovers.

More specifically, you can get *soybeans* themselves fresh, frozen, canned, or dried. You can eat them by themselves, add them to soups or other dishes, or toss them in salads. *Soy sprouts*, which are like regular bean sprouts, are another option; as are *soy nuts,* roasted soybeans, for a quick snack-food way of getting soy. And if you'd rather drink your soy, you can choose *soy milk,* which, like milk, is available regular, low-fat, or nonfat, comes in different flavors (including vanilla and carob), and makes a good base for healthy shakes. Two other traditional sources of soy that will give you a good amount of isoflavones include *tofu,* of course, made from curdled soy milk, which you can eat alone or use as an ingredient in baking and cooking, and *tempeh,* fermented soybeans and grains, which is a great meat substitute.

If you aren't crazy about the taste of soy (and, in fairness, a number of people aren't), there are several soy-based products available that mimic nonsoy foods, including soy burgers and hot dogs, soy cheese, soy ice cream, and soy yogurt. In addition, you can use *soy flour* in your baking.

Finally, you can take soy isoflavones alone, either in capsules that contain the phytoestrogens in soy, or in *soy protein powders,* which come in different flavors and can be added to juice, water, or shakes. This is probably the simplest way of getting some of the benefits of soy, but it may not be the best. As I mentioned before, researchers aren't sure whether you can get all of the beneficial effects of soy from isoflavones as opposed to dietary soy. Yes, the phytoestrogens in soy do produce a number of benefits, but there appears to be more to soy's good works than just the isoflavones. So while popping a few soy isoflavone capsules is certainly easy, it might not be the best way of getting your daily dose of soy. That's not to say you shouldn't take soy isoflavones. But, when possible, it also makes sense to make dietary soy a part of your regular diet.

To make adding soy to your diet easy and appetizing, you may want to look at the different cookbooks available that contain recipes and tips for using soy. Two good ones are: *The Soy Gourmet : The Natural Way to Improve Your Health with 75 Delicious Recipes* by Robin Robertson (Plume), and *Estrogen: The Natural Way, Over 250 Easy and Delicious Recipes for Menopause* by Nina Shandler (Villard Books, Random House). You also can get soy recipes on line at a number of Web sites, including: www.soyfoods.com.

ARE YOU GETTING ENOUGH SOY?

If you want to add soy to your diet, be sure you're eating enough to get all the benefits you're after. You may need more than you think— 200 mg of soy equals 0:3 mg of estrogen. Most studies indicate that you need at least 25 grams of soy a day to see any benefits at all. To reduce your risk of breast cancer, you need about one to two servings of soy; to lower your cholesterol, two to three servings; and to cut your risk of osteoporosis, as much as six to eight servings. Here's a quick breakdown of how different soy products measure up:

Product	Amount	Grams
Soy burger	one	18 grams
Roasted soy nuts	$1/4$ cup	17
Tempeh	4 oz	16
Tofu	1 cake	16
Textured soy protein	$1/2$ cup	11
Soy our	$1/4$ cup	8
Soy milk	8 ozs.	8

FLAXSEED

Another phytoestrogen source, flaxseed, is particularly high in lignans, which have both estrogenic and antioxidant properties. In fact, flaxseed has up to 800 times more lignans than other foods. But that's not all; like soy, there's much more to flaxseed than just phytoestrogens. It's also very high in omega-3 fatty acids (alpha-linolenic acids), containing five times more than any other plant source. These fatty acids can help lower cholesterol levels, fight against heart disease, keep cell membranes elastic and responsive, and more. (For more information on omega-3 fatty acids, see chapter 9.)

Flaxseed has been cultivated in the Middle East for over 7,000 years, yet only recently have researchers begun exploring its role in menopause management. Again, there haven't been numerous studies, but those that have been conducted have shown the following:

- *Flaxseed may help fight breast cancer as well as other cancers*—Several studies have shown that your body converts plant lignans into enterolactone and enterdiol, compounds that appear to help prevent breast cancer. In addition, omega-3 oil, which flaxseed contains, has been shown to have anticancer effects in animal studies. Some studies have shown that flaxseed appears to cut down on the risk specifically of colon cancer.
- *Flaxseed can help with excessive menstrual bleeding*—The linolenic acid in flaxseed helps make prostaglandins in your body, which can help prevent heavy bleeding. But prostaglandins also can cause cramps, so be sure not to take too much if this is a problem with you.
- *Flaxseed can help lower cholesterol and help prevent heart disease*—Studies have shown that flaxseed helps lower LDL cholesterol.
- *Flaxseed may help ease menopausal symptoms like breast tenderness, and other PMS-like discomfort*—The omega-3 acids in flaxseed help reduce pain and inflammation, which can help with the discomfort some women experience with

premature menopause. In addition, since it has an estrogenic activity, flaxseed appears to help cut down on many symptoms that are linked to low estrogen levels.

As for negative reports—there haven't been many. Most studies indicate that when used at the recommended levels, flaxseed appears to have no appreciable toxic effects.

So you can see that flaxseed can help you. Now how and where can you get this? The best source of flaxseed is, logically, whole flaxseed itself. You can buy it in health food stores, most often in the nuts and seeds section. It's best to get whole flaxseeds, not powdered, and grind them yourself at home. You can sprinkle these over cereal, soup, salads, yogurt, and other foods, blend them into fruit shakes or stir them into juice, or use them as an ingredient in cooking. (For recipes using flaxseed, as well as general information, you can check www.flaxseed.com.) By buying the whole seed and grinding it yourself, you get the benefit both of the lignans and of the fatty acids—a double dose of healthfulness. Generally, all you need is about a tablespoonful a day. This small amount gives you the same benefits of one serving of soy. As with soy, the amount you should take goes up depending on the effect you're after. If you want to lower cholesterol levels, you'll need about four tablespoons of flaxseed daily; to help fight osteoporosis, about six tablespoons.

Ground flaxseed is also available in capsules—and flaxseed is also available as an oil, either liquid or in capsules. If you decide to use this form of flaxseed, it's very important that you get fresh, cold-processed flaxseed oil because it can go rancid quickly. It's also a good idea to buy only a little of it at a time and store it in your refrigerator. Like ground flaxseed, you don't need much to get its benefits—only about a tablespoon of oil once or twice a day, or two to three capsules twice a day, in both cases with meals.

VITAMIN THERAPY: THE VITAMINS AND MINERALS THAT CAN ALLEVIATE SYMPTOMS OR HELP PREVENT LONG-TERM CONSEQUENCES OF PREMATURE MENOPAUSE

Vitamins are another part of nature's way of coping with premature menopause. They can help you cope with menopausal symptoms such as hot flashes and vaginal dryness, and help fight against the negative long-term effects of premature menopause such as heart disease and osteoporosis.

Let me say right here that many doctors will tell you it's best to get your vitamins from food sources themselves. And they're absolutely right. Often the nutrients in foods are more helpful than isolated vitamin supplements. But let's be honest: I know from experience that I often don't eat as well as I should and sometimes don't get enough of the right vitamins from my food. And I'm willing to bet it's a similar situation with many of you. This is why it often makes a lot of sense to take vitamin and mineral supplements. Taking supplements doesn't mean you shouldn't make every effort to eat healthfully. Chapter 9 takes a look at the importance of good nutrition when you are in premature menopause. But in this section, we will take a closer look at the specific vitamin and mineral supplements you can use to help ease the symptoms of premature menopause and fight its negative consequences—again, either as a replacement for HRT or as a companion.

Vitamin A

WHAT IT CAN DO FOR YOU

Vitamin A is one of the maintenance workers of vitamins, helping to maintain your eyes, skin, tissues, and mucous membranes. As such, it helps fight the uncomfortable vaginal drying and increased risk of urinary tract and vaginal infections brought about by low estrogen levels. It also helps keep your skin healthy and supple—a help when collagen levels drop due to low estrogen. And as it helps maintain the intestinal walls, it allows for nutrients such as calcium to be better absorbed.

Beyond these benefits, Vitamin A also helps boost your immune system, and some studies indicate that it may help in the prevention of cancer. If you get too little vitamin A, you may get fatigued more often and be more prone to infections, both of which are often side effects of low estrogen levels as well. In addition, several studies found that low levels of vitamin A increased the risk of menstrual flooding, abnormal Pap smears, and even cervical cancer.

SOURCES

Liver, cod-liver oil, or other fish-liver oils; egg yolks; spinach and other dark-green leafy vegetables; cheese and fortified milk products.

RECOMMENDED DOSAGE

Vitamin A palmitate or acetate are the most easily absorbed forms of vitamin A. The Recommended Daily Allowance (RDA) is 4,000 IUs, but research indicates that about 10,000 IUs may be necessary for benefits. Be sure not to take too much vitamin A because high doses can be toxic, and if you have kidney problems, check with your doctor before taking any vitamin A. Because of its toxicity, many doctors and researchers suggest that you get vitamin A through your diet alone or in a small amount in a multivitamin, and take beta-carotene (below) to fulfill any vitamin A needs.

Beta-Carotene, Lycopene, and Other Carotenes

WHAT IT CAN DO FOR YOU

Until recently, many people had never heard of any carotene other than beta-carotene, but research has indicated that the different carotenes may play different roles in the human body, and so in managing your premature menopause.

Beta carotene is converted to vitamin A in your body and works as an antioxidant. Studies have indicated it may help prevent different forms of cancer. However, recent studies have indicated that other non-vitamin-A carotenes may work even better as antioxidants and anticancer agents. One that appears to be particularly promising is *lycopene,* which studies have shown to be particularly useful in decreasing your risk of heart disease. In fact, several recent studies found that the other carotenes, including beta-carotene, had limited effect on reducing heart disease risk, while lycopene was associated with a significantly lower risk. This is an important factor, given the increased risk of heart disease you face as a woman in premature menopause.

Carotenes in general have been shown to help fight tumors and boost your immune system. It appears that carotenes may be involved in a lower risk of uterine and cervical cancer because they are stored in the *epithelial tissues*—the tissues in the linings of internal organs. According to studies, if you eat a high amount of carotenes, you have a much lower risk of these cancers among others. But more research needs to be done before this can be conclusively stated.

Because studies are only now being done focusing on the different carotenoids, you may be best off taking a mixed carotenoid complex. This way, you'll get a number of different carotenes in one supplement, with all of the benefits. One plus is that, unlike vitamin A, carotenes aren't toxic, so when taken at recommended dosages, you'll have no toxicity. One possible side effect, however: If you take a very high amount of carotenes, you may end up with slightly yellow or orange skin, a bit like having a fake tan. This is nothing to worry about, though, and doesn't signal anything more alarming than the fact that your body has an abundance of carotenes in it. Furthermore, the pigmentation will fade if you stop or reduce your beta-carotene intake.

A brief note: This change in pigmentation sometimes happens

to people with hypothyroidism and some with diabetes, as they are unable to efficiently convert beta-carotene into vitamin A. If you do notice this side effect (and are taking beta-carotene within the recommended dosage, that is, up to 25,000 IUs), and haven't been diagnosed with diabetes or hypothyroidism, you may want to speak to your doctor about being tested.

One final note about carotene supplementation: One study found that, in smokers who took high levels of beta carotene, lung cancer rates did not decrease, but actually may have increased slightly. Some scientists speculated that this occurred because smokers normally have low rates of vitamin C—and that this caused a problem with carotenes in the body. So if you smoke and take beta-carotene, make sure you have plenty of vitamin C in your diet (which is good advice anyway) or take a vitamin C supplement.

SOURCES

Fruits and vegetables in general, yellow-orange and dark-green ones, more specifically;

Beta-carotene: yellow fruits such as oranges, apricots, papayas, cantaloupe; sweet potatoes; carrots; dark-green vegetables such as spinach, broccoli, romaine lettuce, kale;

Lycopene: cooked tomatoes, canned tomatoes, tomato sauce.

RECOMMENDED DOSAGE

Beta-carotene—5,000 to 25,000 IUs
Lycopene—2 mg.

B Vitamins

WHAT THEY CAN DO FOR YOU

This family of vitamins can be a big help in coping with premature menopause, both in helping combat symptoms and in fighting negative long-term risks. B vitamins can keep your energy levels up; support your liver function (a definite plus if you're on HRT, as oral estrogen is broken down by your liver); prevent vaginal dryness; increase your resistance to infection; and help maintain your adrenal gland function, which is where the precursor to estrone (the form of estrogen still produced by your body after menopause) is produced. Last but definitely not least, B vitamins help you to deal with the emotional symptoms that crop up during premature menopause, such as anxiety, irritability, mood swings, even insomnia. This is a pretty impressive list of benefits, and there are even more from the different B vitamins individually. Here are a few:

B₆ is particularly important if you're on HRT, since studies have shown that HRT may cause a deficiency of this vitamin, (as well as of B_2, B_{12}, and biotin). In addition, B_6 is another excellent heart-helper. A study of over 80,000 women found that vitamin B_6 with folic acid help prevent heart disease, which women with premature menopause are at a higher risk for. It also helps prevent water retention and bloating (a common side effect of synthetic progesterone and estrogen), and, when taken with vitamin C, improves your sleep and helps with headaches.

Folic acid is another heart-healthy supplement and is particularly helpful in reducing homocysteine levels, which tend to rise on HRT. Homocysteine may damage blood vessel linings and cause artherosclerosis. Furthermore, studies have shown that folic acid appears to help prevent the forerunner to cervical cancer, cervical dysplasia. Possibly most important, it helps your body not only manufacture estrogen, but also use it efficiently.

B₁ (thiamine) keeps mucous membranes moist and helps maintain and strengthen your skin, nails, and hair—again, a plus, since collagen levels often drop when you're in menopause.

B₃ (niacin) helps you with the dilation of your blood vessels—an important benefit if you're prone to migraines or headaches. It also may lower both cholesterol and triglyceride levels, as may *inositol* and *pantothenic acid.*

Choline works to support and maintain your liver function, which, as you know, is important in the breakdown and conversion of estrogen. In addition, it appears to help lower cholesterol levels and strengthen capillary walls (a help if you experience heavy menstrual bleeding), and may help fight against heart disease.

B_{12} is another B vitamin that is affected by HRT: the HRT appears to interfere with its absorption. Some studies have shown that low levels of B_{12} may be linked to Alzheimer's disease. In addition, this is another B vitamin that helps lower your risk of heart disease.

There are other benefits to taking the different B vitamins, but you should have the idea by now: the B vitamins are definitely beneficial to your health!

SOURCES

The different B vitamins are usually found in the same foods, including beans, whole grains, liver, brewer's yeast, egg yolks, and more.

RECOMMENDED DOSAGE

Because the B vitamins work together to perform such vital tasks as helping with glucose metabolization, supporting your liver, and decreasing stress, it's usually recommended that you take the entire B complex, not just one or two of the vitamins. To treat the symptoms of menopause, some researchers recommend you take at least a 50-mg B complex that contains 50 mg of thiamine (B_1), riboflavin (B_2), niacin (B_3), pantothenic acid (B_5), B_6, PABA, choline, inositol; 50 mcg B_{12}, and 400 mg of folic acid.

Vitamin C

WHAT IT CAN DO FOR YOU

Vitamin C is an all-around player—a vitamin that helps fight infections and allergies, one that has antistress properties, and an antioxidant that may play a role in cancer prevention.

As you would guess, then, vitamin C plays a number of beneficial roles when you're in premature menopause. First, it helps to decrease a variety of menopausal symptoms. Studies have found it helpful in helping cut down on hot flashes, especially when taken in combination with citrus bioflavonoids (see below). In addition, it appears to help keep vaginal tissues moist and lubricated. Its anti-infection properties help keep bacterial growth in the intestinal tract down, which can help prevent vaginal and bladder infections that often become more apparent when you're in menopause. It also helps aid the function of the adrenal glands, which are where much of the estrogen your body produces after menopause is made, and in so doing, helps keep estrogen-related symptoms and problems in check.

It also helps prevent long-term negative effects of menopause and simple aging. It appears to help in the prevention of cervical cancer and other cancers. More specifically where cervical cancer is concerned, studies have shown that women with low levels of vitamin C have higher rates of cervical cancer as well as cervical dysplasia (a precursor to cervical cancer) and heavy menstrual bleeding. Vitamin C helps to maintain and build collagen levels, which tend to drop when you are in menopause. This is helpful for your skin and for your bones. As for your heart health, vitamin C helps decrease the rate of LDL oxidation and may help decrease blood pressure. Finally, on the antistress front, taking vitamin C with vitamin B_6 has been shown to help with anxiety and tension, as well as insomnia.

As with certain other vitamins, there's no question that C is a definite asset on a number of health fronts and is a vitamin you should seriously consider adding to your diet if you're not getting enough of it through your regular eating patterns.

SOURCES

Citrus fruits and other fruits such as melon (cantaloupe and honeydew) and strawberries; cruciferous vegetables such as broccoli, Brussels sprouts, cauliflower, cabbage; dark-green leafy vegetables such as spinach, collard greens.

Recommended Dosage

The RDA is 60 mg, but most research recommends up to 500 to 1000 mg daily.

Bioflavonoids

What They Can Do for You

Bioflavonoids aren't technically vitamins, but they're so closely linked with vitamins and are available in the vitamin section of drug and health food stores that I've included them in this section. You often get bioflavonoids in combination with vitamin C, but they're also available by themselves.

Like many other supplements recommended for menopausal women, bioflavonoids have an estrogenic effect in your body. It's a very small one, about 50,000 times weaker than estrogen, but it appears to be enough to help cope with menopausal symptoms, including hot flashes, vaginal dryness, bloating and water retention, even urinary incontinence. More specifically, one study (conducted in the 1960s—unfortunately there have been few more recent studies) found that after only one month, over 50 percent of the 94 participating women taking 1200 mg of bioflavonoids (900 mg of hesperidin and 300 mg of hesperidin methyl halcone along with 1200 milligrams of vitamin C) stopped having hot flashes completely and another 34 percent had a drop in hot flash frequency and intensity. Studies have also shown that bioflavonoids also appear to help relieve moodiness, anxiety, irritability, and other emotional side effects of menopause. In addition, they help in the fight against heart disease and strengthen the capillary walls, so they can help prevent heavy menstrual bleeding. Finally, bioflavonoids help boost and maintain collagen production, which often drops when your estrogen levels are low.

Sources

Found in the pith—the white inner peel—of citrus fruits as well as in black currants.

RECOMMENDED DOSAGE

There's no conventional required minimum allowance for bio-flavonoids, but the typically recommended dosage for women in menopause is 1000 to 1500 mg a day, or a 250-mg capsule taken four to six times daily.

Vitamin D

WHAT IT CAN DO FOR YOU

Vitamin D is a necessity for healthy bones. It helps your body absorb and ultimately use both calcium and phosphorous, the building blocks of your bones. Low levels of vitamin D are linked to both osteoarthritis and, most worrisome for women in premature menopause, osteoporosis. Since premature menopause puts you at such a higher risk for osteoporosis, getting enough vitamin D is a definite must.

As mentioned earlier, recent studies have shown that vitamin D deficiency seems to be more common than thought. Most people are fairly confident they're getting enough vitamin D from the sunlight (generally, 10 to 20 minutes of sun a day is supposed to supply you with "enough" vitamin D) or from fortified milk, and so on. But because it appears that even those people who are sure they're getting enough D aren't, it's a good idea to make sure you're getting enough through a multivitamin, maybe, or careful attention to your diet.

SOURCES

Fatty fish (salmon, sardines, herring); fortified milk and other dairy products; egg yolks; fortified cereals and breads.

RECOMMENDED DOSAGE

400 IUs.

Vitamin E

WHAT IT CAN DO FOR YOU

Vitamin E is another all-around beneficial supplement, helpful both with specific menopausal problems and with overall health.

It appears that it can help prevent and treat vaginal atrophy, especially when used topically. It has also been shown in studies to help reduce breast cysts, to diminish PMS symptoms such as anxiety and moodiness, and to help keep thyroid function regular, which may be particularly helpful for women with an autoimmune basis to their premature menopause. It's also an antioxidant and as such, may be useful in helping prevent cancer and heart disease, as well as in helping to slow the effects of aging.

Finally, for years, vitamin E has been touted as a natural way of reducing hot flashes, but it turns out that it might not be all it was cracked up to be. Doctors have recommended vitamin E as a natural way of reducing hot flashes since the 1940s, which was when the last studies on this aspect of vitamin E were done. Finally, in 1998, a double-blind placebo-controlled study was done specifically to test the effectiveness of vitamin E on hot flashes. Although the results of the study showed that there was what is called a statistically significant reduction in hot flashes, this turned out to be one of those cases where it appeared more significant in the numbers than in actuality. In fact, it turned out that the women on vitamin E had only one less hot flash a day than the women taking the placebo, which doesn't sound like much of a reduction.

But even if this study is correct, it makes good sense to take vitamin E when you're in premature menopause. First of all, many doctors still believe that combining vitamin E with high amounts of vitamin C or bioflavonoids may help combat hot flashes. Moreover, the other benefits of vitamin E are important ones—and shouldn't be overlooked.

SOURCES

Eggs, wheat germ and whole grains, nuts (such as almonds and walnuts), legumes (such as peanuts), vegetable oils (such as corn and safflower).

RECOMMENDED DOSAGE

The RDA of vitamin E is quite low, 8 IUs, but most doctors recommend far more than this, especially to help with menopausal symptoms. Generally, 100 to 800 IUs is the common recommendation, with many doctors recommending a split dosage of 200 to 400 IUs of vitamin E in the morning and another 200 to 400 IUs in the night. But keep in mind that vitamin E isn't safe for everyone. If you have rheumatic heart disease, high blood pressure, or diabetes, or take digitalis drugs, vitamin E can be very harmful. It's best not to take more than 100 IUs in this case. And definitely check with your doctor before even taking this small amount.

Calcium

WHAT IT CAN DO FOR YOU

As discussed in Chapter 3, since premature menopause puts you at such a high risk of developing osteoporosis, calcium is a must!

But calcium may actually do even more for you than help prevent osteoporosis: according to different studies, it may help lower blood pressure and reduce triglyceride levels, help in wound healing and blood clotting, and, in combination with vitamin D, may help prevent colon and rectal cancer. (For more detailed information on calcium and osteoporosis, see pages 87 to 93.)

SOURCES

Dairy products, fish with bones (salmon, sardines), dark-green leafy vegetables; seeds, nuts.

RECOMMENDED DOSAGE

1000 to 1500 mg a day.

Boron

WHAT IT CAN DO FOR YOU

Boron is a nutrient that many people haven't heard much about, but it can be very important when you are in premature menopause. First, boron works with calcium to help fight osteoporosis by preventing bone loss and, possibly, by helping increase bone density. Second, studies have shown that boron may raise estrogen levels in your blood. In fact, if you aren't on HRT, some studies have indicated that it may boost estrogen to the same levels as a woman who is taking HRT.

SOURCES

Fruits, including apples and pears; green and dark-yellow vegetables, including broccoli and carrots; nuts, including almonds and hazelnuts.

RECOMMENDED DOSAGE

1 to 6 mg.

Magnesium

WHAT IT CAN DO FOR YOU

Another coworker of calcium, magnesium is also important for bone health. But that's not all—magnesium also appears to help fight the crashing fatigue that often accompanies the beginning phases of menopause, and it is often recommended by doctors to help boost energy levels. One of the reasons it can help with this is that it aids the processing and metabolization of glucose, converting it into energy. Adequate levels of magnesium also help prevent diabetes mellitus. Magnesium is also a heart-healthy mineral, helping your body to absorb other nutrients and protecting against heart disease and coronary artery problems.

SOURCES

Whole grains; dark-green leafy vegetables; nuts; milk and dairy products; meat and fish; dried cooked beans, especially soy beans.

RECOMMENDED DOSAGE

RDA is 280 mg, but most research indicates that you need 400 mg for maximum benefits.

Potassium

WHAT IT CAN DO FOR YOU

Potassium has a number of roles it plays in your body, including helping keep muscle contractions normal; regularizing your heartbeat; and regulating the fluids and acids in your body. As a natural aid in menopause management, it's most useful as a treatment for fatigue, like magnesium, and studies have found that taking both potassium and magnesium can boost your energy levels significantly. In addition, because it helps regulate the fluids in your bodies, it can help you cope with water retention and bloating. Finally, adequate levels of potassium are necessary to help fight high blood pressure, stroke, and heart disease.

SOURCES

Bananas, potatoes, nuts, citrus fruits.

THE VITAMINS THAT CAN HELP WITH SPECIFIC SYMPTOMS

If you're not on HRT or if you are on HRT and aren't getting relief, you may want to try vitamins to help you deal with the annoying symptoms that come along with menopause. Here's a quick list of different symptoms and the vitamins that may help:

If you're having	you may want to try
Hot flashes and night sweats	Vitamin E (800 IUs/day—400 in the AM, 400 in the PM along with bioflavonoids (250 mg twice or more a day)
	B vitamins
Heavy menstrual bleeding/flooding	Vitamin A, vitamin C and bioflavonoids, iron (take with Vitamin C)
Anxiety, stress, irritability	Vitamin B complex plus bioflavonoids and/or vitamin C
Vaginal dryness and atrophy	Vitamin E (either orally or used as a suppository), bioflavonoids

RECOMMENDED DOSAGE

This is a mineral that you generally get enough of through eating properly; however, if you think you aren't getting enough or if you have low potassium levels, check your multivitamin or multimineral supplement—100 mg should be enough.

Iodine

WHAT IT CAN DO FOR YOU

If you're in premature menopause because of a possible autoimmune disorder, iodine may be especially important. This is because iodine is a key player in your thyroid function. It is involved in the development of your thyroid gland itself, is an important element in *thyroxine,* a principal hormone produced by the thyroid, and, overall, is heavily involved in the healthy function of your thyroid. In addition, several studies have indicated that iodine may also be involved in keeping breast tissue healthy and in preventing breast diseases.

SOURCES

Fish, iodized salt, seaweed, shellfish, kelp tablets.

RECOMMENDED DOSAGE

150 mcg.

HERBS AND OTHER NATURAL THERAPIES THAT WORK (AND A FEW THAT DON'T)

Using herbs, plants, and oils is possibly the most popular and widely covered aspect of coping with menopause the natural way. This is the area of natural menopause therapy that you have probably read about. Herbs such as dong quai and black cohosh, and oils such as evening primrose oil are getting a great deal of attention, some raves, and some criticism. Some of these herbal remedies appear to work extremely well in both relieving physical and emotional symptoms and possibly preventing long-term complications, while others have gotten great press but frankly might not deserve it.

This section should help you take the guesswork out of using herbs, by examining the most popular ones, explaining the claims made about them, and exploring whether or not these claims have been proven.

Herbs have been used for years in treating menopausal symptoms, but much more in Europe than in the United States. As with the other areas of natural menopause therapy, more U.S. doctors and researchers are beginning to pay attention to herbs as a means of treatment. However, there haven't been many studies done domestically. This is beginning to change, but in many cases research has been minimal. Germany has been one of the foremost countries in exploring and studying herbal remedies and has established a panel of experts called Commission E to review the safety and use of over 1,400 herbal drugs. Much of the information below regarding effectiveness and cautions is drawn from their research. When possible, though, I've also included information from recent domestic studies.

You'll note that some of the herbs used in menopause are *estrogenic*—they have phytoestrogens, and so act much like human estrogen in your body. Others are *progesteronic*—they act like or increase progesterone in your body. As you might guess then, these different herbs are often used in different instances, depending upon the symptom you're having and whether or not estrogen or progesterone is the crucial hormone involved; however, in some cases they will help you cope with the same symptoms since progesterone is a precursor of estrogen.

You can get most of these herbs at a health food store or through a naturopathic doctor or herbalist. They are available in tablets, capsules, teas, or tinctures. Some people recommend making your own teas or tinctures from fresh or dried herbs, but it is probably best not to. It's easy to make a mistake and give yourself the wrong dosage, which could cause problems. When in doubt, either have teas or formulas made by a professional herbalist or opt for tablets or capsules made by a reputable vitamin company to insure that you're getting a quality-controlled product.

One important point: because these herbs act like—and actually affect—hormones in your body, you can't take them lightly. It's very important to remember when you consider taking herbs that they are drugs. Yes, they're natural, but they're natural *medicine*. Just as with prescription drugs, certain herbs aren't necessarily safe and may cause serious side effects, especially when taken in combination with other herbs or medicines or if you have a preexisting medical condition. Before you try anything, be sure to consult with your gynecologist or general practitioner. It may also be a good idea to find a doctor or practitioner who specializes in alternative medicine, such as a naturopathic doctor, nutritionist, or herbalist. If you do this, though, review his or her suggestions with your regular gynecologist as well.

The following, then, is a rundown of some of the most popular herbs and oils involved in natural menopause management, what they are supposed to do for you, and how well they do it. For more specific information on these and other herbs, including recommended dosages, you may want to consult other books specifically about natural menopause treatments, speak with herbal experts, and, of course, discuss any treatments with your doctor.

Black Cohosh

CLAIMS

Relieves hot flashes and night sweats, helps fight vaginal atrophy, helps with irritability, depression, and anxiety.

This is an extremely popular natural therapy for menopausal symptoms and a common ingredient in many menopause formulas you find at health food stores.

Black cohosh was used years ago by Native Americans, and has been used a great deal in Germany and other European countries, apparently with great success. While it's been widely touted as a natural way to lower FSH, according to studies conducted in West Germany, black cohosh reduces LH, not FSH, in menopausal women. However, the reduction of LH appears to help cut down on hot flashes and other menopausal symptoms. In addition, because it appears to have relaxant properties, it may help with cramps, heavy periods, and other menstrual irregularities.

One double-blind study compared the effects of black cohosh (in this case, Remifemin, a commonly available capsule that contains 100 percent black cohosh) with Premarin and a placebo. After three months, women on black cohosh were found to have the same drop in menopausal symptoms as those on Premarin, while those on the placebo saw little improvement. Another study compared Remifemin, estriol (a natural estrogen often prescribed in Europe), and Premarin plus progestin, and found all three to decrease menopausal symptoms to the same degree. Still another study found that over 80 percent of the women using black cohosh reported a significant decrease in symptoms, but in this case, it could be due to a placebo effect, since they knew they were taking the herb. Even so, given the positive studies plus the anecdotal evidence, black cohosh is probably a good bet for herbal treatment of menopausal symptoms, especially hot flashes.

In addition, researchers believe that black cohosh may be able to help prevent osteoporosis and reduce bone resorption. While there have been no long-term human studies to substantiate this, a recent animal study found that black cohosh can stimulate bone formation by increasing the body's utilization of calcium, and experts believe that this may be the same in humans.

So black cohosh has a great deal to recommend it and is possibly a good addition to a natural menopause therapy. But don't think that this can replace HRT over the long haul. The German Commission E, as well as other researchers, recommend that you take this for only six months at the most, so black cohosh probably makes the most sense when you're first going through menopause, have bad symptoms, and aren't on HRT yet. Since no studies have been done examining its long-term effects, it is wise to stick with this short-term usage.

Like most herbs, it's available in health food stores from most major vitamin and herb companies. It's also marketed under two brand names: Estroven (which also contains other vitamins) and Remifemin (which is 100 percent black cohosh).

CAUTIONS

May overstimulate the uterus and make heavy menstrual bleeding worse; may cause dizziness, nausea, headaches; may interact badly with drugs used to treat hypertension.

Chamomile

CLAIMS

Helps sleep; fights anxiety.

Chamomile tea has been used for years as a before-bedtime drink to help soothe and calm nerves, and studies have shown that it may have a sedative effect. All in all, this herb appears to be a good choice if you're tense, having troubles sleeping, and want a safe relaxant. Best of all, you can take this even if you're on HRT with no ill effects.

CAUTIONS

May cause allergic reaction in people allergic to ragweed.

Chasteberry, Chaste Tree (Vitex Agnus Castus)

CLAIMS

Hormone balancer; decreases heavy bleeding, regulates period, can help minimize depression.

As you might guess from its name, chasteberry was used in the past to dampen women's libidos—to keep them, yes, chaste. And while it doesn't necessarily do exactly that, it does appear to affect your hormones. Like black cohosh, chasteberry is an herb that appears to act like a progesterone, and one that has been used in Europe for many years to alleviate PMS symptoms as well as menopausal symptoms. It may help diminish both LH and FSH, and appears to affect your pituitary function.

More specifically, some scientific studies have found that chasteberry inhibits the secretion of prolactin by the pituitary gland. High prolactin levels may cause progesterone levels to drop, and so can affect your period. One double-blind controlled study involving women with menstrual irregularities due to high prolactin found that chasteberry raised both progesterone and estrogen levels. Another study found that chasteberry reduced menopausal symptoms in 60 percent of the women using it. But as for the claims that chasteberry is great for PMS-like emotional symptoms including moodiness and depression, especially if used regularly for six months or more, the jury is still out. It's another case where many people believe this and there is anecdotal evidence supporting it, but there's no hard scientific proof. The bottom line, then, is that chasteberry might help certain symptoms, especially irregular periods, but beyond that it is difficult to be sure.

CAUTIONS

Generally considered safe, but may interact badly with dopamine-receptor antagonists or drugs used to treat hypertension. Can cause rash and gastric upset.

Dong Quai

CLAIMS

Helps with numerous menopausal symptoms, including hot flashes, breast tenderness, sore joints, insomnia, and anxiety.

Often called the woman's ginseng, dong quai has long been considered a major herb in helping with menopausal symptoms and has been widely used in China for menstrual problems and menopause for centuries. But does it really do all it's cracked up to do?

As with so many other herbs, it's tough to say unequivocally if dong quai really works. Research has indicated that dong quai contains a number of pharmacologically active substances, including chemicals that are vasodilative, or involved in the control of blood vessel dilation, which is linked to hot flashes. In addition, it has anti-inflammatory and analgesic properties, which should help lessen the pain of sore joints or breasts. But there have been few definitive studies done on dong quai. Most studies were conducted in China and aren't standardized, so it's difficult to determine how valid the claims are.

A 1997 double-blind study conducted in the United States showed that dong quai wasn't any more effective than a placebo. More specifically, about 33 percent of the women taking dong quai (4.5 grams a day for six weeks) said that it helped their hot flashes, but 29 percent of the women taking the placebo said the same thing, which means that there was no real statistical difference. In other words, the women who report feeling better with dong quai may actually be feeling the benefits of the "placebo effect." Another study of 71 menopausal women found that even after six months, there was no statistically significant change in vaginal dryness or number of hot flashes.

That said, it's difficult to say whether dong quai really works or not. It's a case of not having enough evidence to really draw a conclusion. Given the number of claims about dong quai and the anecdotal evidence, there is a chance that it does work, but since several studies have indicated the opposite, it's definitely not a sure thing.

CAUTIONS

May cause sun sensitivity; however, generally considered a relatively safe herb.

Evening Primrose Oil

CLAIMS

Long used to help with PMS symptoms; also believed to help the body produce estrogen and/or enhance estrogenic activity.

Evening primrose oil is a particularly good source of gamma-linolenic acid (GLA), which your body makes from essential fatty acids. GLA is a precursor of *prostaglandins,* which do a number of things in your body, including regulating the stickiness of blood platelets, helping keep blood vessels toned and elastic, aiding in the function of your gastrointestinal tract, keeping salt and water levels in your body balanced, and much more.

As such, it is usually used to help fight PMS symptoms, which are often the same as many menopausal symptoms such as bloating, water retention, breast tenderness, and cramps. It also appears to help fight vaginal dryness and improve the condition of your skin, and may help combat insomnia. Where hot flashes are concerned, it doesn't work as well as many herbs; it may help make hot flashes less intense, but it doesn't eliminate them.

In addition, because of the GLA, evening primrose oil can help you fight the long-term possibility of heart disease by lowering your cholesterol and improving blood vessel elasticity.

CAUTIONS

While there has been no evidence showing any major problems with evening primrose oil, some studies have shown that it aggravates epilepsy and may also cause negative effects in people suffering from bipolar depression. In addition, because it appears to have strong estrogenic properties, many doctors recommend that anyone at risk for estrogen-dependent cancer steer clear of this.

Feverfew

CLAIMS

Reduces migraines and joint pain.

Feverfew has been used for hundreds of years as a headache and joint-pain reliever, and recent studies back this up. It appears to be especially helpful in reducing both the number and severity of migraines. One study found that migraines were reduced by 24 percent in people taking about 80 mg of feverfew daily, and other studies have resulted in similar (sometimes even better) findings. In addition, several studies showed that even lower amounts of feverfew—as little as 60 mg—worked equally well in cutting back on the frequency and intensity of migraines. This is especially good news if you're one of the women who suffers from migraines while on HRT.

CAUTIONS

None.

Gamma-Oryzanol

CLAIMS

Relieves hot flashes.

Gamma-oryzanol, or ferulic acid, is a nutritional element found in rice bran oil that appears to have an effect on your pituitary: it promotes the release of endorphins (the "feel-good" enzymes that give people runner's highs) by the hypothalamus, and has been shown to lower both cholesterol and triglycerides—both definite positives when you're in premature menopause.

It may be especially helpful if you're not on HRT and if you're suffering from hot flashes. Gamma-oryzanol was first studied as a menopausal symptom reliever in the 1960s, when it was concluded that 300 mg of gamma-oryzanol reduced hot flashes by 50 percent or more in 67 percent of the women studied. Later studies found even better results, with over 85 percent of the women on 300 mg of gamma-oryzanol reporting a reduction in symptoms.

But these results aren't as conclusive as they sound. The studies were very small, so it's difficult to determine whether or not gamma-oryzanol is really as good as it sounds. On the plus side, though, it seems to be completely safe to take, as clinical studies and laboratory experiments haven't found any side effects from this supplement.

CAUTIONS

None found as yet.

Garlic

WHAT IT CAN DO FOR YOU

Garlic is good for your heart, which is a definite plus because premature menopause increases your risk of cardiovascular disease. Garlic lowers LDL cholesterol and triglycerides, and raises HDL cholesterol. In fact, eating just one clove of garlic a day has been shown to lower cholesterol by 10 to 15 percent in most people. Garlic also appears to have immune-enhancing properties and anticancer effects.

SOURCES

In general, you're best off getting garlic in your diet. Raw garlic has the best effects but, since many people would rather not deal with a raw clove, cooked garlic will give you some of the benefits. You can also get your garlic the easy way—in capsule or tablet form. Again, this isn't as effective as popping a raw clove, but it's a good way of getting at least some of the benefits of garlic, and it's a lot less smelly!

RECOMMENDED DOSAGE

At least one raw clove a day or, for those who would rather get their garlic in a less odiferous way, take the equivalent of that in a capsule form. The exact amount should be specified on the bottle.

Gingko

CLAIMS

Helps memory; helps get rid of menopausal "brain fog"; may boost libido.

Gingko is known as the memory-booster herb and, since low estrogen levels may cause fuzzy thinking and memory lapses, it's often used to combat these. Apparently it works by increasing the dilation of blood vessels and overall blood flow. Studies have shown that it does appear to help memory loss, but these studies were of older people who were already suffering from memory problems and/or dementia. However, observational studies have indicated that it may help sharpen your mental processes.

In addition, gingko was recently shown to help perk up a lagging libido. One study found that 91 percent of the women treated with 60 to 120 mg of gingko three times a day reported a resurgence in libido. These women were taking antidepressants, however, and weren't necessarily going through menopause; however, these results are interesting. Since gingko doesn't appear to be toxic, it may be a good herb to try.

CAUTIONS

May cause headache, gastric upset, and, in some cases, allergic skin reactions.

Ginseng

CLAIMS

Boosts energy; reduces stress; helps with lagging libido.

Another Chinese herb that has been used for thousands of years, ginseng is used for a wide range of health conditions, including depression, insomnia, anemia, asthma, nervousness, and sexual problems such as impotence. It's also considered a energizer, used to fight fatigue, increase your mental sharpness, and combat the effects of aging.

So much for all the claims—what about its efficacy? The good news is that ginseng is one herb that has been studied quite a bit. Studies have shown that it does work well to decrease anxiety and ease stress, which can help you cope with the tensions of going through premature menopause and the emotional upheaval that changing hormone levels cause.

In addition, ginseng is often recommended for women in menopause because it has estrogenic properties and so can boost estrogen levels in your body. But a 1997 research study found that ginseng wasn't any more effective than a placebo in terms of replacing estrogen. However, women using the ginseng reported a greater feeling of well-being than those on the placebo, again underscoring its use as an antistress remedy. One important note to add: Commission E found ginseng to work well in fighting both fatigue and loss of concentration but recommended that it be used regularly for three months at the most.

Finally, you should be aware that there are a number of different ginsengs available. If you want a ginseng that will have more of an estrogenic effect to help alleviate menopausal symptoms, opt for *panax ginseng* (also known as Chinese or Korean ginseng). If you are already taking estrogen and want ginseng just to boost your alertness and combat fatigue and stress, choose *Siberian* or *American ginseng,* which has less estrogenic activity.

CAUTIONS

Too much ginseng was reported to cause a number of side effects, including increase in blood pressure, diarrhea, sleep disruptions, and more, but this occurred only with very high doses of 3 grams or more daily. Because of its estrogenic properties, it may also cause bleeding, ovarian cysts, and breast tenderness.

Kava Kava

Claims

Good for anxiety, restless sleep, depression, the general blahs—all common symptoms of premature menopause.

Kava kava is a Polynesian herb that has been used for hundreds of years in religious rites. Recently its use has began spreading to the West, where it has been said it could treat anxiety. And here's a case where the claims appear to be true and were proven so quite recently. One recent placebo-controlled, double-blind study conducted on women with menopause symptoms found that the women taking 100 mg of kava kava three times a day reported a difference after only one week, with much less anxiety and depression. It also appears to help reduce fatigue, another common aspect of premature menopause.

Cautions

Should be used only on an occasional basis; regular or heavy use may cause side effects such as diarrhea, skin problems, dizziness, and so on.

Licorice

Claims

Relieves hot flashes; fights vaginal dryness; relieves sore joints.

Okay, this isn't licorice *candy,* but licorice *root,* so eating extra licorice sticks won't help you cope with premature menopause. But taking licorice root capsules or drinking licorice tea may help with a number of menopausal symptoms. According to researchers, licorice helps balance the ratio between estrogen and progesterone in your body. By so doing, it may help alleviate both hot flashes and vaginal dryness, but since there haven't been any extensive studies done, it's difficult to be sure how effective it may be. However, it has been proven to have anti-inflammatory properties and acts much like hydrocortisone, which can help relieve muscle aches and sore joints that many women experience. In addition, licorice appears to have some antidepressant qualities as well.

To ease menopausal symptoms, herbalists often suggest 500 to 1000 mg or one to two cups of licorice tea, daily. One added bonus is that this tea actually tastes good!

CAUTIONS

Can deplete potassium and raise your blood pressure. If you have high blood pressure or any other cardiovascular disorder, you should avoid this herb.

Motherwort

CLAIMS

Relieves hot flashes and night sweats, may help vaginal lubrication.

It is difficult to be certain whether or not motherwort works, because it hasn't been subject to scientific testing. However, herbalists and naturopaths have long recommended motherwort for hot flashes and night sweats and to help fight sleep disruptions. It's also said to help fight vaginal dryness. It's possible that it works because it has slight estrogenic properties, but this hasn't been proven. All in all, though, it appears relatively safe and possibly effective.

CAUTIONS

May increase menstrual bleeding.

Red Clover

CLAIMS

Fights hot flashes, prevents irregular bleeding, can be used as an estrogen replacement.

Red clover is rich in phytoestrogens, particularly coumestans, and also is one of the few plants that contains all four types of isoflavones. In addition, it is high in bioflavonoids. As you might imagine, since it packs such a potent punch in terms of ingredients, red clover is thought to be a help in alleviating a number of menopausal symptoms.

Because it is so phytoestrogen-rich, red clover can help balance your estrogen levels, boosting them when they're low, and blocking stronger estrogens when they're higher. Studies have demonstrated that red clover can help ease hot flashes and other symptoms linked to estrogen levels. One doctor who felt the claims were overstated ran a double-blind study herself and found that red clover did work well to relieve symptoms. It is also reportedly helpful in dealing with ovarian cysts, fibroids, and endometriosis. Finally, because it has such a high level of isoflavones, it also may be a cancer fighter. All in all, red clover looks like an excellent choice, especially if you aren't currently on HRT.

In fact, this is one herb that has recently begun getting a lot of attention. Because of this, an Australian company introduced a red clover tablet with the brand name of Promensil.

CAUTIONS

No adverse effects reported.

Sage

CLAIMS

Reduces hot flashes, night sweats; may also work as a tranquilizer.

Sage is another herb containing phytoestrogens and it's another herb that hasn't been studied scientifically in terms of its effect on menopausal symptoms. However, because it contains both phytoestrogens and bioflavonoids, it has estrogenic properties and progesterogenic qualities as well. As such, it may work to reduce hot flashes and night sweats. In fact, one study found that it helped relax muscles and appeared to lower blood pressure, both of which could contribute to decreasing hot flashes.

CAUTIONS

Excessive dosages can cause kidney or liver damage.

St. John's Wort

CLAIMS

Natural tranquilizer, helps relieve irritability, depression, fatigue.

Another success story in the herb world, St. John's Wort has long been used to fight depression, and recent studies have confirmed this, making this herb one of the best-known herbal remedies.

According to over 23 different studies, St. John's Wort was over twice as effective as a placebo in helping fight depression. Since depression and moodiness are often symptoms that come with premature menopause, especially when your hormone levels plunge suddenly, as they do after surgical menopause, this is an herb that can be a great help.

CAUTIONS

Rare side effects include dry mouth, dizziness, gastric upset. In addition, many experts advise avoiding this herb if you're taking prescription antidepressants.

Valerian

CLAIMS

Natural tranquilizer—helps relieve anxiety; natural sleep aid.

Valerian has been used as a tranquilizer for over 1,000 years and is still getting a great deal of attention for its sedative effects. It is used widely in Europe to treat insomnia, as well as for nervousness and menstrual problems. Where menopause is concerned, it is generally used to help fight sleep disturbances that arise when estrogen levels are low, as well as the jittery, tense feeling some women experience.

How well does it work? Here is another case where it is difficult to be completely positive, because studies on valerian have turned up mixed results. Some have indicated that it does work well as a sleep inducer—a natural sleeping pill with no hangover effects the next morning—as well as an antianxiety agent. In one double-blind study conducted in 1989, almost 90 percent of the valerian users reported improved sleep. However, other studies haven't substantiated these claims, but even these studies found that several components of valerian have a relaxing effect on the intestine, which could translate into an overall calming effect. And there have been numerous nonscientific studies that have indicated that valerian works well as a tranquilizer with no real side effects. All in all, then it may be a good choice for you if you suffer from insomnia or tension.

CAUTIONS

Can cause liver and cardiac damage, although this appears to be rare; generally not recommended for anyone with kidney or liver problems. In addition, it is usually recommended that you don't use valerian as a regular supplement but only on occasion, when you need it.

Wild Yam

CLAIMS

Reduces hot flashes, helps reduce heavy bleeding.

Wild yam has been the source of debate primarily because some companies have claimed that it can be used as a natural progesterone in place of a progestin or prescription natural progesterone. But this doesn't appear to be the case. Although a

---

TREATING SPECIFIC SYMPTOMS WITH HERBS

Just as certain vitamins are often recommended to help you cope with different menopausal symptoms, so too are certain herbs and oils. Here's a quick rundown of what you may want to try to help you deal with different symptoms—but, again, check with your doctor before trying any of these . . . especially if you're currently on HRT:

If you're having	you may want to try
Hot flashes/night sweats	Black cohosh; evening primrose oil; gamma-oryzanol, motherwort; licorice
Heavy bleeding/flooding	Chasteberry (Vitex); flaxseed; wild yam root
Vaginal dryness/atrophy	Chasteberry
Insomnia	Chamomile; evening primrose oil; kava kava; motherwort; valerian
Moodiness, anxiety, irritability	Black cohosh; ginseng; kava kava; motherwort; passion flower
Depression	Kava kava; St. John's Wort
"Brain fog"/ forgetfulness	Gingko; ginseng; sage

component of wild yam, *diosgenin,* is the precursor of estrogen, progesterone, and testosterone, and most plant-based hormones used in HRT are actually made from wild yam, there is no proof that diosgenin can be changed into any of these hormones in your body. Given this, wild yam isn't recommended as a replacement for any hormones, not even natural progesterone. However, wild yam can help with some menopausal complaints.

More specifically, because it appears to have estrogenic and progestogenic properties, it may help minimize some symptoms linked to low estrogen levels, such as hot flashes, and others linked to progesterone, such as excessive bleeding. In addition, it is an anti-inflammatory and can help combat the achy joints and muscles some women experience in menopause.

CAUTIONS

None reported.

Chapter 7

Finding and Working with the Right Doctor

The first gynecologist I saw about my premature menopause seemed genuinely concerned about my condition, but he didn't seem to know much about it. I had dozens of questions, and while he really tried to answer them, he didn't know about the implications of premature menopause, only normal menopause. So I decided to try a second doctor, one who was supposed to be well versed in natural therapies. To put it bluntly, it was a total disaster.

His office seemed like a baby factory—the waiting room was crowded with pregnant women, the wait was long, and the place was a zoo. When I finally got in to see him, he spent only a few minutes chatting with me, then sent me to the examination room, where, draped in the little paper gown, I waited . . . and waited . . . and waited . . . while he saw other patients. Twenty-five minutes later, he finally came in to examine me—a procedure that lasted about five minutes. He commented on how atrophied my vagina already was with little concern for my feelings, told me to go on HRT immediately, then, when I asked why HRT was necessary, just said that anyone who didn't go on it would be crazy. When I said I was interested in exploring natural HRT, he wrote me a prescription for

Estrace (which is natural) and Provera (which isn't). Finally, I had to ask *him* to test my FSH and estrogen levels, which are typically tested before you go on HRT to establish a baseline measurement.

This was an unpleasant enough experience, but it got even worse when I finally called back for my test results. The woman I spoke with on the phone first checked my results and said that I was completely normal. I remember holding the phone, thinking for one crazy, wonderful moment that everything was okay after all. But when I told her to double-check, she asked me my name again, then discovered she had been looking at the wrong chart. As it turned out, my FSH was over 150 and my estradiol was 12 (both definitely in the menopausal range). She was completely dumbfounded because of my age, and I had to tell *her* that I was already aware that I was in menopause. Needless to say, I didn't return to that doctor.

Finally, after talking with other women and asking for referrals, I tried another doctor. During my first office visit, she spent nearly an hour taking notes about what I said. She knew about premature menopause, she encouraged me to ask questions, and, best of all, she listened to me. When I went home, I was so relieved. For the first time since I had been diagnosed with premature menopause, I felt like I was finally in good hands. I had a doctor whom I really trusted, one I felt I could work with.

My story isn't unusual. In fact, I was one of the luckier ones. After talking with other women in premature menopause, I've heard dozens of horror stories—doctors who insist that a woman isn't menopausal even though she's been complaining of hot flashes, irregular periods, and infertility; doctors who prescribe inappropriate medication; doctors who just don't seem to care.

There are also the good experiences, of course—the doctors who genuinely listen; those who know the whys and wherefores of premature menopause; those who can help and offer the support that is necessary in going through such a difficult change in one's life.

The trick, then, is finding one of those doctors.

Unfortunately, it's often difficult. It's tough enough for anyone to find a doctor who can work well for and with you, and it's sometimes even more difficult when you're going through premature menopause. Many ob/gyns seem more interested in the obstetrics side of their practice and don't seem to have as much time to spare for someone in menopause. In addition, speaking from experience, it's sometimes uncomfortable sitting in a waiting room filled with other women your age who are pregnant, when you're dealing with the unwelcome fact that your reproductive system has shut down. Other doctors, even those who specialize in menopause, often aren't used to dealing with a *young* woman in menopause. They don't understand the emotional fallout you're going through; or are too quick to assume that your situation is just the same as that of a woman in her fifties. Then there are the doctors who just won't listen. They'll dispense bits of information along with prescriptions and tell you to come back in six months; you leave the office feeling somehow dissatisfied.

And you *should* be dissatisfied. Premature menopause is a special situation that demands a good relationship between patient and doctor. It's crucial that you don't give up and settle for a doctor you aren't happy with. Remember, premature menopause isn't a one-shot deal. It's something you'll be living with for years, so you need a doctor you can work with over time. Because this condition combines both physical and emotional issues, you need to feel you can talk honestly to your doctor, ask questions, and get clear explanations. You need a doctor who understands that premature menopause isn't a walk in the park, that there is emotional fallout, and it isn't "all in your head," as some women have been told.

You need a doctor who knows the consequences of premature menopause, as opposed to regular menopause, and can explain to you what long-term consequences you face, why you need certain therapies, and what will happen if you choose not to take them; a doctor who will be there to answer the inevitable questions that will crop up along the way.

The good news is that it is possible to find such a doctor. I know because, after a couple of misses, I found a doctor whom I could work well with. And other women with whom I've spoken have similar stories.

> I met a lot of stupid doctors who didn't care enough to listen. . . . I finally found a gynecologist who seemed reasonable. At least she didn't argue with me, tell me I'm not in meno, I'm just being silly, etc.
> —Amy, age 35

The key is not giving up and knowing what to look for and how to look for it. This chapter should help. It is designed to help you determine what you want in a doctor and the ways to go about finding and evaluating doctors. And it will also help you become a good patient. Remember, the doctor-patient relationship is two-sided. Just as you want to find the best possible doctor to work with you, you need to be the best possible patient to keep the lines of communication open and the partnership working.

CHOOSING A DOCTOR

> All in all, I am happy with the care my doctor has given me. She is the same gynecologist I have had since I graduated from college in 1984. She delivered my two sons. And she was heartbroken to have had to deliver the bad news to me in her office in 1994 about the brain tumor. I trust her and I respect her. I am comfortable enough to make appointments just to discuss a problem. She's very direct and doesn't mince words! I really don't need the niceties when I'm there for a reason!!
> —Susan, age 36

It's very possible you already have a gynecologist whom you like and trust. However, often after a woman is diagnosed with premature menopause, she discovers that her current gynecologist isn't the best choice. Maybe his or her office is primarily focused on obstetrics, or perhaps he or she doesn't seem to know much about premature menopause (a very common problem). Whatever the reason, you may discover that you've got to start looking for a new doctor.

The problem is that you're so busy dealing with the shock of a premature menopause diagnosis and so eager to get help that you don't stop and think about what you want and need from your doctor. That's what happened to me; I just wanted to get a doctor quickly, one who was part of my HMO and who would tell me what I could do to help me cope with the incredible hot flashes and night sweats I'd been having. I did no research whatsoever—just opened my HMO handbook, called a few doctors who were in my neighborhood, and made an appointment with the first doctor who was accepting new patients.

I very quickly learned that was definitely the wrong way to go about it! I did ultimately find a doctor who worked well for me, but only after I started researching doctors, examining what I wanted from a doctor, and asking for referrals.

In short, then, finding a doctor should be a carefully thought-out process. You shouldn't choose a doctor blindly from a directory or based on location. It's your body that's at issue here, and premature menopause is a condition with many short-term and long-term consequences. As an informed medical consumer, you deserve the best care possible—and it's up to you to seek it out.

Decide What You Want from a Doctor

The best way to begin finding the right doctor for you is to start with the basics: Who do you consider to be a good doctor for your situation?

Of course, everyone wants a good doctor, but what constitutes the right doctor for you varies from woman to woman. It's a matter of personal preferences.

I would recommend a female physician, as all of mine are. I don't feel men, no matter how many books they've read and women they've talked to, appreciate a woman's feelings. My feelings are very strong in this regard.
                              —Susan, age 36

A doctor with an open mind (a big trick in itself!) and who communicates well. Someone who seems to give a damn in general, and not just "going by the book" and cramming four patients into a half-hour time slot.
                              —Bryana, age 38

I don't care if the doctor is a woman or a man—I just want someone who will listen to me and who will let me be involved in my treatment. I'm not saying I want to diagnose myself. But I think I should have some input.
                              —Alicia, age 34

I've had negative experiences with doctors—being treated like my problems were all due to stress, they were all "in my head," if I talked to a psychiatrist I'd feel better. That's the worst! [The best doctor would be] someone who listens and understands that you know your body better than anyone else in the world, no matter how many degrees they may have!
                              —Steph, age 28

Since you'll be coping with premature menopause for years, it's important that you think honestly about what you need and want from a doctor—personality style, medical orientation, and so forth. If you don't feel comfortable with a doctor, you won't be able to talk honestly and openly, which is crucial in treating your condition. Take the time to give it some serious thought. You may want to ask yourself the following (and keep in mind that there are no right or wrong answers):

- *Do I feel more comfortable with a man or a woman?*—Some women want only a female gynecologist, reasoning that only a woman can truly understand what another woman is going through. And when you're going through premature menopause, you will often have to talk about many extremely personal aspects of your life and body, such as your sex life. It's important that you feel able to be totally honest and forthcoming about these issues. Some women feel uncomfortable talking with a man about topics like vaginal dryness or discomfort during sex; others have no problem with this. Would your doctor's gender make a difference to you?

- *Do I want a doctor with a traditional practice or one who is open to alternative medicine?*—This is an important point to think about. More traditional doctors tend to be wedded to the tried-and-true forms of HRT (Premarin and progestins). Others are open to prescribing newer forms of HRT, including natural hormones, and still others incorporate alternative treatments such as acupuncture or herbal supplementation in their recommended therapies. Think about the course of action you would feel best taking. If you think you will be happy with traditional HRT, then a traditional doctor makes sense. However, as more research indicates possible problems with long-term exposure to synthetic hormones, and, since premature menopause treatment generally requires many years of HRT, you may be better off seeking a doctor who is open to prescribing natural HRT, that is prescription hormones that are bioidentical to those your body makes. Finally, if you are interested in exploring alternative therapies, such as incorporating herbs and other supplements into your treatment, it makes sense to seek out a doctor who is open to this—perhaps a holistic doctor or other alternative practitioner.

- *Do I want a doctor who specializes in menopause, or, even more specifically, in premature menopause or hormonal disorders, a gynecologic or medical endocrinologist, or will I be just as happy with a regular gynecologist or GP who specializes in women's health?*—Frankly, this can get a little problematic since premature menopause isn't a common speciality. However, many large medical centers (especially in larger cities) do have doctors who specialize in hormone disorders. And as more baby boomers enter menopause, more gynecologists are focusing on menopause as a specialty. You may feel more comfortable seeing a doctor who specializes in menopause (premature or otherwise), as opposed to a regular ob/gyn, because you don't have to deal with the "baby factory" feel of many doctor's offices. More importantly, a menopause specialist is often more up-to-date in terms of HRT, and usually has a hands-on knowledge of menopause. In general, then, you are probably best seeking a menopause specialist, if not a premature menopause specialist.

- *Should I see a reproductive endocrinologist, who specializes in infertility and hormonal disorders, because I want to explore the possibilities of pregnancy?*—This is a very specific specialty, and one that may fit the bill for your needs. If you are eager to pursue a pregnancy, you may want to begin seeing a reproductive endocrinologist, as opposed to a regular ob/gyn, from the outset of your premature menopause.

Beyond these more technical questions, also think about such things as *personality*—would you feel comfortable with an authoritarian doctor or prefer one who is more flexible?—*age*—would talking with a younger doctor enable you to establish better rapport? Or does age not matter to you at all?—*size of practice*—would you rather see a doctor in an individual practice or one in a larger practice or clinic?

All in all, at this stage of the game, you should try to get an idea of what you consider to be the ideal doctor for you. This way, when it's time to meet with a doctor, you can determine whether he or she meets your criteria.

How to Find the Best Doctor for You

Once you have an idea of the type of doctor you're seeking, it's time to start looking for that doctor. Consider trying one or more of the following:

- *Ask other women, especially, if possible, others who are also going through premature menopause*—Friends and family can often give you the best recommendations based on their personal experiences. They've got a unique perspective from the examining table itself, and can give you an idea of how a doctor treats her patients, her bedside manner, her medical philosophy, and so forth. However, don't blindly assume that just because a friend recommends a doctor, he or she will be right for you. Does the person who recommended the doctor have needs similar to yours? Does she like the same sort of things in a doctor as you? If you don't know the answers to this, don't be afraid to ask your friend or relative, and ask about the doctor she's recommending as well. It's best, of course, to get recommendations from other women in menopause and, even better, from women in premature menopause.

- *Ask for referrals on-line on one of the many menopause message boards or Web sites available*—This is the high-tech version of getting personal recommendations, and one that's especially helpful if you don't know anyone personally going through premature menopause or even menopause. For example, AOL and the World Wide Web have a number of menopause message boards. You can post a message asking if anyone can suggest a doctor in your area. (For a listing of menopause sites on line, see Resources, page 367).

- *If you're happy with your primary care physician, ask her for suggestions*—Because your primary care physician, general practitioner, or internist knows you and your needs as a patient, he or she can often give you the names of doctors who will fit in with your patient style.

- *Ask medical professionals which doctors they see*—Sometimes one of the best ways of finding a good doctor is to speak with people who work with doctors—nurses, physician's assistants, and other doctors. Often they'll have insight into how a doctor works with patients, what type of medical orientation he or she has (open to natural alternatives or strictly traditional, for example), and so forth.

- *Call local hospitals to get names of doctors who specialize in menopause*—Another tried-and-true method of locating prospective doctors, this method is especially helpful because you can be sure that doctors are affiliated with hospitals in your area.
- *Contact the North American Menopause Society for a list of doctors in your area who have registered as menopause specialists*—The North American Menopause Society (NAMS) is a group that offers information on menopause, including answers to frequently asked questions, updates on news and studies, and lists of menopause centers and doctors. While NAMS doesn't make any claims for these doctors, since these doctors have chosen to register with NAMS as menopause specialists, the chances are good that you'll be able to locate several doctors in your area who are well versed in treating menopause. One caveat: since there are no requirements for the doctors who list themselves as menopause specialists, you aren't guaranteed that these doctors are actual specialists or just general gynecologists with some menopausal patients. So if you do use this resource, do be sure also to interview the doctors or their office staff by phone to determine whether they fill your needs. You can reach NAMS by calling 216/844–8748 or by requesting a directory on-line at the NAMS Web site—www.menopause.org.
- *Check whether major medical centers in your area have specific menopause or hormonal disorder clinics or group practices*—This is often a great way of finding doctors who have experience in premature menopause. In addition, sometimes these centers conduct studies, and if you qualify, you may get free care.
- *Don't necessarily limit yourself to gynecologists*—Many women have had good luck with other health care providers, such as physician assistants, nurse practicitioners, and general medicine MDs. Of course, if you do opt for one of these other health care providers, be sure he or she is a woman's health specialist. There are too many potential consequences

of premature menopause to take the risk of seeing a health care provider who isn't well versed in women's care.

- *If you're part of an HMO, consider going out of network—* You may find that the doctor you want or one who's recommended highly isn't part of your HMO. In this case, it makes sense to consider paying for optimum health care if possible. More and more specialists are in practices that accept no insurance at all. Keep in mind that your body is worth the extra expense!

- *Read menopause books and articles, and check on-line Web sites to find the name of doctors who are menopause, premature menopause, or surgical menopause experts—*Books and articles often interview doctors, which can give you a great idea of those doctors' views on HRT, menopause management, and their general medical philosophy. In addition, many doctors and practices have set up Web sites that list their backgrounds, philosophies, the types of treatments they endorse, and more. By doing a simple search using ''menopause'' or ''premature ovarian failure'' as your keywords on one of the major Internet search engines (such as Yahoo, Lycos, or Infoseek), you can locate doctors who specialize in these areas on-line. (Incidently, this is also a good way of finding doctors who specialize in infertility problems—a help if you're interested in pursuing a pregnancy either through donor eggs or more experimental treatments.)

- *Check reference books and magazine articles that list top doctors—*One book that is often available in library reference sections is *The Best Doctors in America*, by Woodward/White, Inc. This lists doctors across the country who were chosen as tops in their field. Also, often regional magazines put out special ''top doctors'' issues—for example, *New York* magazine publishes an annual issue listing top doctors in the New York metropolitan area as chosen by other doctors.

CHECKING UP ON PROSPECTIVE DOCTORS

If you want to be particularly careful or well informed, you may want to check the credentials and backgrounds of those doctors you're considering. Here are some suggestions on how to proceed.

For general information The American Medical Association maintains a Web site (www.ama-assn.org) that has a section called "Doctor Finder." In this you can find general information on doctors, including office address and phone number, fax number, medical school(s) attended, information on any specialties the doctor practices, where he or she trained as a resident, hospital affiliations, and other background information.

To check about board certification Most experts agree that the best doctors are board-certified, which means that they got extra training in a specific area after medical school. Generally you can simply ask doctors if they're board-certified. But if you want to check on your own whether a doctor is board-certified and has completed post-medical school training, you can call the American Board of Medical Specialists at 800/776–2378.

To check if the doctor has had any disciplinary actions taken against him or her, has been sued for malpractice, or has had a license revoked You can call your local state medical society to check if a doctor's license has ever been revoked. In addition, you can check your local library for the Public Citizen Health Research Group's *Questionable Doctors: Disciplined by State or Federal Government,* which lists doctors who have been disciplined, why they were disciplined, and what action was taken against them.

For both general and disciplinary information A company called Medi-Net offers medical consumers information on doctors nationwide. For $15, you can find out if there has been any disciplinary action taken against the doctor, as well as such information as schools the doctor attended, fellowships, residencies, licensing, and American Board of Medical Specialists (ABMS) certification. You can get information on any additional doctors for $5 more. (For more information, you can contact Medi-Net at 800/972-6334 or 888/275-6334).

One important note to keep in mind: Malpractice lawsuits are more and more common these days . . . and are often not an indication of incompetence on the doctor's part. The key is determining whether there has been a pattern of complaints or problems. In general, doing this sort of credential checking is simply another way of getting enough information about a doctor or doctors to help you find the best one for your situation.

Let Your Fingers Do the Walking: How to Evaluate the Doctors You're Considering Before You Make an Appointment

Once you've put together a list of doctors who interest you, call the doctors' offices to do a little background digging. This will take you only a few minutes and it could save you a lot of time and trouble over the long term. A few phone calls can give you a lot of information, can help you see if the doctor's practice fits in with your needs, and can help you make up your mind about what doctor will work best for you. It's simple, painless, and very productive.

I was a bit of a skeptic about this approach until I tried it myself. I had chosen my first two doctors pretty much at random. But, determined not to go through yet another doctor switch, I decided to try the phone interview method before making an appointment—and I learned that it worked well. I had a list of doctors' names, some from referrals, some from research, but all of whom seemed to be great choices for me. But when I sat down and started calling, I was able quickly to tell which ones seemed like pretty good bets and which weren't. In my case, I knew that I was interested in trying natural hormones— not vitamins or herbal supplements (although I did want a doctor who would be open to that as well), but natural forms of HRT. So one of my first questions was: ''Does the doctor prescribe natural hormones to any of her patients?'' Usually I'd be put on hold, then the receptionist would come back and tell me what the doctor had said. And in a number of cases, I immediately learned that the doctor thought that Premarin and Provera would be my best choice—something I didn't agree with. This way, instead of making an appointment, going to see a doctor, and then learning that she and I wouldn't see eye to eye on hormone therapy, I was able to strike her name from my list of possibilities.

At other times, the receptionist would be so busy that she didn't even want to answer my questions, something that bothered me. And still other times, I'd get a stunned: ''You're *sure* you're in menopause?'' Again, not quite the sort of response that impressed me! Finally, at other times, I'd learn that the doctor was most certainly open to prescribing natural hormones, but also recommended special nutrition supplements that I could buy only from her, or believed in health treatment that was a little *too* alternative for me! When I called the doctor whom I ultimately chose, I got a great deal of help from the receptionist, the ''right'' answers to my questions, and a good ''vibe'' overall from the conversation.

So by calling the doctor's office and asking several questions, not only can you learn general information about the office—its hours, how busy it seems, and so on—you may also be able to get a feel for the doctor herself and her medical philosophies to see if she will be a good match for you. Here's a quick rundown to give you an idea of what you may want to cover:

Start by explaining that you're a woman in premature menopause who is looking for a new doctor, and ask if the doctor is accepting new patients. Obviously if she isn't, it's a done deal, but, in this case, you may want to ask if she has any associates who are accepting new patients.

If the doctor is accepting new patients, then it's time to find out a few things. Ask the receptionist if she has a few minutes to answer some questions. You'll be asking two types of questions: some about office procedures, and some about the doctor and her practice.

Where office procedures are concerned, find out:

- *What are the office hours?*
- *How long does it normally take to get an appointment?*
- *How long does the doctor usually spend with patients?* This is a good way of determining whether the office is so busy that you get whisked in and out in no time, or whether you'll have time to sit and seriously discuss your case with the doctor.
- *What insurance (if any) do they accept?*
- *How does billing work—does the office bill patients or do they expect payment at the time of the appointment?*
- *When a patient calls with a question, does the doctor call back?* Or does she have a nurse or other assistant return the call?
- *What kind of facilities do they have?* Can you get blood tests on the premises or will you have to go to a lab? What about other procedures such as ultrasound, biopsies, or bone density testing?

You can also learn a lot about the office not by the answers to your questions, but by the feel of the conversation in general. What does the person answering the phone seem like? Helpful? Harried? Abrupt? The attitude of the staffers on the front desk can give you a real insight into the "feel" of the doctor's office, and possibly into the doctor's personality as well. Is the receptionist friendly or does she seem irritated by your questions? Are you put on hold immediately? Does the office seem superbusy? Remember, you'll be dealing with the receptionist or others on the office staff when you call with questions and so forth. Moreover, the personalities of the front desk staff can often give you a clue as to how the office is run and so what the doctor is like.

Finally, ask if it's possible to speak with the doctor herself for a few minutes. This is a great way of discovering if the doctor sees eye to eye with you about the type of treatment you're interested in, and can give you an idea of her personality. Often you won't be able to speak directly to the doctor, however, so try to find out what you can about the doctor, the types of treatments she'll be open to, and so forth from the receptionist.

Try to find out the following from either the doctor or the desk staffer about treatment:

- *Does the doctor have other patients in premature menopause?* Obviously, this would be a positive thing, but there's a good chance the doctor won't have other patients in your situation.
- *If the doctor is an ob/gyn, what is the ratio of the practice in terms of obstetrics to regular gynecology?* If it seems as though the bulk of the doctor's practice is obstetrics, the doctor may not be up on the most recent developments in menopause. Moreover, you may be uncomfortable in a doctor's office that is geared to pregnant women.
- *Most important, what is the ratio of patients in menopause in relation to the rest of her practice?* Again, you're probably best seeing a doctor who has a relatively high ratio of patients in menopause.
- *If you're interested in natural HRT as opposed to traditional, is the doctor open to prescribing this form of therapy?* This one question can save you a great deal of wasted time. By discovering whether the doctor would prescribe the form of HRT you want, you can quickly see if there will be a conflict between your desires and the doctor's proclivities.

If you get good "vibes" from the phone conversation and if the answers to your questions seem positive, you have two choices: you can either select a doctor based upon your phone conversation, or you can set up a consultation or interview appointment with the doctor. The latter makes sense if you have narrowed your list of possible doctors to two or three and need more information to make a final selection. The point of the meeting is to get acquainted and determine whether the doctor will meet your criteria. If, however, you are quite sure that you have found a doctor you feel comfortable with, then you can go ahead and set up a regular office visit that will include both an interview/medical history consultation and a physical exam.

In either case, the first meeting with a doctor is an important one. You'll be able to discover if indeed you've found the right doctor—the one you need and deserve!

The Final Step in Choosing a Doctor: The First Face-To-Face Meeting

When you first go to a new doctor's office, you can start evaluating from the minute you walk through the front door. All sorts of seemingly minor components add up and can give you an idea of whether this doctor is right for you or not. Notice such things as how you're greeted by the front desk staff, what the office environment is like, how comfortable the waiting room is, how office staffers interact. If you have to wait a while before you can see the doctor, did you receive an explanation and apology? Obviously, what you want is a professional, yet friendly, environment, one that makes you feel comfortable.

But the real nuts and bolts of the matter arrive when you finally sit down to talk with the doctor. Here's when you can see how well you believe you'll be able to work with this particular doctor.

As I mentioned earlier, because premature menopause affects you both physically and emotionally, it's more important than usual that you feel you have a rapport with your doctor. The issues involved in the treatment of premature menopause are often highly personal, for one thing. In addition, if you go on HRT, you'll be seeing your doctor fairly frequently, especially initially, so it's vital that you feel able to talk.

In your first interview with your doctor, you'll of course be talking about yourself—your health history, symptoms, and so on. (A little later in this chapter, I'll explain what you can expect in your first office visit.) But you should also be determining if the doctor is right for you. Here are some questions to either ask or think about during your first meeting with your doctor—whether it's a "scoping-out" interview on your part or a full-fledged office appointment:

- *If you haven't had any tests that are commonly run to indicate menopause (FSH and estrogen blood levels), how does the doctor react when you say that you think you are experiencing premature menopause?*—This is probably the one most important indicator of whether or not this is the right doctor for you. As I've said repeatedly, all too often, women in premature menopause are handed the "you're too young" line when they explain to a doctor that they believe they're entering menopause at a young age. If the doctor immediately says this, the chances are extremely high that this is definitely not the doctor for you!
- *What is your doctor's philosophy?*—You don't necessarily have to come out and ask the question point-blank (although you can, if you want!). You should be checking whether the doctor is an authoritarian type who doesn't want input from you and just gives you instructions and procedures to follow, or whether she is one who welcomes discussion, patient input, and questions. How does the doctor react if you mention that you've read books or have done research on your condition? It's also wise to ask about the doctor's attitudes toward HRT, hysterectomies, natural supplementation, and so on. You're trying to get the most accurate picture of the sort of treatments the doctor normally prescribes to see whether they mesh with your preferences.
- *How much time is the doctor willing to spend just talking with you?*—You shouldn't be whisked out of the consultation room into an examination room in only a few minutes flat. Treating premature menopause isn't solely a hands-on proposition. It also requires that the doctor know what your body has been going through, what your lifestyle is, the symptoms you've been experiencing, your personal health history and that of your family, and your emotional well-being as well.

If the doctor is too quick to cut off the talk and head for the physical examination, you probably won't wind up with the care you deserve.

- *Ask if you'll be able to keep copies of your medical records, test results, and the like*—In general, it's a good idea to keep a file at home with these records in case you switch doctors, need ready reference for emergencies, and so on. Furthermore, if a doctor is unwilling to give you your own records, this should send up a red flag. It may mean the doctor doesn't want you to be involved in your own health care (not a great sign) or that he or she is uncomfortable having you see your own test results.

Finally, take a few minutes to think about how you feel during the entire meeting with the doctor. Usually you'll know deep down if you feel at ease, if you feel you can trust the doctor and work well with her—in other words, if this is the doctor for you. If you're not pleased with the doctor, or if everything seems fine but you just don't feel quite satisfied, there's nothing wrong in continuing your search. It's not uncommon for women in premature menopause to try out a few doctors until they find the right one. So remember, it's up to you to keep looking for that right doctor, one you can feel comfortable with, feel secure with, and trust. It's worth the time, effort, and thought. Speaking from experience, I believe that when you do find the right doctor, it makes a huge difference in how well you can cope with the unpleasant surprise of premature menopause.

WORKING WITH YOUR DOCTOR

Choosing a doctor you think is right for you is one thing. Actually working with that doctor is another. To get the best possible health care, it's important for you to know what you can expect when you see a doctor for premature menopause, and what you can do to ensure that you get the care you deserve.

Your First Office Visit: What to Expect

When you first see a doctor as a patient to discuss your premature menopause, you'll go through both a medical history interview and a physical exam. Both are vital components of the office visit, each supplying different information to the doctor. It is also likely that you will undergo certain tests if you haven't had any done recently. All of this will enable your doctor to get a picture of your current menopausal status and begin evaluating what form of hormone replacement therapy or other menopausal management therapy would work best for you.

THE CONSULTATION

This is essentially the "get-acquainted" portion of your visit in a number of ways. Your doctor will begin getting acquainted with you, your medical history, and your symptoms, and you'll begin getting an idea of how your doctor will be handling your menopause. Because your doctor needs to know just what you've been experiencing as well as important facts about your past health and your family's medical history, it's important to be prepared with all necessary information—and extremely important to be as explicit and forthright as possible when answering questions.

You should be prepared to tell your doctor about:

- *Your family medical history*—When your mother entered menopause and any diseases that run in your family, including breast cancer, osteoporosis, and cardiovascular disease. This will help your doctor evaluate whether or not HRT is a good choice for you, and the form of HRT that may work best.
- *Your own medical history*—Again, this is important, especially when it comes to prescribing HRT. If you've had a history of blood clots, for example, this will affect the form of therapy the doctor recommends. If you're in premature menopause due to breast cancer or other cancer treatments, your doctor will need to know the type of treatment you had,

the duration, and so forth. And if you're in surgical menopause, again, your doctor will need to know the specifics
about your disease and the treatment you followed.

- *Your lifestyle*—General information on your habits, including
exercise, diet, smoking, and drinking. And be completely
truthful! All too often, women feel uncomfortable admitting
to bad habits to a doctor—for example, if they smoke, they
don't want to mention it because they know it's bad. But this
isn't the time to make yourself out to be a saint! All of this
information is important in terms of evaluating HRT options
and possible long-term risks from premature menopause. Unless you're honest, you won't get the help you need.

- *Your menstrual cycle over the past few months*—Frequency
of periods, any skipped periods, duration, flow, and so on.
As mentioned earlier, it's a good idea to have this all jotted
down to be sure you don't make any mistakes.

- *Physical symptoms*—What symptoms you've been experiencing, how often you get them, severity of the symptoms. And
tell the doctor about them in order of importance, which will
enable her to understand what your priorities are.

- *Emotional symptoms*—Something that often isn't a factor in
regular gynecological exams, but one that does play a part
in premature menopause. Because of the emotional toll that
premature menopause causes, not to mention the very real
mood swings and depression brought on by depleted hormone
levels, it's important to discuss emotional symptoms you've
been going through. This will help the doctor determine
whether to put you on an antidepressant or other medication
or herbal supplement (such as St. John's Wort).

- *Your sex life*—Not the easiest topic to chat about with someone you've only just met, but a necessary one. For example,
if you've been experiencing pain during sex, you may already
be suffering from vaginal atrophy; or if you've lost interest
in sex, you may have low testosterone levels. Again, be as
frank as you possibly can.

- *Your future plans for pregnancy*—Another topic that is specific to women in premature menopause. If you're consider-

ing pursuing the use of donor eggs or other more experimental treatment for premature menopause, let your doctor know. This may affect the type of therapy you can get, or she may be able to tell you about infertility clinics or reproductive endocrinologists. In fact, even if you're considering adoption, it's a good idea to mention this. She may have information on adoption agencies or private adoption lawyers that can help you.

If possible, it's an excellent idea to bring copies of any pertinent medical records such as blood tests you've recently had (not only FSH or estrogen levels, but also cholesterol tests or general blood chemistries). Your doctor may want to retest you, but even in this case, it's helpful for her to have a record of your past tests.

It's hard to say exactly how long you can expect this initial consultation to last because it can and does vary according to your specific situation, what you need to cover, and so forth. But all in all, expect to spend from 15 minutes to as much as 30 to 40 minutes just talking. If the doctor talks to you for less than 15 minutes, or if you haven't covered the points listed above, don't hesitate to offer subjects yourself—and think about looking for a new doctor!

The Physical Exam

Once your doctor has had a chance to talk with you and learn about your case, it's off to the examination room—the dreaded stirrups and examination gowns.

Even though you're seeing the doctor specifically because of premature menopause, the physical exam itself is pretty much the typical gynecological exam you've been through dozens of time before. Expect the doctor to check your weight, pulse, blood pressure, and heart; feel your thyroid—the gland in your throat—to check for swelling or abnormalities; give you a breast examination; and palpate your abdomen. Then it's on to the pelvic exam, in which your doctor will check for vaginal atrophy (a sign of low estrogen), give you a Pap smear, and view your vaginal walls and cervix.

Unless you've had more than one recent blood test to check your hormone levels, you will probably get a blood test taken at this time as well, to run hormone level tests and, possibly, other blood tests such as thyroid antigen.

TYPICAL COMPONENTS OF A PHYSICAL EXAM

Here's a list of the procedures and tests you receive when seeing a doctor, as well as what the doctor is checking for, and why these procedures are important.

Physical Exam

Cardiovascular checkup (blood pressure measurement, listening to heart, and so on)—Checks for signs of cardiovascular disease, high blood pressure, varicose veins, which helps the doctor determine whether you're a good candidate for HRT.

Pap Smear—Part of your usual gynecological exam; checks for possible cancerous or precancerous cells in your vagina, cervix, and uterine lining. If a Pap test comes back positive, your doctor will probably order other tests.

Thyroid—Checks for enlargement or lumps. If there appear to be abnormalities, you'll probably also get a thyroid blood test.

Breasts—Checks for lumps, thickening, cysts, and nipple or skin changes.

Abdomen—Checks for swelling and tenderness.

Pelvic exam—Checks for cancer of the vulva, size and condition of your reproductive organs, strength of your pelvic muscles, uterine cancer signs, vaginal dryness and atrophy, uterine or bladder prolapse.

Blood Tests

Blood tests are done to determine the levels of different hormones you are producing (which are used to diagnose menopause), and to measure other components such as cholesterol and thyroid hormone. Most common is testing of:

Follicle stimulating hormone (FSH) levels—Usually drawn on the first, second, or third day of your cycle; usually tested for at least two successive months; high FSH (over 30) is considered a signal of menopause or ovarian failure.

Estradiol level—Also usually tested more than once; low levels are usually considered a sign of menopause or ovarian failure.

Depending on your symptoms and health history, the doctor may also check your:

Testosterone level—Typically measured if you're complaining of symptoms such as very low libido, and so on; levels less than 30 nanograms per milliliter are typically considered low.

Progesterone level—Levels greater than 5 mg/ml on day 20 of your cycle indicate that you are still ovulating.

Luteinizing hormone (LH) level—High LH to FSH levels can signal polycystic ovarian disease (PCOD), which can cause stopped periods without menopause.

Prolactin level—Often measured if you have stopped having periods, but aren't experiencing menopausal symptoms, and/or if your FSH and estradiol levels are normal.

Lipid profile (blood cholesterol and triglyceride levels)—Measures your LDL and HDL cholesterol as well as your triglycerides; given to determine your cardiovascular risk, which often increases with low estrogen levels; if you have high levels before going on HRT, your doctor may want to check it a few months after taking HRT to determine if the HRT has had a positive impact.

Thyroid—Measures the levels of thyroxine (T4) and T3; often tested because premature ovarian failure is often linked with autoimmune disorders and because many thyroid disease symptoms mimic menopausal ones.

If you haven't had a recent physical or blood chemistry test, your doctor may also test your blood sugar levels, liver function, and blood count, all to help determine your overall health and condition.

Special tests given for specific circumstances:

Bone mineral density test (BMD)—Covered in detail in Chapter 3; checks for signs of osteoporosis or osteopenia.

Vaginal sonogram (also called a pelvic ultrasound)—Measures the thickness of your uterine lining; shows if you have uterine or ovarian cysts, endometrial hyperplasia, fibroid tumors, uterine or ovarian cancer, sometimes even endometriosis. Typically given if you have unexplained or excessive bleeding, especially if you are on HRT.

Endometrial biopsy—Small scraping of tissue taken from your uterine lining; typically given if you have unexplained bleeding and if your sonogram showed possible abnormalities.

Follow-Up Visits: How Often, When, and Why

As you'd expect, you'll go back to see your doctor once the results from your blood tests are in. At this point, you and your doctor will discuss the results and come up with a course of action. Usually you will be given a prescription for HRT and begin taking it immediately. You may also be sent for a bone mineral density test, since premature menopause puts you at such a high risk for osteoporosis.

Your doctor will probably recommend that you schedule a follow-up visit in two to three months to see how the HRT is working. This gives your body time to adjust to the hormones, and allows you to see if your symptoms subside and if you have any difficulty with the HRT. Again, it's a good idea to be prepared when you go in for the follow-up, armed with information about how you've adjusted to the HRT. Be prepared to explain when and if you are bleeding, any symptoms or side effects you've noticed, and the like. And don't ignore emotional symptoms. As mentioned in Chapter 5, some women experience PMS-like symptoms from HRT, including depression and moodiness. It's important for you to let your doctor know what is happening to you, so she can evaluate your treatment. If the HRT doesn't seem to be doing its job, you may go through another blood test to see where your hormone levels are and try another form of HRT, until you end up with a therapy that works well for you. Your doctor may recommend that, during your first year on HRT, you go in for follow-up exams every three months.

Your doctor may suggest that you get your bone density checked after a few months of taking HRT if you showed bone loss in your first scan. This will show how well the HRT is working in combating osteoporosis, and will signal if you need any further intervention, such as increasing your calcium intake or even taking Fosomax or another bone-builder.

Once it appears that you have adjusted to HRT, your doctor will usually tell you to come in for a checkup every six months. You should have a pelvic exam, a breast exam, and any blood or urine tests necessary, depending upon your symptoms, and once a year, you should have a Pap test.

WHEN SHOULD YOU CALL YOUR DOCTOR BETWEEN VISITS?

While you may have no trouble adjusting to HRT and will see your doctor only during appointments, there are certain times when you should *always* call your doctor to explain what is happening and possibly arrange an interim checkup. Call your doctor if:

• *You are on HRT, have an intact uterus, and experience any unusual bleeding*—including extremely heavy bleeding, bleeding when it isn't expected (after six months of continuous HRT, for example), breakthrough bleeding, and so on. This may signal fibroids, endometriosis, polyps, or something more serious such as endometrial hyperplasia or uterine cancer. In this case, your doctor should order a pelvic ultrasound and/or an endometrial biopsy.

- *You notice changes in your symptoms*—perhaps you had stopped getting hot flashes and are getting them again, are noticing a change in your periods, or are experiencing strong cramping. Your doctor needs to know about these changes and may want to change your HRT.
- *You develop uncomfortable side effects from HRT*—such as migraines.

Finally, if you have any questions at all—about treatment options, new prescriptions that have been introduced and that interest you, minor side effects, anything that affects your quality of life—you should feel free to call your doctor and ask. If you're with the right doctor, you should be secure in the knowledge that she will answer your questions and take interest in your menopause management.

The 10 Rules of Being a Good Patient

Having a good doctor-patient relationship is a two-way street. To get the best care possible, you have to be a good patient.

Being a good patient doesn't mean accepting the doctor's word blindly or staying completely quiet throughout an examination. It does mean being involved, interested, and informed.

1) Be Prepared The old Boy Scout motto applies just as well to medical patients. When you see your doctor for a regular appointment, call with a question, or come in for a special problem, you should always be ready to explain exactly what your complaints are, what symptoms you've been having, and so on. As I've mentioned before, it's often a good idea to keep notes on symptoms or jot down questions you have. This way, when you speak to your doctor, you'll have the pertinent information at hand. It's also helpful to list your complaints or questions in order of importance, so you'll be sure to get the most important points covered if you run out of time.

2) Be Organized When you call for appointments, let the receptionist know why you need to see the doctor, and be as specific as possible. This will help her schedule enough time for you. And be sure you know what you need to bring with you for insurance purposes.

3) Be Prompt Don't show up late for appointments. It sounds simple, but many people do this, and it doesn't make for the best doctor-patient relationship! If you're worried that you'll be stuck reading magazines in the waiting room for a long time, call before your appointment and ask the receptionist if the doctor is running behind schedule and if you should arrive later.

4) You Expect Your Doctor to be Professional Yet Friendly, So Be the Same A good doctor-patient relationship is a professional one, so you should be professional yourself. Don't overdo the small talk, little niceties, and jokes. A little of this goes a long way. Yes, it's good to feel at ease and to chat a bit. But you don't want to waste the doctor's time on subjects that don't relate to your medical situation, nor do you want to detract from the real business of your appointment—your health.

5) Don't Underplay Symptoms or Physical Complaints All too often, when you're sitting in a doctor's office, you get an attack of the "it's not really that bad" syndrome and either don't mention problems you've been having or mention them as an afterthought, as if it's really not a big deal. Well, when it comes to premature menopause—or anything about your health, actually—it *is* a big deal! Some symptoms can mean you're adjusting poorly to HRT, or worse, that you've developed complications such as fibroids, or even cancer. Your doctor won't be able to help you if you don't clearly and honestly present any physical complaints to her. Do her and yourself a favor by speaking up. A confident patient who is forthright about her problems gets the best care.

6) Ask Questions This is one of the toughest areas for many women . . . including me. While I'm a forthright person in general, put me in a doctor's office and suddenly I find myself keeping my mouth shut, listening, and nodding my head—even if I have a million questions. But it's important to ask questions of your doctor—questions about treatments, prescriptions, tests, and so on. Again, being a good patient means keeping yourself informed and understanding what is going on in your body. If you don't ask questions, you won't be able to get a clear picture of your medical situation.

7) In a Similar Vein, Be Sure You Understand the Doctor's Answers and Don't Be Frightened to Ask for Further Explanations Just because your doctor may think she's answered your questions, this doesn't necessarily mean she has where you're concerned. If your doctor explains something to you, but you're still unclear about it, simply say so, and ask for further explanation at that time. Don't go home and wonder, or call later. Asking follow-up questions at the right time saves time for both you and the doctor.

8) If You're Confused, Ask for Information in Plain English, Not Medicalese Often a doctor will tell you about procedures or treatments using technical language, and you have only the vaguest idea of what she's talking about. Speak up! Ask for a translation in simple, layperson's terms. If you don't understand what is being said, you can't make an educated decision, which in the long run won't help the doctor or you.

9) Before You Leave, Be Sure You Understand the Whys, Hows, and Possible Side Effects of Tests or Medications Again, it's a matter of speaking up and asking questions. Before you leave your doctor's office, before you fill that prescription or schedule a test, make sure you know what to expect, what the test entails, and why it's being recommended, or what the prescription is for, why you need it, and whether you can expect any side effects. This way you'll know what you're in for and you won't need to call the doctor later with questions.

10) Finally, If You're Dissatisfied With the Care You're Getting, Speak Up! Your doctor won't know that you have a problem with her care unless you point it out. So let her know— diplomatically. Be clear, honest, and explicit. Then, if the problem isn't rectified, start looking for a new doctor.

Chapter 8

Having a Baby

It's Still a Possibility

One of the most difficult aspects of learning I was in premature menopause was being told I couldn't have a child—at least not my own biological child from one of my own eggs. I first thought that there had to be some mistake, that there was some way around it, taking fertility drugs to force ovulation, or harvesting whatever eggs I might have. But a reproductive endocrinologist at a fertility center gave me the facts as honestly and compassionately as she could: with premature menopause, the chances of getting pregnant were slim. It could happen, she said, but it would be somewhat of a miracle. My best chances of having a child were either opting for a donor egg or adoption. And if I wanted to go the donor egg route, I could start immediately. I was already so confused, trying to grapple with my diagnosis and come to grips with the huge change that was being wrought in my life, that I decided to wait . . . and think . . . and research all the options open to me.

Most women who learn they're prematurely menopausal, whether naturally or through surgery, find the loss of fertility one of the toughest things to handle about their condition. Even those women who already have children find this very difficult to deal with.

The idea that you are infertile is a very painful concept to digest when you are in your twenties or thirties. Your peers are talking about having children. Friends and family may be pregnant or happily anticipating a time when they will be. Ads on television show glowing women excitedly checking at-home pregnancy tests. Magazine articles about women's health assume that you are in your childbearing years and focus on this aspect of your health. Yet in the back of your mind is the terrible fact: you are unable to have children.

But if you really want to, you can. Having a child isn't an impossibility.

No, it's not as simple as you may have wished. When you are prematurely menopausal, you can't just bank on regular biology as your friends can.

Actually, some women with premature menopause do become pregnant the old-fashioned way. Some studies show that about 8 percent of women with premature ovarian failure spontaneously ovulate and get pregnant. Of course, you can't predict if you will be one of those lucky women. And if you are in surgical premature menopause and have no ovaries, this can't happen to you. But there are options open to you that will enable you to become a mother.

This chapter explores these different options. It covers the most popular form of assisted reproductive technology for women in premature menopause, egg donation, which allows you to be pregnant, carry, and deliver a baby that can have a genetic link to your husband. It also examines immunosuppression, a more experimental way of getting pregnant with your own eggs. Finally, it looks at adoption, another fulfilling option that enables you to experience motherhood. It examines what each method of having a child entails, what you can expect, what you should know to help you begin making a decision, and specific sources to help you learn more.

More than anything, however, this chapter is designed to let you know that premature menopause doesn't mean you have to give up your dreams of having a child. It may have changed how you go about having that child, but motherhood is still a definite possibility. You may have to readjust your expectations and seriously think about the many issues that arise of not being able to have children naturally. You may need time to mourn the fact that you won't be able to have a family as simply and naturally as you had expected. But if you choose to pursue the different paths open to you, remember that motherhood is within your reach.

SPONTANEOUS OVULATION AND PREGNANCY: IT'S NOT COMMON, BUT IT CAN HAPPEN

My family doctor, whom I'd gone to originally, said wait for one year until all bleeding completely stops. The gynecologist said start HRT at once. You're much too young and your heart is too vulnerable to be without estrogen. Since I have a family history of cardiac disease, I started HRT. I went on Prempro and felt much saner. I went off Prempro a few months later. I was having breakthrough bleeding (which is normal on Prempro) and I just wanted to see what would happen if I left my body alone. I suppose I was still hoping it would all go away and I'd be normal again. I did use a progesterone cream. Actually, I think I overdid it—the cream had a relaxing effect on me. I stopped the cream after about two months because my breasts were very tender and swollen and I was getting really weird. I then had a period from hell that lasted about a week and spotted for the rest of the month almost nonstop. I went to the gynecologist, had a normal Pap. Meanwhile, I was feeling much more myself, so out of curiosity, I had my FSH redrawn. It was down almost 70 points. The doctor's office said not to worry, the FSH does fluctuate even in meno. I refused to restart the HRT. I was feeling much more myself and I wasn't really convinced I needed it. I continued to spot almost every

month, and was getting worried. I knew that postmeno
bleeding is a sign of cancer. So I went to a new MD and
a new gyne, who both insisted I have an endometrial biopsy done just to be sure it wasn't cancer. It wasn't.
There was a benign polyp that may have been a contribu-
tor. But just for the hell of it, I had my FSH rechecked.
It was 5.9! I was impossibly, but surely, back in the fertile
range! And that's where I am. It's been three months
since I had the biopsy, and this month my period came
right on my old schedule. So maybe I can get pregnant?
                                    —Amy, age 37

It is rare, but it does happen: women who have been diagnosed with premature menopause—those who still have ovaries—suddenly begin ovulating again and get pregnant naturally.

Doctors are not sure why this happens or how to predict it.
Here are the facts: research has shown that as many as 50
percent of women with premature ovarian failure have what
appear to be ovarian follicles when their ovaries are examined
by ultrasound. Depending upon which study you read, either
fewer than 5 percent or up to 8 percent of women diagnosed
with premature ovarian failure suddenly revert back to normal
for no apparent reason. Their FSH levels drop to premenopausal
levels, and they begin ovulating again.

Could you be one of these lucky women? There is little way
of telling. According to the studies and reports, this spontaneous reversal of premature menopause often happens when a
woman is on estrogen. Some doctors hypothesize that this may
occur because the estrogen makes the FSH receptors on the
follicles more responsive to the FSH your body is circulating,
but this is only a theory with no scientific data to back it up.
In addition, because pregnancies after premature menopause
haven't been closely studied, it is unclear whether being on
estrogen actually helps cause a remission of premature menopause, or if it's just that the women who report this reversal
are ones that have been tracked because they are on HRT. All
in all, it's impossible to be sure at this point. Other women

have reported great success with herbs that have estrogenic properties. Still others say that they've done nothing, but suddenly they began getting their period again and continued as if nothing had ever happened in the interim.

The problem is that no one is sure why and how this happens. A number of factors may be involved: some researchers theorize that traumatic stress—anything from the death of a spouse or parent to an accident to low-grade constant stress from a job or bad relationship—may cause temporary menopause, and that, after a while, when the body is relaxed again, it returns to its normal menstrual cycle. Another possibility is that when you are in the beginning stages of premature menopause, your body periodically reverts to normal hormone levels. So you may ovulate on and off when you are first in premature menopause even if your FSH tested at a high level, because in certain months your FSH may have slid back down to "normal" levels. Yet another possibility is that ovulation occurs if the ovarian failure was caused by an autoimmune disease, and the autoimmune disease goes into remission.

One thing, though—and on this one, I speak from experience—having a period again, even for an extended amount of time, doesn't necessarily mean that you'll be able to get pregnant. In my case, I started having my period again for over six months, and assumed that everything was completely normal again. However, during that time, I also had my FSH levels retested and discovered that, although I was getting my period, I didn't seem to be ovulating, since my FSH levels were still well over 100. And I didn't get pregnant.

But for all the negative stories, there are positive ones as well. I personally know of one woman who got pregnant after several years of premature menopause (she was on estrogen and Chinese herbs) and another who got pregnant after having done nothing for her premature menopause at all.

So it is possible. The general rule of thumb: pregnancy may happen to you if you've still got your ovaries and follicles. The odds aren't with you, but sometimes miracles do happen—and one could happen to you!

DONOR EGGS (OOCYTE DONATION): A TRIED-AND-TRUE WAY OF HAVING THE CHILD YOU DREAM ABOUT

Having a child—actually carrying the child for nine months and being able to bond with it—really matters to me. So my husband and I have finally decided that egg donation is the right choice for us. I'm very excited about the prospects. I know that this way I have a real chance of being the mother I have always wanted to be.
—Sarah, age 28

When I went to a reproductive endocrinologist (RE) for a second opinion about my premature ovarian failure diagnosis, the first thing she told me was, yes, I was definitely menopausal. The second thing she told me was that if I wanted to have a child, I should consider donor eggs. Given my health and my age, the odds were excellent that I would be able to bear at least one child, possibly more—"an instant family!" as the RE enthusiastically put it.

More often than not, if you're prematurely menopausal, still have a uterus, and want to have a child, you will hear the same thing. Your doctor will tell you to think about going through *in vitro* fertilization with a donor egg. This is a tried-and-true way for a woman who doesn't have working ovaries or viable eggs to be able to carry and bear a child—often a child who has a genetic link with her partner, since his sperm can be used.

Egg donation was initially available only to women with premature ovarian failure. Now it's also offered to a wide range of infertile women, including those who have failed other attempts at assisted reproductive techniques, older postmenopausal women, and women with genetic diseases.

For many women in premature menopause, this is the best answer to their infertility for a number of reasons:

• *While there is no guarantee, you do have a very good chance of getting pregnant and delivering a baby through donor eggs*—This method has one of the highest success rates of all assisted reproductive procedures, about 30 to 40 percent, which means that for every five donor egg cycles attempted, two are successful—that is, they result in the birth of a baby. When you get a fresh egg transfer (as opposed to having a frozen embryo implanted), the success rate should be the same as you would have had if using your own eggs. One key point, however, you should be aware of is that different clinics have different success rates, so if you decide to follow this procedure, be sure to find out the success rate for the particular clinics you are considering.

• *You have the opportunity to actually carry a baby*—You can be the baby's "gestational" mother, as it's scientifically called. This allows you to bond with the child throughout your pregnancy, to experience the birth of your child, and to breast-feed.

• *Because you are carrying the child, you have control over prenatal care*—You can be sure to do all the right things: follow the best possible diet, not smoke or drink, everything and anything you think would be best for your baby.

• *The child can have a genetic link to your husband*—This is often a great comfort to both father and mother, since their child can have a biological bond with at least one of them.

• *Although the child will have no genetic link to you, he or she may resemble you*—If you use a donor such as a sister, your child will have genes from your family gene pool. And in most cases, if you are using an anonymous donor, efforts are made to find a donor who "matches" you physically. In other words, if you're short, brunette, and olive-skinned, the fertility clinic will match you with a donor who is also short, brunette and olive-skinned. This is one of those factors that may not matter to some women, but does make a difference to others, especially those who feel that it's easier for the child if he or she physically "fits" into the family, and those who would prefer not to tell people that they had their child through egg donation.

How It Works

Egg donation is a relatively straightforward procedure. To boil it down to its most basic, a donor, a woman usually no older than 34 or 35, donates eggs to be used by a donor recipient, a woman who can't produce her own healthy eggs. These eggs are fertilized *in vitro* and the embryos implanted in the recipient's uterus. The recipient's partner's sperm is usually used for fertilization, but it can also be done with donated sperm.

More specifically, a known donor (usually a close relative, such as a sister or first cousin) or an anonymous donor screened by the fertility clinic is given hormones to ovulate and produce a number of mature eggs. In the meantime, the recipient takes hormones to synchronize her menstrual cycle with the donor's cycle and to prepare her uterine lining for the egg.

When the donor's eggs are mature, they are harvested, usually by a method called "aspiration," in which a long needle withdraws the eggs from the donor's ovaries. The eggs are then fertilized in a laboratory, and finally implanted into the recipient's uterus. For the first three months of pregnancy, the recipient continues taking progesterone and estrogen. After the first trimester, though, the placenta takes over and the pregnancy proceeds like a normal one.

What Will Happen: The Steps Involved in Egg Donation

That's the scientific side of things. But, of course, there's a bit more involved in the entire process. Here is a quick rundown of what you can expect if you choose to pursue donor eggs as a way of having a child—from choosing a clinic to having donor eggs implanted in your uterus.

CHOOSING A REPRODUCTIVE CENTER

Your first step will be choosing a reproductive center to work with. Depending upon where you live, you may have a number of centers to choose from. You can find out about different clinics by asking for referrals from your gynecologist or RE, checking with support groups such as RESOLVE, looking on-line for geographic directories and Web sites, and talking with other people who have used fertility clinics.

It's a good idea to research clinics carefully, to be sure you find the one that seems best for you—one that you feel comfortable with, that has a high success rate, and that has doctors whom you trust. Going through a donor egg cycle can be emotionally draining, so it's important to find a center that suits your individual needs and expectations. Here are some questions to ask and points to think about to be sure you're getting the best possible clinic for your situation:

- *What were the clinic's success rates for egg donation over the past year?*—Be sure to get as specific information as possible. Find out how many donor egg cycles were completed, how many women got pregnant, and most important, how many babies were successfully delivered. This is the only way to find out an actual success rate, since a number of donor egg cycles may result in miscarriage.

- *How often does the clinic perform egg donation for women in your age group and with premature menopause?*—This will give you an idea of how accustomed they are in treating someone like you, and will indicate their expertise. Clearly, you will do best with a fertility clinic that has a substantial number of egg donation patients.

- *How much will the treatment cost, and what, if any, insurance plans does the clinic accept?*—An obvious question but one that can get a little confusing. Some clinics may quote you a cost that doesn't include certain elements such as tests, drugs, even initial consultations. Make sure you get the total cost for everything involved in the whole donor egg procedure. Also find out about insurance coverage. If you are an HMO member and can't get coverage for the procedure, can you have your HMO ob/gyn or RE prescribe the necessary drugs for you and so be covered at least for that portion of your treatment?

- *How long a waiting list is there for donor eggs?*—If you are supplying your own donor, this question obviously doesn't apply. But if you are going to use an anonymous donor, you need to know roughly how long you can expect to wait for eggs. Many clinics have a waiting list, some for as long as two years or more; others may have a shorter wait.
- *Does the staff seem supportive?*—Going through a donor egg cycle can be nerve-racking, so it's important that you feel comfortable, confident, and secure with the clinic and its staff members. Do you feel that you're being treated well? Are you getting full explanations when you ask questions? Are there counselors available to help you through the procedure? Does it feel "right" there?

THE INITIAL SCREENINGS

Once you've decided upon a center, you and your husband will attend orientation meetings. You'll usually meet with several different people—the medical doctor, a mental health professional, and an office manager or administrator to discuss the financial side of things. This will enable the reproductive center to screen you both psychologically and physically and be sure you understand what will happen, the different elements involved, and the cost.

The psychological evaluation is important, as the center wants to be sure you and your husband are emotionally ready to go through the egg donation cycle. You will be asked your feelings on a number of issues, including how you have handled your inability to have a child with your own eggs, your thoughts on raising a child, and so on. In some instances, they will decide that this doesn't seem a good time to proceed. This usually occurs when you haven't had time to mourn your infertility adequately. Sometimes you just need some more time to put the past in the past, and then move on. It doesn't mean, however, that donor eggs are out of the question, just that, in the eyes of the psychologist or center social worker, you should wait until you are mentally prepared to go through the sometimes emotionally draining egg donation procedure.

The medical screening is relatively straightforward. You and your husband will supply the doctor with an extensive genetic and medical history background on both of you—covering everything from your genetic ancestry to your family health history to your own health history.

If your husband's sperm will be used for fertilization of the donor egg, your husband will undergo a semen analysis to be sure his sperm is viable. And both you and he will be screened for HIV and other sexually transmitted and infectious diseases such as hepatitis. You will also go through a general physical examination, checking your uterus and other factors that could affect your ability to carry the child. If you aren't "officially" menopausal—that is, if you haven't stopped having periods for at least a year—you will also undergo an ovarian exam. This way, the doctor will determine whether or not you have a risk of getting your period spontaneously and disrupting the donor egg cycle.

Once it looks as though you are both able psychologically and physically to handle egg donation, it's often a waiting game. If you're not using a known donor, you will have to wait until the center finds an anonymous donor to supply you with eggs. This can take anywhere from a few months to a year or two, depending upon the specific reproductive center. But eventually the call will come—there's a donor for you! And then it's on to the actual donor egg cycle.

THE EGG DONATION CYCLE

The egg donation cycle can be broken down into several major elements: getting the eggs, which is a matter of preparing the donor to ovulate, then actually harvesting the eggs; getting you ready to receive the eggs, which entails synchronizing your cycle with the donor's and preparing your uterus for egg implantation; fertilizing the eggs with your husband's sperm; then finally, egg implantation.

First, let's look at how the reproductive center will get both the donor and you ready for ovulation.

The first step, of course, is screening. Whether she is known or anonymous, the donor is tested for HIV, hepatitis, and other infectious diseases, and undergoes both physical and psychological evaluation just as you and your husband do. Because ovulation usually produces just one egg per cycle, the donor is given hormones to ripen more than one follicle and so produce more than one egg. This "controlled superovulation," as it is technically called, is very important because the chances of pregnancy rise with the number of fertilized eggs you receive. Your reproductive specialist will want to harvest a number of eggs, then implant two or more (usually no more than four) of them in your uterus, in the hopes that at least one will attach to your uterine lining and launch a successful pregnancy. (Granted, this also increases the chance that you will have twins or even triplets!)

For about two to three weeks, the donor remains on a combination of hormones, which will make the follicles ripen and the eggs mature. Throughout this time, the center tests her hormone levels and tracks the growth of the eggs on ultrasound to be sure everything is proceeding well. Finally, when the eggs are ready to be harvested, the donor gets a shot of human chorionic gonadotropin (hCG). About 36 to 38 hours later, the eggs are retrieved by "ultrasound aspiration," which simply means that an ultrasound-guided needle is inserted, usually through the vagina, to remove the eggs.

Throughout this entire process, you, the recipient, also take hormones. If you were still getting periods, you may get hormones to be sure your own cycle is completely suppressed. Depending upon the particular program, you will be put on estrogen as long as weeks before egg retrieval is due or only days before. The estradiol, taken as a pill, patch, or injection, will start building your uterine lining; and for about two weeks, your uterine lining will be tracked by ultrasound to be sure it is building enough, and you may also get blood tests to monitor your hormone levels. When the donor gets her hCG injection, you begin taking progesterone (pill, vaginal suppository, or injection) to prepare your uterine lining for egg implantation. So by the time the donor is ready to ovulate, your body should be prepared for pregnancy as if you yourself had naturally ovulated.

The next major step is fertilizing the eggs. The eggs retrieved from the donor are taken to a lab, checked and graded for maturity, and prepared for fertilization. (This may mean the eggs are shaved, to make their linings more easily penetrated, among other things.) The same day the eggs are collected, your husband, if you are using his sperm, supplies it by masturbating. The sperm is checked and treated in the lab to be sure that only the best samples are used, and sperm is put with each egg from the donor. By the next day or so, you will usually know how many eggs were successfully fertilized.

Only two to three days after the eggs are fertilized, it's time for implantation of the fertilized eggs (or pre-embryos) in your uterus. This is a simple procedure and takes only about ten minutes. It's similar to the egg retrieval process. The eggs are sucked up into a long, slim catheter which is then inserted through your vagina up to your uterine entrance. The eggs are then released into your uterus. For about 12 days to two weeks after this, it's another waiting game; you'll take both estrogen and progesterone while you wait to see if one or more of the eggs has successfully implanted into your uterine lining. If everything works well, you will be pregnant, and you'll stay on both estrogen and progesterone for the first trimester of your pregnancy.

If for some reason you don't get pregnant, you have another option. Usually the reproductive center will freeze any unused fertilized eggs from your donor egg cycle, so you can have these eggs thawed and used later. However, there is a bit of a downside: typically there is a higher success rate with a fresh transfer than a frozen.

SURROGACY: USING A SURROGATE MOTHER
TO HAVE A CHILD

Another option for building a family when you are in premature menopause is for a surrogate mother both to provide an egg and carry the child to term. Since egg donation is the usual choice of women who have uteruses, this option is usually considered primarily by women who are in premature menopause due to a complete hysterectomy and oophorectomy.

Just as with egg donation, using a surrogate mother gives you the opportunity to have a child who is genetically related to your partner. His sperm can be used to artificially inseminate a surrogate who will carry the fertilized egg through the pregnancy. As you might expect, the success rates for surrogacy vary widely, depending on both your partner's and the surrogate's fertility.

You can use either a known surrogate, typically a relative, or an anonymous surrogate arranged for either privately or through surrogate programs. If you opt for an anonymous surrogate, you may or may not have contact with her, depending upon the program you're in. Different surrogacy programs have different rules about this. In some cases, you'll be given her personal history, but never meet her; in others, you can interact with her throughout the pregnancy; and others maintain total confidentiality—you know nothing about the surrogate other than the fact that she is carrying your child.

Although there aren't set guidelines as with donor eggs, there are general rules that most surrogacy programs will follow in choosing a surrogate. A surrogate will be a younger woman (again, typically no older than 35), one who has already successfully gone through at least one full-term pregnancy, and one who passes certain health standards such as no smoking, drinking, or drug use. The surrogate should be screened for infectious diseases and any other medical disorders, should undergo a thorough physical examination, and—something that is very important in this scenario—should also undergo psychological evaluation. This is particularly important because, unlike an egg donor, a surrogate mother will carry a child for the entire pregnancy.

By the same token, it's highly recommended that you and your partner also be sure that surrogacy is a method you can handle. There are a great deal of emotional and psychological issues involved in this method—and it's wise to be sure before you proceed that you fully understand them. There also have been controversies associated with surrogacies including several well-publicized cases in which surrogates sued to keep the children they carried. For this reason, it's vital you also understand any legal ramifications as well.

What Is Involved

All in all, this process is a bit less technical than donor eggs, chiefly because the surrogate mother will be using her own eggs, which means there is no *in vitro* fertilization involved. Because you aren't involved biologically, you won't require any physical testing or follow any procedures. Instead both the surrogate and your partner (if his sperm will be used) undergo thorough testing.

The surrogate's reproductive cycle will be tracked, and near the time of her ovulation, she will be inseminated with your partner's sperm. And if the egg is successfully fertilized and all goes well, she will carry the baby until birth.

EXPERIMENTAL ATTEMPTS TO REVERSE PREMATURE MENOPAUSE

If you are in premature menopause and still have ovaries, there may be a chance—a slim chance—that you can ovulate and get pregnant with your own eggs.

More doctors have been exploring ways of either inducing ovulation or suppressing premature ovarian failure in prematurely menopausal women who have working ovaries. If you're prematurely menopausal, your ovaries aren't working, but some doctors claim that some women may have a chance to get their ovaries working again, at least temporarily.

Here's why. According to several studies, the pelvic ultrasounds of about 40 percent of women with premature ovarian failure show what appear to be viable ovarian follicles. In other words, they do have eggs in their ovaries. So the question is: What can be done to stimulate the follicles and cause ovulation in these women?

Many researchers believe that it shouldn't be an impossibility. As mentioned earlier in this chapter, some women in premature menopause spontaneously ovulate with no intervention whatsoever or while on estrogen. But this is unpredictable and, unfortunately, uncommon. The goal of the researchers, of course, is making ovulation controllable, predictable, and, if not common, at least more common.

But there is bad news: so far, the different methods briefly explained below haven't had a great success rate—at least none that has been proven by controlled studies. Some researchers point out that the success rate may be just the same as getting pregnant with no procedure. Others, though, claim that they have been more successful, and that pregnancy is more common than the naysayers are willing to admit. While no controlled studies have proven that these methods work, anecdotal reports suggest otherwise, they say.

In truth, the jury is definitely out.

However, if you are in premature menopause, have ovaries, and want a child, you may want to explore these different methods. Do keep in mind that these are experimental treatments, so there's little way of knowing how well they work. In addition, treatment may be costly, physically taxing, and emotionally draining. Furthermore, many reproductive endocrinologists or ob/gyns won't offer these treatments. If you are interested in pursuing these, your best bet is to check for clinical research studies or specific doctors who specialize in experimental infertility treatments.

A few important points:

- *You may have a better chance if you receive treatment early on*—Some doctors believe that your chances of pregnancy decrease the longer you are in menopause and advise women who want to get pregnant to explore infertility treatments as soon as possible. This is because you may still have eggs in your ovaries, and your hormone levels may still be only on the borderline or may periodically bounce back into the normal ranges. Again, however, this doesn't necessarily mean you will be able to ovulate.

- *You will probably be tested to see if you have viable follicles*—You may need to have a pelvic ultrasound so the doctor can take a look at your ovaries. In addition, you may have to have your hormone levels measured two to four times.

- *It is also important to be tested for an autoimmune disorders*—Researchers recommend a "double bridged enzyme linked immunosorbent assay," or more simply ELISA, as a way of screening which women with premature ovarian failure may respond well to temporary treatments. In addition, some doctors recommend that you have skin tests for estradiol, progesterone, and hCG as well.

Ovulation Induction through Fertility Drugs

This is an area that has been explored for years. But so far, attempting to get a woman with premature ovarian failure to ovulate by giving her hormones or fertility drugs has met with very limited success. This sort of treatment has resulted in ovulation, but the ovulation has been unpredictable and not all that common. Researchers continue to explore different methods, doses, and procedures, hoping to come up with a more consistently successful treatment.

At this point, it appears that you have a better chance of ovulation induction if:

- your LH levels are higher than your FSH levels; and/or
- your estradiol levels are higher than 40 pg/ml.

Most commonly, a doctor who tries to get you to ovulate will put you on estradiol plus fertility drugs such as Clomid and Humegon. Several doctors have claimed that this works; however, the successes reported by this method are anecdotal.

Studies have also been conducted using growth-hormone-releasing hormone. In one successful case, a 29-year-old woman, who had failed to ovulate on human menopausal gonadotropin and FSH, ovulated after growth-hormone-releasing hormone was administered. Other methods that have been tried but haven't been proven to work include gonadotropin-releasing hormone (GnRH), human menopausal gonadotropins (hMG), and Danazol.

On the bright side, as research continues in this area, infertility experts hope to develop a successful approach to inducing ovulation in prematurely menopausal women in the near future.

Autoimmune Suppression: Treating the Underlying Autoimmune Disease to Temporarily Reverse Premature Ovarian Failure

Autoimmune suppression is a newer method of enabling a woman to ovulate and get pregnant even if she has been diagnosed with premature ovarian failure. This method has received a great deal of attention, some positive, some negative.

The theory behind this is fairly simple: if a woman has gone through premature menopause due to ovarian failure brought about by an autoimmune disorder, then it might be possible to suppress the autoimmune disorder and so temporarily reverse the ovarian failure, allowing the woman to ovulate and get pregnant.

As you would expect, the first step in undergoing this approach is to determine if an autoimmune disorder is indeed the cause of your ovarian failure. You undergo autoimmune testing (the ELISA, as mentioned above, or, depending upon your family history and own medical history, other immunological testing). If these tests are positive, then the hope for temporarily reversing your ovarian shutdown and restoring them to normal function lies in suppressing the autoimmune response in your body.

To do this, you are put on a high daily dose of prednisone, a corticosteroid, to kill the autoantibodies that are preventing you from ovulating. This is designed to put your premature ovarian failure into remission, so enabling you to ovulate. Several doctors have claimed a very high success rate with this treatment. However, the results have not been subject to a double-blind research study comparing the results with those of women on placebos. In addition, there is another problem to be aware of: the high doses of prednisone you need to take over a long period can cause a number of serious side effects, including necrosis of the bones.

The National Institutes of Health have been conducting a clinical research study to determine if a lower-dose, shorter-term, alternate-day prednisone therapy would enable a woman to ovulate, while avoiding those health risks. As of this writing, however, the results of the study were not available. For more information on this study, you can contact:

PATIENT RECRUITMENT AND REFERRAL SERVICE, CC
Quarters 15D-2, 4 West Drive MSC2655
Bethesda, Maryland 20892–2655
301/496–4891
800/411–1222
Fax: 301/480–9793
E-mail: prrc@cc.nih.gov

Ovarian Tissue Transplant

This is a very new—and highly experimental—treatment, one that some reproductive specialists believe may be a break-through. But, as of this writing, the jury was still out.

The theory behind ovarian tissue transplanting is relatively straightforward: if you have still-healthy ovarian tissue—that is, ovarian tissue that is still generating hormones and containing viable eggs—it can be surgically removed and preserved. Then, later, it can be reimplanted into your pelvis to take over for the ovaries that may have been damaged because of chemotherapy or other treatments, ovaries that were surgically removed, or ovaries that have failed due to premature ovarian failure. The key, of course, is in having ovarian tissue removed *before* you undergo ovarian failure, whether naturally, due to surgery or cancer treatments. It is hoped that by implanting the frozen healthy ovarian tissue, a woman will begin to generate the normal level of hormones (and so not suffer from menopausal symptoms), and may even produce viable eggs—that could be used in in vitro fertilization . . . allowing her to become pregnant with her own egg.

In February 1999, the first ovarian tissue transplant was performed in the United States and it was unclear as to how successful the procedure would turn out to be in terms of restoring fertility. Briefly put, a young woman who had lost first one ovary, and was due to lose her second to surgery due to a non-cancerous pelvic disease had ovarian tissue removed and cryogenically preserved before removal of the second ovary. A reproductive endocrinologist and surgeon tested the frozen ovarian tissue and, finding that some of the tissue was still producing hormones and also contained viable eggs, surgically reimplanted the tissue in her pelvis—in the hopes that it would continue to generate hormones . . . and eggs. At the time of writing, it was impossible to determine whether the procedure had worked, since it takes about six months for eggs to grow. However, many doctors felt that the procedure appeared very promising—and could signal a breakthrough, especially for women with still working ovaries who would have to undergo chemotherapy or radiation treatments that destroy the ovaries. On the flip side, though, other doctors were more cautious, pointing out that the real test was whether normal blood supply would be restored to the implanted ovarian tissue—and whether the new tissue would generate enough hormones.

So the jury is definitely still out—but, even if this particular procedure fails to work as well as hoped, it is an area that should see continued research over the near future.

ADOPTION

I have finally come to terms with all my issues about not being able to have a biological child of my own, and now my husband and I are ready to proceed with adoption. It took me a while before I felt I could actually handle this course of action, but I know it's the right time now. We've gone to several agency meetings to see what they were like and have decided to look for a private adoption. We've already begun dealing with a ton of paperwork, are talking with some adoption lawyers, and hope to find a birth mother within the next year.
—Leah, age 27

We will definitely adopt! We haven't begun researching it because at the moment we are happy devoting all of our time to each other. We both *love* children and look forward to being parents one day.
—Steph, age 28

Another way to have the family you have dreamed about is to adopt. This is a very popular choice among prematurely menopausal women. While it is often difficult to come to terms with the fact that you can't have a biological child, you may find that adoption is the answer to your prayers. Many women say they find great comfort in the thought that they will be a mother to a child who doesn't have one of her own.

Of course, deciding to adopt is a serious decision and one you shouldn't undertake lightly. As is the case with assisted reproduction, you need to take time to think about this choice and to be sure you are ready to make the step.

If you are interested in exploring adoption, the best thing you can do is to start researching it to learn exactly what is entailed. There are a number of excellent sources available to you. Adoption associations and organizations offer general information about adoption, as well as providing directories to agencies and other groups. You can call them or check their Web sites for extensive information on line. Two good bets are:

* *Adoptive Families of America* (612/535–4829 or 800/372–3300; www.adoptivefam.org);
* *National Adoption Information Clearinghouse* (703/352–3488 or 888/251–0075; www.calib.com/naic).

The Internet in general is a wonderful place to begin exploring adoption. There are numerous support groups, message boards, and organizations on line that can offer you information, referrals, and leads. Support groups and message boards are particularly helpful, because they give you the opportunity to speak with other people like you—people looking to adopt a child, or thinking about it—and can give you real insight into the personal side of things.

There are several excellent books that cover adoption in general, as well as those that focus on specific areas such as international adoption. These can give you an in-depth look at both the practical and emotional side of adoption and help you with your initial decision about adoption, as well as telling you the best ways to proceed and negotiate your way through the adoption process.

The Different Ways to Adopt

If you decide that adoption is right for you, you face another decision: How do you go about it? There are several options open to you: private agencies, public agencies, private adoption, international adoption. Here is a quick rundown of these different options to help you better understand your choices.

ADOPTION AGENCIES

Using an adoption agency is the most traditional way of going about adoption, and still the most popular method used. But all agencies are not created equal. First, there are two basic types of agency: public and private.

Public adoption agencies are state-run agencies. Generally, each state has a number of these agencies. Typically, they have children who were taken from their biological parents due to abuse or neglect. Most state agencies are less likely than private agencies to have infants and usually more likely to have children with special needs, as well as older children. While public adoption agencies are usually cheaper than private agencies, you often have a longer wait for a child.

Private adoption agencies, as you would expect, are run by private organizations, but are licensed by the state. Because they are private, they can vary greatly. A private agency can be non-profit or for-profit; large or small; traditional or less traditional. Some are geared more to specific groups such as single mothers or gay couples; others are less open to anything but the most traditional couple (working husband and stay-at-home wife). Because of this wide range, you need to research individual agencies to be sure you have found one that will work well with you. Your best bet is to attend meetings the agency holds; call and ask for literature; and, if possible, speak with other people who have used the agency. Private agencies are more likely to have babies than public agencies, but they also usually cost much more.

Whichever type of adoption agency you choose, you will go through a similar procedure. First, you will have to fill out an application and go in for an initial screening interview. Many agencies will decide whether or not you can proceed with them based only on these two elements. If you aren't turned down, you next go through a "home study"—you supply the agency with extensive information about you and your husband, including medical history, employment background, financial status, and information on your marriage, how you feel about parenting, why you are adopting, and what kind of child you would like to adopt. You often also have to write a biographical statement about your life from childhood on, and give the agency recommendation letters from references. Next comes a series of interviews, both as a couple and individually, in which a social worker evaluates you as prospective parents, and usually a final interview in your home, so the social worker can get an idea of how you live and whether your home is suited for a child. Once you have gone through this, you will finally learn if you have been approved, and then begins the wait for the agency to provide you with a child. You may have to wait a long time, depending upon what you told the agency you were looking for in a child. For example, waits for infants are often much longer than for older children. Once the agency has found the "right" child for you, you meet again with the agency workers to learn about the child and often to meet the child. If all goes well, you meet with the child a few more times, then he or she is finally placed with you—in other words, you can take the child to his or her new home. It's still not legal, though; you still have to go through the formal court proceedings to finalize the adoption, a process that can take as much as six months or more.

PRIVATE (OR INDEPENDENT) ADOPTION

To put it as simply as possible, a private adoption is an adoption conducted outside the agency system: you or your lawyer finds a child who is up for adoption, you set up a preadoption agreement; and finally, the child is placed with you and you go through formal adoption proceedings.

There is, of course, more to the process than that. To begin with, although it is a private adoption, most states require a "home study" in which a social worker interviews the prospective adoptive parents in their home, and most birth parents will not consider adoption until they see a home study as well. There also is a lot involved in finding a child to adopt. While an agency provides the child for you, in private adoption, it is up to you. Many people use their adoption lawyer to locate a child; others hire adoption facilitators—people who help put birth mothers together with adoptive couples; others advertise.

Because there are many legal aspects to private adoption (ones that an agency takes care of in an agency adoption), you need to find a lawyer who specializes in private adoption. To do this, you can ask for referrals, check with adoption support groups, and contact the American Academy of Adoption Attorneys (202/832–2222) for names.

Private adoption is, in some ways, more difficult than agency adoption. It can be complex and time-consuming, as well as costly, since you usually have to cover medical care and legal costs for the birth mother. And, of course, there have been cases where the birth mother changes her mind and, after all the time and effort, the adoption doesn't go through. But there are also many advantages to this method. It is sometimes the only option open to people who have been rejected by agencies. It is often quicker than going through an agency. Finally, it is probably your best chance at getting a baby, as opposed to an older child.

INTERNATIONAL ADOPTION

International adoption is an option that is becoming more popular, particularly because it is so difficult to get an infant domestically. But it is also a great choice for nontraditional adoptive parents such as singles, gay couples, older couples, or those who have been rejected by agencies.

There is no set way of arranging an international adoption. It can be done privately, through an agency, or even a little bit of both, by using a private agency for assistance in some aspects of the adoption but doing the rest on your own. In addition, different countries have different criteria.

If you are adopting internationally through an agency, you will have a home study to evaluate your fitness as a parent just as you would in a domestic adoption. Once you are approved, though, you have to file papers with the Immigration and Naturalization Service (INS) and wait for approval by the government. The agency then finds you a child and you have to be approved yet again, this time for that specific child. Next, the agency handles the legal matters necessary for the foreign country to give approval for the adoption. Once this is completed, you file another INS form and apply for a visa for the child, as well as for citizenship. And, finally, after this time-consuming process is complete, you will be able to take the child home.

Private international adoption is usually more difficult than agency adoption. You need to find the child on your own and make all legal arrangements with both your state and the country from which you are planning to adopt. Usually you will need both a foreign contact to help you locate the child, and a foreign lawyer to handle all the legal aspects of the adoption in the country from which you intend to adopt. As with agency adoption, you will need to file the pertinent forms with the U.S. government—getting approval for the adoption, getting a visa, and filing a citizenship request. Because there is so much involved in private international adoption, your best bet is to contact support groups for independent international adoptive parents, such as Americans Adopting Orphans (206/524–5437; www.orphans.com).

Chapter 9

Taking Charge of Your Body through Diet and Exercise

> One of the things that was extremely upsetting about pre-
> mature menopause was the changes in my body. I'm not
> talking about the hot flashes or the night sweats now, but
> the *visible* changes—weight gain, a thicker waistline, more
> fat through my midsection, the loss of elasticity in my
> skin. It was bad enough knowing that my reproductive
> system was acting as if I were 30 years older; it was even
> worse thinking that I would be stuck looking older as
> well—that I would be a walking advertisement for prema-
> ture menopause. But then I learned that premature meno-
> pause didn't have to mean premature aging—that there
> were actions I could take that would reverse the negative
> effects of premature menopause and make me look (and
> feel) my age again. What a relief. . . .

As if you don't have enough to cope with when you're going
through premature menopause—the knowledge that your reproductive system is effectively shutting down, the emotional ups
and downs, the mood swings, hot flashes, insomnia, and all the
other symptoms—you also have to face another distressing reality: more often than not, you're beginning to look different.
Your body's appearance is changing as your reproductive system changes.

You might not notice it initially because the changes are slow. In my case, the changes occurred over several years before I even knew I was entering premature menopause. Over time, I noticed that my waistline seemed to be, well, disappearing. My tummy, which I had religiously put through hundreds of crunches and situps a day, was rounding. I was putting on weight without changing my eating or exercise habits. Worse, people were telling me I looked older. And when I looked in the mirror, I had to agree with them.

I couldn't figure out what was going on.

Only when I learned that I had been going through perimenopause in my early thirties did the scenario begin to make sense. Suddenly there was a reason for the changes I had noticed: lagging estrogen levels were causing the weight gain, the thinner skin, the shift in body fat.

But being in premature menopause doesn't mean you have to resign yourself to looker older or different. You can fight the effects of menopause on your body. You can keep your body looking your chronological age even when your hormones have essentially fast-forwarded to the age of 50. To a great degree, going on HRT will most definitely help reverse the effects of menopause. But in addition to this, it's a matter of diet and exercise.

Perhaps you've always followed a good diet and exercise regularly. That's great, but with premature menopause, you may want to adjust your regimens somewhat to be sure you're getting the maximum benefit. And if you're not the most healthy eater or if you exercise rarely, then this is the time to start a new nutrition and exercise program—specifically geared to help reverse the effects of premature menopause, to help cope with your changing body, to work with other therapies you're using, and to help stave off the unpleasant side effects of menopause as well as the health risks of osteoporosis and coronary heart disease.

This chapter discusses the nutritional and exercise programs you can follow to jump-start your metabolism and keep your weight down, your muscles toned, and your body looking and feeling great.

By coping with premature menopause through diet and exercise, you can be healthier than you've ever been. In an odd way, premature menopause can become a positive in your life— it can be the catalyst that launches you into a healthier lifestyle and a healthier you.

YOUR NEW BODY: HOW PREMATURE MENOPAUSE CAN CHANGE YOUR BODY AND WHAT YOU CAN DO ABOUT IT

Let's start with something that drives me and many other women in premature menopause crazy: many books and articles insist that women put on weight during menopause because they're older. It's not a function of menopause, they argue. It's a function of aging. Your metabolic rate drops as you age, which accounts for the weight gain. In addition, older women are often more inactive.

Well, perhaps this applies to the average woman in menopause who is in her fifties. But what if you're in your twenties or thirties—and you start noticing the creeping weight gain and new thicker body contours?

Dozens of prematurely menopausal women I've spoken with have seen it happen to them. They're not middle-aged. They're still young. So, regardless of what the books say, it can't be age that causes these changes. And it isn't. It's *menopause*, plain and simple.

It doesn't happen to everyone, but here are some of the changes that are common to women in premature menopause:

- *Weight gain*—with no change in your diet or exercise habits.
- *Change in your body fat distribution from a "pear" to an "apple"*—weight shifts from your hips, thighs, and buttocks to your abdomen.

- *Rounder stomach*—in line with the above shift in fat distribution.
- *Disappearing waistline*—again, part of the change in body fat distribution.
- *Dry skin with a crepey, thinner texture*—especially apparent around your mouth and eyes.
- *Loss of muscle tone and skin elasticity*—sagginess in your skin, often apparent in your face, stomach, around your knees, and so on.
- *Saggy, droopy breasts*

These changes are not life-threatening but they do affect your ego at a time when you least need it. They also affect older women in menopause, of course, but it's often worse for women in premature menopause. The biggest difference? When you're in premature menopause, the changes in your appearance are often more apparent than the changes an older woman in menopause goes through (especially to you), simply because most other women your age aren't experiencing the same thing. Other women in their twenties and thirties aren't getting the so-called "middle-aged spread" that women in their fifties experience, but you are. Other women your age aren't suddenly discovering that the skin around their eyes is beginning to look thinner and more crepey, much like that of an older woman. And other women your age aren't noticing that weight is piling up.

> **I have had weight gain, and of course it is in my tummy. Makes me look like I am pregnant. Why there? So people can ask: Are you pregnant? and then you have a reason to tell them your sob story about being in meno at this early age. They have no clue about it and how hard it is for you.**
>
> **—Stacey, age 33**

The key culprit, as you may have guessed, is your hormone levels. Many of the body changes women go through during menopause appear to be directly linked to low estrogen levels. Others are linked to progesterone levels. And still others may be an offshoot of the emotional ups-and-downs you're going through as a result of changing hormone levels.

More specifically, as stated earlier in this book, lower levels of estrogen may cause a variety of physical side effects. First, because estrogen is stored in fat, many researchers believe that when you enter menopause, whether naturally or through surgery, your body responds by holding onto fat cells in an effort to boost the lagging estrogen levels. The result? It's tougher to lose fat and much easier to keep the pounds on.

Second, as estrogen levels drop, your level of androgens, the so-called "male" hormones, increases in relation to the estrogen. Unopposed by the higher levels of estrogen your body used to have, the androgens produce male characteristics—in this case, the shift in body fat from your hips, thighs, and buttocks to your midsection, resulting in the "apple" shape that is more common in men and in postmenopausal women, and incidently, also increases your risk of heart disease.

Third, low estrogen levels affect the production of collagen, which results in drier, thinner skin, sagginess of tissue, and lack of muscle tone.

Low progesterone levels in relation to estrogen, which is popularly called "estrogen dominance," also cause a number of side effects. Among the more common ones are increased bloating and water retention, which may not be actual fat, but makes you look heavier, and blood sugar fluctuations, which can increase your appetite and slow your metabolism.

Finally, there's the mood connection. As you know, declining hormone levels can cause mood swings, depression, and anxiety. This is because the levels of serotonins and endorphins in your brain apparently drop in the face of fluctuating hormones. What raises serotonin levels in your brain? Certain foods such as chocolate. When you go through premature menopause, you may notice you have food cravings, much as you did when you had PMS. But unlike PMS, your hormones don't bounce back to regular levels, so you may have food cravings longer than in the past, and you may cave in and eat more of the foods you shouldn't, such as fats, salty snacks, and sweets.

Regardless of what some people have claimed, then, there does appear to be a biological basis for the changes in your body. It's not in your mind; it's in your hormones.

So that's the bad news. But all is most definitely not lost! There are three things you can do to help fight the changes in your body brought on by changing hormone levels:

1. Raise your hormone levels through HRT and/or natural supplements.

2. Eat correctly.

3. Exercise regularly.

It's a simple prescription, and one that makes a difference. Since HRT and natural supplements have already been examined in previous chapters, this chapter will focus on the nutrition and exercise plans that can turn back the clock for your body. And as an added plus, by switching to healthy eating and exercise habits now, you'll not only regain your premenopausal body, you'll also get in the habit of healthy living for the years to come.

EATING WELL, EATING HEALTHY: GOOD EATING IS MORE IMPORTANT THAN EVER

By following basic rules of healthy eating, you can rev up your metabolism, protect your body against such menopausal-related diseases like osteoporosis and heart disease, and level your moods. You will be on the track to a healthier, slimmer, leaner body not only now, but for the rest of your life. Best of all, it's easy to eat well. It just takes a little knowledge, a little forethought, and a little discipline.

The most important point to make is that eating well and, incidently, eating to lose weight and keep your body looking its best, doesn't mean dieting. It should be a lifestyle change, not a quick-fix crash diet. It's basically a matter of opting for nutrient-rich, lower-calorie foods, cutting down on saturated fats and empty calories (like sugar and alcohol), and getting enough of the nutrients that make a difference to a menopausal body.

To get you started, here are the rules to follow:

Rule #1: Think Low Fat to Keep Your Weight Down and to Cut Down on the Risk of Disease

This is one of the best things you can do for the overall health of your body. First, as you know, premature menopause increases your risk of heart disease. By cutting down on fat, you can help shift the odds in your favor and help prevent heart disease. Saturated fats raise your blood cholesterol level, so a low-fat diet will help you keep your cholesterol levels down. A low-fat diet also appears to help prevent cancer. If you're on HRT and concerned about breast cancer, this is particularly important, as studies have indicated that both breast and ovarian cancers are linked to a high-fat diet, particularly one high in fats from dairy foods such as butter and whole milk products.

As for weight control, cutting down on fat is a definite help. More often than not, high-fat foods are also high-calorie foods, which certainly don't help you keep your weight down. Typically one gram of fat has over twice the calories as a gram of protein. And not only is fat usually more caloric, it also converts quickly and easily to body fat.

But don't think that you have to go crazy and cut all fats from your diet. Recent studies have indicated that an extremely low-fat diet may be harmful to your health. Your best course of action? Be aware of fats; opt for lower-fat foods; and cut saturated fat from your diet.

Rule #2: Keep Your Fiber Intake Up

Fiber is your friend when it comes to healthy eating. It fills you up, keeps your digestive tract healthy, and helps you eliminate some of the fats you eat. In addition, it can help prevent certain types of cancer and lower your cholesterol. You need both insoluble and soluble fiber. Insoluble fiber helps keep your

elimination regular and helps protect against cancers of your
intestinal tract. Foods high in insoluble fiber include *whole
grains, fruits, and vegetables.* Soluble fiber keeps your blood
sugar levels stable, and is metabolized slowly, a real help in
keeping from overeating. Foods high in soluble fiber include
apples, barley, beans, flaxseed, prunes, rolled oats, oat bran.

Rule #3: Be Sure to Get as Much Calcium as Possible

You already know that you're at a great risk for osteoporosis,
so calcium is a must in a good premature menopause diet. Low-
fat dairy products supply you with calcium along with needed
protein, and keep your bones strong without adding too much
fat. And calcium-rich vegetables, such as broccoli, are another
excellent source. In fact, recent studies have indicated that non-
dairy calcium foods may provide the body with more bio-available
calcium than dairy products.

Rule #4: Don't Forget Protein for Overall Health and Weight Loss

Protein can help you build your body and burn calories—quite
an effective one-two punch! But all too often, especially recently, people tend to overlook the benefits of protein, especially
as a way of keeping weight in check.

In recent years, the emphasis has been on high-carbohydrate
eating. Books and doctors extolled the virtues of carbs and
claimed that a high-carbo diet was the best thing for you. But
the pendulum is shifting back, and more books have been coming out asserting that high-protein/low-carb is the way to go.

Regardless of whom you believe, there is no question that
protein is a necessity in your diet. It is made from amino acids,
some of which your body makes and others of which you can
get only by eating protein. It is, in one form or another, present
in every cell of your body. It makes, maintains, and repairs
cells—from muscle to other tissues. It is a crucial ingredient in
everything from your bones to your hair, and makes up such
vital substances as hormones (such as insulin) and disease-
fighting antibodies.

It's clear, then, that protein is a must in anyone's diet. But it's especially important if you're going through premature menopause, and here's the big reason why—*you can actually jump-start your metabolism with protein.* Protein's thermic effect is higher than that of carbohydrates or fats. In other words, you burn more calories when you digest a high-protein meal than one high in fats or carbs. So you're getting more bang for your buck when you eat protein. One other big plus: because it is used in the manufacture of insulin, protein helps keep blood-sugar levels stable, which helps in preventing both mood swings and food cravings.

Rule #5: It May Be Easier to Add or Keep Weight On, So Keep an Eye on Calories

For a while there, it seemed as though everyone forgot about calories. Articles, books, and nutrition experts were focusing on low-fat eating as a way of keeping your weight down. Well, that is true to a large degree; higher-fat foods do usually help you pack on the pounds, especially because they're usually higher in calories!

It's a simple scenario: calories are energy units. They're what your body burns as fuel, and if you take in more calories than you burn, you gain weight. It's that simple. On the whole, it doesn't matter if they're "good" calories or "bad" (although some nutritionists believe it's easier to pack on pounds if you eat too many carbohydrates because it affects your insulin levels). But on the simplest level, if you're trying not to gain weight, you have to burn the calories you eat, so make sure you don't take in too many calories in the course of a day's eating.

How much is too much? It really depends on the individual—your height and weight, your body build, your fitness level, and how active you are. But it's good to keep in mind that only 3500 calories add up to one pound of added weight, and those 3500 calories can add up over time, especially if you're not exercising.

So calories count, but (here's the good news!) you don't have to count calories. If you follow the good eating guidelines

QUICK, TRIED-AND-TRUE WAYS OF CUTTING CALORIES THE HEALTHY WAY

- *Eat fewer fats*—A gram of fat is higher in calories than either protein or carbohydrates, so if you cut down on fats, you're usually cutting down on the most caloric foods.

- *Increase your fiber intake*—Not only is fiber good for your digestive system, it fills you up so you're not tempted to eat more. An added plus is that high-fiber foods such as whole grains, fruits, and vegetables are packed with nutrients and naturally low in fat.

- *Try to eat more before 5:00 PM—and nothing after 8:00 PM*—Many studies have shown you're best off eating large meals earlier in the day. You're more active, so you can burn off some of the calories you've taken in. In fact, to put it more scientifically, many studies have shown that it takes about four hours after eating for your blood triglyceride levels to rise. So if you have a large dinner at 7:00 or so, your triglycerides will hit their height at 11:00, just as you're going to bed or lying on the couch watching television, which means you'll probably store them as fat.

- *Drink water whenever you can remember to, and definitely before meals*—Water not only is good for your system, it also fills you up, so you'll eat a little less.

- *Stay active*—Exercise will burn calories and increase muscle mass, which burns more calories than fat.

included in this section, you're well on your way to keeping your calorie intake in check painlessly.

Rule #6: Finally, Give In to Your Cravings a Little
Eating well and healthily doesn't have to mean depriving yourself. You are going through premature menopause so you have a lot going on already—there's no need to punish yourself.

Often allowing yourself a little something you crave can help you keep eating properly.

For example, according to several surveys, chocolate is the number one food craved by women with PMS and women in menopause. A key reason? It increases the levels of serotonin and endorphins in your brain, making you feel better. So having a little chocolate may help you stabilize your moods and chase away the blues, which is well worth the small amount of fat and sugar you're eating. Of course, you shouldn't overdo it.

Good Food Choices for Good Health

To keep you in line with the rules listed above, here is a quick rundown of the types of food that can do the most for you, and how they fit into your premature menopause diet.

WHOLE GRAINS: HIGH-ENERGY AND FIBER-RICH FOOD

Whole grains offer you the carbohydrates your body needs for energy, plus high fiber, and, as a great added bonus, they taste great!

More specifically, whole grains are one of the best forms of *complex carbohydrates* you can eat. In comparison with simple carbohydrates (essentially sugars, including refined sugar, honey, molasses, or fruit), complex carbohydrates are metabolized more slowly, circumventing the sugar-rush-then-crash you often get with simple carbs. And when you opt for whole grains as opposed to refined complex carbs such as white bread or white rice, you also get a great deal of fiber.

This combination of slow metabolization, high fiber, and the good "mouth" feel of carbohydrates makes whole grains a wonderful choice when you're in premature menopause. The fiber in whole grains can help you keep your weight down. It fills you up quickly and keeps you feeling satisfied for a longer time than other foods, which is a definite plus when you're trying to avoid overeating.

How can you get more whole-grain fiber into your diet without much of an effort? The general rule of thumb is to go with the darker starches. In other words, switch from white flour to whole wheat in baking. Eat whole-grain breads instead of white breads, whole-grain crackers instead of refined processed ones. Opt for brown rice instead of white rice, and whole wheat pasta instead of regular. And be sure to read labels: sometimes processed foods such as breads and crackers that you think are whole grains aren't.

Good sources of whole grains include *whole wheat, rye, barley, millet, buckwheat, quinoa, rolled oats* (not instant oats), *polenta, kasha, corn, brown rice.*

One warning, however: a number of women may be allergic to whole wheat and may suffer from bloating and digestive problems. If you notice this sort of effect, it's a good idea to stick with the other whole grains instead.

FRUITS AND VEGETABLES: VITAMINS, FIBER, AND CARBS ALL IN ONE

Fruits and vegetables offer a lot: they're nature's way of providing you with needed vitamins and nutrients; they're high in carbs to give you energy; many are low in calories, and they're all low in fat. And since fruits are sweet and contain fruit sugar (which is metabolized more slowly than refined sugars), you can eat fruit to satisfy your sweet tooth and get vitamins and minerals at the same time.

Different fruits and vegetables offer different positive benefits, so it's important to eat a variety. Here are a few specific benefits you can get from fruits and vegetables. This isn't a comprehensive list, just a brief rundown to give you an idea of the many benefits you can get by making fruits and vegetables an important part of your diet.

Many fruits and vegetables contain high amounts of potassium, a mineral that assists in lowering blood pressure, which is particularly helpful when you're on HRT. *Bananas* are particularly high in potassium, as are a number of other fruits. On the vegetable side, other good sources include *beans, leafy greens, potatoes,* and *squashes.*

Cruciferous vegetables are also important. These are vegetables in the cabbage family that contain phytochemicals called indoles that protect against cancer. The vegetable highest in indoles is *broccoli;* other good choices include *Brussels sprouts, cabbage, cauliflower,* and *kale.*

You also should eat vegetables that are naturally high in vitamin A, which has been shown to help prevent cancer, including breast and cervical cancer, and immune deficiencies. In this case, the easy tip-off that a vegetable is high in vitamin A is its color. Most vitamin-A-rich vegetables are yellow, orange, red, or dark green. Good choices in this family include *carrots, dark-green lettuces* (such as *romaine* or *green leaf), kale, peppers, squash,* and *sweet potatoes.*

Vitamin-C-rich fruits and vegetables are a good choice because vitamin C can help with hot flashes, protect against cancer, and may prevent excessive bleeding. Good choices include *apricots, berries, broccoli, Brussels sprouts, cabbage, cauliflower, citrus fruits, melons, peas, peppers, potatoes,* and *tomatoes.*

Calcium, magnesium, and iron are important for a woman in premature menopause; you can get these naturally from eating *leafy green vegetables.*

Many fruits and vegetables are also great sources of soluble fiber, which helps keep your blood sugar stable and can help with food cravings, mood swings, and weight control. Good sources of this include *apples, prunes,* and *beans.*

Finally, to help keep your cholesterol levels down, opt for *onions* and *garlic.*

LEAN PROTEIN FOR A LEANER YOU

As mentioned before, protein not only gives your body necessary amino acids that it can't make on its own, it's also a help in losing weight or in keeping weight down. But, unfortunately, many foods that are high in protein, such as red meat, are also high in fats. In addition, certain studies have shown that animal protein may increase the risk of heart disease and can leach calcium from your system.

But you can and should still get the benefits of protein in your diet. It's simply a matter of choosing the right protein.

First, let's tackle these negatives head-on. Red meats and high-fat dairy products do have high levels of saturated fat; but you can get around this problem by opting for lower-fat meats or by choosing plant proteins instead. As for the calcium-leaching problem, many studies have indicated that the actual amount of calcium lost from your body is relatively low. As long as you are getting enough calcium, either through your diet or through supplementation, this shouldn't be a problem.

So how can you get the protein you need while still avoiding saturated fats?

It's not as difficult as you might think. Animal proteins can be a good choice. They're complete proteins, which means they contain all of the essential amino acids. Good sources of protein are *low-fat and nonfat milk* and *dairy products* such as *cottage cheese, low-fat* or *nonfat yogurt, reduced fat cheeses* (all of which pack a double-punch since they're high in calcium as well); *chicken and other poultry* (preferably skinless and white meat), *fish; lean meats* (as long as you remember that a little red meat goes a long way, since it is higher in fat than other sources of protein). As for meats, you can eat them in moderation as long as you look for cuts that aren't too fatty. Your best bets? Opt for meats graded "select," choose lean cuts such as sirloin, loin, round, and leg, trim fat before cooking, and eat smaller portions. In addition, to avoid the possibility of getting too many xenoestrogens and other xenobiotics, you may want to choose organic or natural meats and dairy products.

Another good source of protein without the negative of saturated fat is plant proteins. These are "incomplete" proteins—in other words, they don't supply all of the amino acids you need—but if you combine plant proteins, that is, eat different ones throughout the day, you can get all the protein you need. Good sources of plant protein are *dried cooked legumes* (beans, peas, and lentils); *nuts* (also a great source of magnesium, calcium, and potassium) and *seeds; tempeh, tofu, and other soy products* (also a good choice because of the phytoestrogens they contain): *rice;* certain grains such as *quinoa* and *amaranth.*

THE RIGHT TYPE OF FATS

In spite of its bad press, fat is necessary. It supplies essential fatty acids to your body, which help produce hormones and other substances in your body that regulate inflammation, blood clotting, and blood pressure, help with cell growth, and lower cholesterol and triglycerides. Fat also helps your body to absorb and use fat-soluble vitamins such as vitamin D, which is necessary for the use of calcium and helps convert beta-carotene into vitamin A. Fat cushions your bones and organs, keeps your body warm, provides energy, and it vital in the maintenance of healthy skin, hair, and nervous system.

It's clear, then, that you do need fats in your diet. The key is getting the right fats. The rule of thumb: try to limit your intake of saturated fats as much as possible. Saturated fats increase your risk of coronary disease and may raise your cholesterol levels more than dietary cholesterol does. Saturated fats are chiefly found in animal products such as meat (beef, lamb, veal, pork, chicken, and turkey) and whole or low-fat dairy products. But some vegetable fats are also saturated fats—so be sure to avoid palm oil, palm kernel oil, coconut oil, and hydrogenated oils.

Instead, opt for unsaturated fats. Your best bet is *monounsaturated* fats, such as *olive oil, peanut oil,* and *canola oil,* as well as *olives* and *avocados,* which lower your bad LDL cholesterol while keeping your HDL cholesterol the same.

Polyunsaturated fats also lower LDL cholesterol but unfortunately lower the good HDL cholesterol as well. Even so, these are a better bet than saturated fats, as long as you don't overdo your intake of them. Polyunsaturated fats include vegetable oils such as *corn oil, safflower oil,* and *sesame oil.* And soybean oil and wheat germ oil are good sources of vitamin E, which some studies show as controlling hot flashes. Another good source of polyunsaturated fats is fatty fish, such as *salmon, mackerel, sardines,* and *tuna.* The fat found in fish oils may help decrease your risk of blood clots—a positive especially if you are on HRT and concerned about the risk of stroke or other blood-clotting disorders.

One final note: even these "good" fats should be limited. As a rule of thumb, try to ensure fat calories make up only between 15 to 30 percent of your daily intake.

WATER

Water is often overlooked but is a definite necessity for a healthy diet. About two thirds of your body is water, and while you can live without food for weeks, you can't live without water for more than a day or so.

Take a look at everything water does for you: it is vital in blood formation, removes toxins from your body, and transports nutrients through your system. It's a key component in digestion, absorption, circulation, and excretion. It keeps your joints lubricated, regulates your body temperature, and moisturizes your skin.

In addition, it's fat- and calorie-free, so you can drink as much of it as you want! One added plus is that drinking water often helps you cut down on your appetite, making it a great weight-loss aid.

Aim to drink at least six to eight glasses of water a day. (If this seems difficult to you, remember that you can get your water not only from plain old water, but also from noncarbonated beverages like herbal tea.) And if you're not sure if you're getting enough water, here's a simple tip: check the color of your urine. If it's dark yellow (and you're not taking vitamins that change the color), you need more water; if pale yellow, it's fine.

What to Avoid, Cut Down on, or Just Be Aware Of

Part of eating right is not eating certain things or at least, cutting back on them. The following aren't great choices for anyone, but they are even more problematic for women in premature menopause.

Some of them increase your risks for diseases that premature menopause already puts you at an increased risk for, such as osteoporosis. Others intensify menopausal symptoms, and others offer you empty calories and the prospect of weight gain. All in all, then, these are the bad guys in a prematurely menopausal woman's diet.

CAFFEINE

Caffeine is one of the bad guys in premature menopausal nutrition.

First, caffeine works as a diuretic—you urinate more frequently because it increases the blood flow through your kidneys. While this may help you feel temporarily thinner (especially if you're retaining water), it does have a distinct negative: if you overdo a diuretic, you may become slightly dehydrated and retain more water, resulting, of course, in more bloating.

More important, caffeine leaches calcium from your system, which increases your risk of osteoporosis. In addition, it taxes your adrenal glands, which are key players in the production of hormones, both before and after menopause. So excessive caffeine consumption may lower your body's production of estrogen. This may be why caffeine often causes hot flashes in some women. It also may increase breast tenderness, which is common if you're taking a progestin. Finally, there are the well-known side effects of caffeine—nervousness, jitters, general anxiety. If you're already suffering from these symptoms as a result of premature menopause, the last thing you need is something that makes them worse.

But here's some good news if you can't imagine life without

that morning cup of coffee: most doctors and nutritionists seem to agree that a little caffeine won't put you at risk for most caffeine-related problems. Just limit yourself to about 150 mg of caffeine a day—about two cups of coffee—and you should notice no negatives.

SUGAR

Sugar has a few strikes against it. First, and most obvious, it's high in calories but empty of nutritive value. So you're getting no benefit from your sugar consumption other than a good taste (which, I realize, is not a bad thing, so you don't have to cut sugar completely out of your diet—just cut down on it!)

To digest sugar, your body uses calcium, magnesium, manganese, and other minerals, all of which are important, especially to fight osteoporosis. It also leaches your body of phosphorus, which is necessary in the utilization of calcium, and this is another way it may interfere with your fight against osteoporosis. It also increases your risk of getting vaginal infections because it increases the alkalinity in your vagina; stresses your adrenal glands (which make postmenopausal estrogen); and can make any blood-sugar imbalances you have more intense.

All in all, then, sugar has a lot of negatives and only one positive: its taste. Your best course of action is to try to be aware of what you're eating. Sugar is in more foods than you may think—everything from ketchup to baked potato chips. Make an effort to trim back your sugar consumption. Don't necessarily deprive yourself of sweets, but try to opt for fresh or dried fruit, or cookies and cakes sweetened with fruit juice. And when you get a major craving and can't go on unless you have a little sugar, do remember that a little should go a long way. Indulge yourself but don't overdo it!

ALCOHOL

Alcohol has a good side and a bad side. Let's start with the positives: alcohol in moderation has been linked to decreased risk of heart disease, chiefly through its apparent ability to raise HDL cholesterol. And it does have a relaxing effect, something that can be a help if you're tense or stressed out.

On the negative side, it has been linked to an increased risk of breast cancer, liver disease, and—if you drink too much—heart disease. It also appears to lower estrogen levels if you're not on HRT and increase them if you are on HRT—a bit of a paradox, but one that several studies have borne out. This is what causes women often to notice an increase in hot flashes if they drink. In addition, it's high in calories and offers no nutritive benefits. Finally, it acts as a depressive, which can make your frame of mind worse if you're already in a funk.

So what's the upshot? A little alcohol doesn't seem to be a bad thing, and in fact may be a good thing. But the key is to drink a little—one drink a day seems to be the consensus among most doctors, although some say two a day is all right. Your best bet? Talk to your own doctor and see what input she can give you, based on your personal health history.

SALT

Salt is a particularly bad choice when you are in premature menopause because it increases water retention and bloating, which are both common especially in women taking progestins as part of their HRT. In addition, it may increase your risk for high blood pressure.

The problem is that it's very difficult to avoid salt, especially if you eat a high amount of processed foods. Even so-called "healthy" frozen foods that are low in fat and calories often have an incredibly high amount of sodium. So it's important to read labels carefully if you eat processed foods. Try to avoid fast foods (which are usually high in fat as well as salt content) and salty snack foods.

It's a little easier to limit salt when you're preparing your own meals. In this case, try substituting herbs for salt if you need a little extra zing of flavor. And put down the salt shaker when cooking. If your family wants salt in their meals, let them add it at the table.

Supplements to Be Sure You're Getting What You Need

It would be wonderful to be certain that you're getting all the essential vitamins and minerals through your diet. But the chances are that you're not. The average modern diet often has major voids, even if you try to eat healthily. So in addition to eating smart, it may make sense to take certain vitamins and minerals, especially those that are often difficult to get through your daily diet.

Chapter 6 talked about the supplements you can use to help raise your hormone levels and fight the symptoms and long-term risks of side effects. But beyond these specific recommendations, there are other vitamins and minerals you need for your overall health.

A FEW WORDS ABOUT MULTIVITAMINS AND MINERALS

Your body needs about 13 different vitamins, from A to, well, not Z, but K, to function at its best. To get all of these from your food takes an enormous amount of careful eating, which would also add up to an enormous amount of calories. And even then, there's a good chance you won't get exactly what you need.

This is why it is probably a good idea to take a multivitamin and mineral supplement to be sure you're getting enough vitamins in the proper amounts. If you are willing to do the research, you can take individual supplements, but be sure you're not getting too much of one thing and not enough of another. Certain vitamins and minerals should be taken together, and if you're not getting one, you're not getting the benefit of the other and may even be hurting yourself.

There are two general types of vitamins: *water-soluble* vitamins, such as vitamin C and the B vitamins, which are quickly absorbed and the excess flushed out in your urine. Because of this, you need to replenish these vitamins daily, as they are not stored in your body. On the other hand, *fat-soluble* vitamins, such as vitamins A, D, E, and K, are stored in your body fat and can build up to toxic levels if you take an excessive amount. Again, this is why it's important to know what you are taking and talk to your doctor about any supplements you decide to add to your diet.

Minerals are also a must when you're in premature menopause. As mentioned earlier, minerals such as calcium, boron, magnesium, and others are especially crucial in the prevention of osteoporosis. But minerals are also important for a range of other functions, from regulating your nervous system to aiding in the transport of oxygen through your system. Just as there are two general categories of vitamins, there are two main types of minerals: *primary or major minerals*—calcium, phosphorus, chloride, sodium, potassium, sulfur, and magnesium, which are found in higher amounts in your body—and *trace minerals*— which include such minerals as copper, chromium, iodine, manganese, and zinc and are found in much smaller amounts in your body (less than five grams). But less, in this case, doesn't mean less important. Many of the trace minerals are extremely important.

Most women can get an adequate supply of many minerals in the course of regular eating. But there are some minerals that you may not be getting enough of. *Calcium*, of course, is possibly the most important mineral to get when you are in premature menopause. But in addition, here are some other important minerals and what they can do for you:

- *Chromium*—Helps metabolize fats and carbohydrates, keep blood sugar levels stable, and maintain good cholesterol levels. Has been claimed to help burn fat and increase muscle, but this is still unsubstantiated.
- *Iron*—Helps transport oxygen in your red blood cells; prevents anemia. One important point: if you are not getting your period anymore, then you may be best off not taking

an iron supplement. In fact, several studies have linked excessive iron to an increase in cancer and heart disease if you also have high LDL cholesterol levels.

- *Magnesium*—Helps prevent osteoporosis; also helps metabolize blood sugar.
- *Manganese*—Another bone helper; also helps the body use vitamin C and the B vitamins; regulates insulin; and is involved in the production of hormones.
- *Potassium*—Helps prevent water retention and bloating; involved in the regulation of the heart, thyroid, muscles, nerves, and kidneys; important in the prevention of high blood pressure and heart disease.

Beyond these general guidelines, it's especially important to be sure you're getting the following two major groups.

ANTIOXIDANTS: THE FREE RADICAL FIGHTERS

You've probably heard a great deal about antioxidants. This is a nutritive family that is in the news a great deal and for good reason: antioxidants help protect your body against major risks such as cancer, heart disease, and diabetes, as well as helping to prevent other aging-related problems.

They do this by fighting the damage caused by *free radicals*. Your body makes free radicals all the time as a natural offshoot of living. When you digest food, metabolize nutrients, or just breathe, your body produces free radicals. And they actually serve a good purpose in your body. They're used to fight bacteria and viruses. But if you make too many free radicals or if they're not counterbalanced by antioxidants, they can cause cell damage, speed up the aging process, and cause a variety of diseases. You are also exposed to free radicals through smoking, pollution, and synthetic chemicals.

Because free radicals are so prevalent, it's clear that antioxidants are a necessity for your good health. You can get antioxidants through the foods you eat—fruits, vegetables, and soybeans are all good sources. In addition, you can take supplements to insure that you're getting as many antioxidants as you need. The key antioxidants to take are:

- *Beta-carotene*—Found in carrots, spinach, broccoli, and other vegetables, the most famous antioxidants, but recent studies have shown that other carotenes or carotenoids (such as alpha-carotene, lycopene, and lutein, to name a few) may offer better protection against free radical damage. So you may instead choose to take a *mixed carotenoid complex* that includes beta-carotene as well as the other carotenoids.
- *Vitamin E*—Considered the key antioxidant vitamin, this helps repair damaged cell membranes, supports the immune system, blocks certain cancer-causing substances, and helps fight heart disease by keeping plaque formation down and lowering LDL cholesterol.
- *Vitamin C*—According to studies, appears to be a cancer fighter, especially breast, cervical, and gastrointestinal cancer.
- *Selenium*—Also supports your immune system and fights against cancer and heart disease by producing an antioxidant called glutathione. It is found naturally in brewer's yeast, garlic, broccoli, cabbage, cucumbers, organ meats, onions, and radishes, among other foods.
- *Zinc*—Another immune system supporter, also reduces cholesterol while raising HDL and is involved in stabilizing your blood sugar levels.

In addition, there are other antioxidant supplements of phytochemicals that occur in foods and that you may want to take if you feel your diet isn't providing enough of them. Among them are *broccoli extract,* which provides *sulphorphane; lycopene* (if you're not taking a carotenoid complex that contains it), which has recently been shown to have potent cancer-prevention properties, according to several studies; *grapeseed extract,* which provides *proanthocyanidins;* and *bioflavonoids,* such as a complex including rutin, hesperidins, and more.

ESSENTIAL FATTY ACIDS (EFAs)

Essential fatty acids do a number of good works in your body—they protect arteries, lower cholesterol and triglyceride levels, and also appear to help fight against autoiummne diseases. Most important, they are one of the key elements in keeping your cell membranes strong and efficient, and are crucial in aiding the function of prostaglandins, which help reduce inflammation and regulate your hormones. The problem is that most of us don't get enough essential fatty acids in the course of our day-to-day diets.

There are two main types of EFAs: *omega-3 fatty acids* and *omega-6 fatty acids*. The best sources of these are *fish oil* (also called MaxEPA) found in fatty fish like salmon and tuna; and *flaxseed oil*, explained in depth in Chapter 6, not only supplies fatty acids but also phytoestrogens.

Most vegetable oils also contain fatty acids, but in varying amounts. Among them are: *borage, evening primrose, hazelnut, pumpkin* and *sunflower oils*.

EXERCISE: NOT JUST FOR GOOD LOOKS, BUT FOR GOOD HEALTH

Exercise is the other change you can make to cope with your premature change of life. It can help you slim down by burning calories and fat and increasing your muscle mass. As mentioned earlier, it can make your heart and bones stronger. And it can help you cope with the moodiness that so often accompanies premature menopause.

The problem is that it's often tough to get motivated, especially when you've first been handed the information that your body is changing.

I know this all too well. In my case, I had been an exercise fiend—a once-avid runner until I developed knee problems, I lifted free weights at home, rode a stationary bike, and used a cross-country ski machine at least five days a week, usually more. But when I first learned I was in premature menopause,

I did exactly the wrong thing: I got depressed and stopped exercising. I was so upset about the diagnosis and so disgusted with the physical changes I saw in my body that I basically gave up. I figured that there was no hope. I was gaining weight even while exercising, so why not just quit? I reasoned.

Well, it was pretty bad reasoning on my part, I now realize. My hormones were against me, or so it seemed, but exercise can and does help you get rid of the weight you may have begun packing on. I learned this when I stopped exercising and watched my weight go up even more while my body looked lumpier, saggier, and generally worse. Finally, I started exercising again. I started slowly since I was out of the habit. I started doing the cross-country ski machine for 20 minutes three or four days a week, and began walking every day. I added sit-ups and crunches for my abdominals. And slowly, I started seeing changes, positive changes this time. I've kept it up, and I'm looking much more like myself again. In all frankness, I don't look exactly as I used to. I'm not quite as thin as I once was, and I am still having a definite hate-relationship with my stomach, which isn't as flat as I'd like. But I've lost a lot of the weight I had put on, my waistline is back again, and I feel good again—probably the best side effect I could have hoped for. I feel like me again, a fairly fit 39-year-old woman, not a menopausal woman!

So, speaking from personal experience, exercise can make a huge difference both in your looks and your outlook. And you don't need to go out and run marathons. The key is getting your metabolism revved up again, getting your body active to fight against the physical changes that your hormonal changes are creating. It's doable and it's not as tough as you might think. Just start moving—you'll be glad you did!

How and Why Exercise Can Make a Difference

Enough of the pep talk—let's take a look at the practical side of things. What can exercise do for you, and what forms of exercise work best for women in premature menopause?

Exercise is important to anyone in terms of health and looks, but it is an especially crucial element in coping with premature menopause for a number of reasons. First, as has been mentioned before, there are the major health reasons—the fact that exercise can help you build bones and prevent osteoporosis, as well as help fight heart disease. But there are also other effects that exercise can have that can make you look and feel better and erase the obvious physical side effects of premature menopause:

- *It raises your metabolic level, which often drops with your hormones*—This is an important plus: by exercising, you're able to reset your metabolic "set-point," the calories you burn while at rest. This helps you keep your weight down over the long term.
- *It increases your muscle mass, which not only makes you look better, but also helps you burn more fat and calories*—Muscle burns calories more quickly and efficiently than fat, which means that the more muscle you have, the more fat you'll be burning off even when you're just sitting around doing nothing.
- *It's a natural appetite suppressant*—You may think that activity makes you more hungry, but in the short term, exercise depresses your appetite. For a while after exercising, you'll usually feel less hungry, which helps you keep your weight in check. And when you finally do get hungry, you'll be able to eat more with no weight gain, since you've already burned off calories!
- *It helps make your skin more supple and moist, fighting back against the drying and aging often caused by low estrogen*—Exercise has two great skin-enhancing effects: it helps increase the production of collagen, which often drops when your estrogen levels drop, and it increases blood flow to your skin, which keeps it softer and more youthful.
- *It raises the levels of endorphins in your brain, which are often lower when your estrogen levels sag*—Just 20 to 30 minutes of moderate activity will cause your brain to release

more endorphins, the natural "feel-good" chemicals in
your brain.

* *It improves your body's ability to use blood sugar and insulin*—This stabilizes your blood-sugar levels, helps prevent or
  manage diabetes (which has been linked to premature menopause), and helps you avoid the mood swings associated with
  blood sugar ups and downs.
* *It can make your sleep more regular, a help if you're suffering from premature menopausally induced insomnia*—And if
  you exercise regularly, you get a deeper, more restful sleep,
  which also can help you look and feel better.
* *It's a natural stress-buster*—Premature menopause is a stressful condition to deal with, and exercise can help alleviate
  some of the stress you feel, not only by releasing endorphins,
  but also by increasing oxygen flow to your cells. In addition,
  a number of women have found that exercise is one of their
  best ways of coping with symptoms such as hot flashes,
  which helps relieve stress as well.
* *It can help your sex life by boosting your energy levels and
  increasing your self-confidence*—Many women find that regular exercise results in a healthier libido, because they feel
  more energetic, toned, and confident.

There's no question about it: exercise is a must when it
comes to getting your body back in shape after going through
premature menopause. Eating properly alone just won't do it.
You need exercise to tone and trim. It's the only way you can
burn calories and lose body fat.

Perhaps most important of all, it helps you reclaim your body.
Premature menopause often makes you feel as though you're
out of control—your hormones are haywire, your body is acting
as if it's older than it is, and you feel as though you're being
dragged along for a ride you didn't want to go on. But exercise
can help reverse the visible and psychological effects of premature menopause by enabling you to take charge of your own
body again.

Getting Started

There are dozens of excuses why you can't get started on an exercise program: "I'm too busy." "I can't spend enough time to get myself in shape." "I feel terrible. The last thing I want to do is exercise." "I look terrible. The last thing I want to do is go to a health club filled with fit people." And so on and so on.

But for all the excuses, there are compelling reasons to start exercising. The real key is to focus on the positive: exercise can and will help you cope with premature menopause. It is that simple.

So for every excuse you come up, come up with an answer. You're too busy? Then you can develop an exercise program that fits into your busy schedule. Start walking instead of driving everywhere. Walk up stairs instead of taking an escalator. You feel terrible? Exercise will help you feel terrific. You don't want to go to a health club? Exercise at home.

The important thing is to start, and if you haven't been exercising in years, just take it step by step. You don't need to commit a huge amount of time or effort initially. More studies and organizations have reported that you can get benefits from exercising in small increments—10 minutes here and 10 minutes there, adding up to 30 minutes or more daily. This means you can take a brisk 10-minute walk with the dog in the morning, walk around the block during your lunch hour, and rake the leaves in the evening, and you've done it!

If you get just 30 minutes of moderate exercise each day, you'll increase your oxygen consumption (in other words, you'll be getting aerobic benefit) and you'll burn four to seven calories each minute. It might not sound like much, but this is a great beginning and a way of becoming "moderately fit," as the Centers for Disease Control and Prevention and the American College of Sports Medicine determined in 1995 when they formed a committee to develop fitness recommendations for Americans.

This is the *minimum* amount of exercise you should get. And little things like cleaning your house, mowing the lawn, and such actually count.

Since this is the minimum, though, you probably won't see dramatic results. This is enough to keep your heart healthy and, depending on how much you eat, to keep your weight and body as it is now. If you want to increase your fitness level, lose weight, and add muscle, you have to work a little harder. You will need to do more strenuous exercise for longer, uninterrupted periods of time five to six days a week.

Whichever you opt for, it's obvious that you can easily fit exercise in your life. To make it work for you, follow these basic rules:

Rule #1: Set a Goal for Yourself that Isn't Ridiculously Tough to Reach Decide what you want to do initially: Lose a few pounds? Increase your fitness level? Then figure out how long you think it will take. This gives you a framework to build your exercise program around and gives you something tangible to aim for. Don't aim too high though. You want to set a reasonable goal so you can reach it—and be inspired to keep on going!

Rule #2: Commit Yourself to a Certain Amount of Exercise You need to decide that you will do enough exercise to reach your goal. This may mean you'll have to set aside half an hour a day, six days a week, or 20 minutes a day three days a week. But whatever it is, promise yourself that you will meet your time commitment.

Rule #3: Set up a Formal or Informal Exercise Schedule You may decide that every Monday, Wednesday, and Friday, you'll run or go to the gym for aerobics, and every Tuesday and Thursday, you'll do weights and calisthenics. Or you may be a little more free-form and decide that every day from Monday through Friday, you'll get 30 minutes of exercise whenever you can fit it in. As long as you have an idea in your head of what you want to do and when you want to do it, you'll be better able to stick to your exercising.

Rule #4: Start Slowly You don't want to burn yourself out at the very beginning. Remember, this is the start of a lifestyle change. You're going to want to exercise for the rest of your life, so take your time. You don't have to make up for lost time by jumping in and going crazy with too strenuous or too intensive a program. You have a lot of time in which you can build up your body and increase your exercise program, so don't rush!

Rule #5: Keep Reminding Yourself of the Positive Benefits Whenever the thought of putting your body through exercising seems particularly annoying, conjure up a mental image of how you'll look in a few months time. Remind yourself that you'll be able to fit into the jeans that are too tight now, or that your energy level will surge. Keep focusing on the positive end results and it will help motivate you.

Rule #6: Don't Expect Overnight Results but Be Aware of Small Improvements It often takes about six weeks or so to really see major results in your body, but even before that, you can notice little things that are improving. Maybe you'll notice that you just feel better—you're not getting as stressed out or your hot flashes are less annoying. Or you feel more energetic. Maybe you can see a new muscle cut in your arm, or your waistline is a teeny bit smaller. Remember, all these little victories add up!

The Components of the Best Workout for Women in Premature Menopause

To get the most out of your exercise program, it's important to get both aerobic and strengthening exercise. This combination is unbeatable when it comes to fighting heart disease and osteoporosis, not to mention burning fat as well as building muscle, which also helps you burn more fat.

You should talk with your doctor before starting any exercise program. This is especially important if you have a heart condition or any family history of heart disease, diabetes, or high blood pressure. In addition, if you haven't been physically active in years, it's a good idea to get a checkup before you begin, to determine how much you can push yourself initially.

AEROBIC EXERCISE

This is (literally) the heart of your exercise program. Aerobic exercise creates an oxygen demand in your muscles. Because they need more oxygen, your heart needs to beat harder and more efficiently, sending more blood into circulation to deliver the oxygen to your muscles. Over time, this strengthens your heart, improves your circulation, and makes your respiration more efficient. It also raises levels of HDL cholesterol and lowers LDL, and appears to help lower high blood pressure. And these are just the cardiovascular benefits! There are weight-control benefits as well: because your body is working hard and using up oxygen, your heart rate rises and you burn calories. Finally, aerobic exercise is a mood enhancer and a great way of working out stress. All in all, it's a very important aspect of your premature menopause exercise program.

The key to effective aerobic exercising is to get your heart into its target range. This is the point at which your body is pushing itself to the point where it will raise your breathing rate and increase your oxygen demand by working your heart at about 60 to 80 percent of its maximum rate. It's simple to figure out your target heart rate range: just subtract your age from 220 and multiply that figure by 0.6 and 0.8. For example, if you are 35, subtract that from 220. This gives you a maximum heart rate of 185 beats per minute. Multiply this first by 0.6, then by 0.8, giving you a range of 111 to 148. This means that, to get the ideal aerobic workout, your heart should be beating within this range as you exercise.

You can check your pulse rate while you exercise to be sure you're reaching your target heart rate range. After about five minutes of exercise, take your pulse in your neck for 10 seconds and multiply this by 6. This will give you a rough idea of your heart rate and will let you know if you're taking it a little too easy or, for that matter, pushing a little too hard. Another good trick to check if you're working out strenuously enough is to try singing one line of a song. You should be able to get through one line before taking a breath. But if you can sing more than one line, you need to work a little harder.

To get the maximum cardiovascular benefit and really start burning fat, you should work out aerobically for at least 20 minutes, although 30 minutes is considered much better. If you haven't worked out in a while, though, start small and work your way up. Begin with a brisk walk or the equivalent for 10 minutes a day. Each week add five or 10 minutes, depending on how you feel while exercising. By the end of a month, you should be up to 20 to 30 minutes.

Aerobic exercise three days a week for 20 to 30 uninterrupted minutes is enough for you to maintain your current fitness level and weight. If you want to increase your fitness level, and in so doing lose weight, you'll need at least 30 minutes a day, five to six days a week, doing more vigorous exercise. This should raise your heart rate even more, to the upper end of your heart rate range, and will burn over seven calories a minute.

One beauty of aerobic exercise is the range of different activities you can do. And even better, you don't necessarily need any equipment, other than a pair of sneakers and a little energy! Any of the following will fulfill your aerobic exercise requirements: brisk walking (a great choice if you're just beginning an exercise program, jogging, running, biking (stationary or outdoors), cross-country skiing (on a machine or outdoors), swimming (although this tends to burn fewer calories than other forms of aerobic exercise), rowing, aerobic dancing, jumping rope.

Here are a few tips to get the most out of your aerobic workout:

- *Split your aerobic workout into three sections*—First a warm-up of five minutes of slower exercise to warm your muscles and get your blood flowing; then if you choose, you can do a few minutes of easy stretching to get your muscle elongated and ready to work out. Next, the core of your workout—the high-intensity portion in which you exercise at your target heart rate range. And finally, a cool down of a few minutes of slower exercise to get your heart rate to return slowly to its resting rate.

- *If you get bored with one activity, try switching between different ones*—This will keep your interest level up and your fitness level as well. One day, try brisk walking for 30 minutes, the next, ride your bike, the next, run . . . and so on. Not only will this keep you from being bored, but you'll work different muscles, which can result in a more balanced fitness program.

- *If the tried-and-true forms of exercise seem dull, be creative!*—You don't have to stick to the basics, walking, running, biking. You can also get a good aerobic workout by in-line skating, ice skating, even dancing. As long as you're getting your heart rate up for a set block of time, it counts!

- *Set aside a particular time each day for exercising*—So you can make it a habit.

- *If possible, get your aerobic exercise first thing in the morning*—This will often help you burn more fat: if you exercise before eating breakfast, you'll be burning off calories already stored in your body. In addition, it's not as easy to put it off and wiggle out of exercising if it's the first thing you do each day. You don't have as many excuses. And it's a great way to begin your day. You'll start off feeling healthy and fit, which can help you keep disciplined about food for the rest of the day.

WEIGHT TRAINING

Weights, as mentioned earlier in the book, are one of the best ways of strengthening your bones, aiding in your fight against osteoporosis. But lifting weights doesn't only help your bones; it also can make you look great. Weight training doesn't burn body fat like aerobic exercise does, but it can help you increase muscle mass, which burns more calories than body fat, and so helps you lose weight. Here's an encouraging fact: every pound of muscle you add to your body burns 50 to 100 calories more each day. Clearly, this is a number that can really add up. Weight training can also help you trim your body by toning the sagginess that may have come with premature menopause. And it is also a great body shaper—a wonderful way to help make your body look young and well proportioned again.

For example, many women have weaker upper bodies, which contributes to their pear shape. They're smaller on top and wider on the bottom. When you go through premature menopause, you'll often see even more weight pad out your thighs. (I speak from experience on this one!) So working out with weights, building and strengthening your upper body, can help you balance out your figure and give you a more attractive proportion.

You can also use weights to target other problem spots. Lower estrogen levels often cause droopier, saggy breasts. By doing weight lifting that works your pectoral muscles, you can build the muscle under your breasts, making them firmer and even making them look larger.

Weight training works because it is a *resistance* exercise. You use your muscles against a resisting force—the weight or machine—and by forcing your muscle to exert itself to lift or push the weight, you increase its strength. This tones and shapes the muscles. And it doesn't make them bulky, no matter what you may fear. You won't end up looking like a body builder. You will, however, wind up with a fitter, leaner body.

As with aerobic exercise, you have a few options open to you. You can use free weights, weight machines, or other forms of resistance such as bands. And you can work out in the privacy of your own home or at a gym. In general, you may be best off beginning by working with a fitness trainer or in a class to be sure you're doing all exercises properly. At the least, it is wise to watch a video that demonstrates the different exercises. This will give you a clearer idea than simply looking at static pictures in a book or magazine article, and will ensure that you know how to do each exercise. Improper weight training can hurt your muscles and won't give you the benefits you're after.

You should do weight training two to three times a week— *no more than this*—for about 20 to 30 minutes a session. Two times a week is enough for you to maintain your current level;

three times a week to increase your strength and see changes in your body shape. And always take a day off between sessions to give your muscles a chance to relax, rebuild, and repair. You can get your aerobic exercise in on those days off, so you're still working on making your body better than ever!

A few other tips:

- *The general rule of thumb: Don't start with too heavy a weight*—It's safest and best to begin with weights you can lift or move comfortably and are able to do eight to 15 repetitions with. Keep in mind, also, that you should generally be able to do two to three sets of these repetitions. Most experts recommend that you start with three- or five-pound weights and work your way up.
- *As you find the weight becomes easy to lift, start adding weight in 5-percent increments*—If you can't do 10 repetitions, decrease the weight and work back up to the heavier weight.
- *Don't forget to warm up before you begin*—This will help you to avoid muscle injury. Something as simple as running or walking in place for five minutes will warm your muscles and prepare them for activity.
- *Stretch the muscles you've worked after you have finished*— Stretching keeps your muscles long and lean—the look you're after.

CALISTHENICS

With all the attention paid to aerobic exercise and weight lifting, it's easy to overlook plain old calisthenics. But when you're in premature menopause, calisthenics can be a real help in making your body look the way you want it to.

Done properly, calisthenics help strengthen muscles in particular problem spots. They're not spot reducers, as you probably know. Calisthenics won't burn fat; only aerobic exercise does that. But strengthening the muscles in a problem area can help that area look better. In addition, if you can't or won't use weights, you can use calisthenic exercises to strengthen certain areas of your body. For example, you can do bent-knee push-ups to work your chest, shoulders, and upper arms; body dips (raising and lowering your body with your arms) to work your arms, and so on.

Some general tips:

• *If you've noticed that your stomach has become rounder, try crunches or bent-knee sit-ups, and don't forget your lower abs!*—Yes, crunches or sit-ups are a good choice. But often it's your lower abdominals that really need work when you're in premature menopause. So, in addition, to your normal routine of crunches, add reverse crunches or similar exercises for your lower abdominal muscles. (Check with a fitness trainer or look in an exercise book for ones that specifically target your lower abs.) These are often worked very little, so it may take a while before you can work up to a number of repetitions, but you will notice a difference after about six weeks.

• *To regain your waistline, remember to work your obliques*— These are the muscles that run diagonally across your abdomen, and they can help you trim your waistline.

• *Keep your abdominal muscles tight whatever exercise you're doing—aerobic, weights, or calisthenics*—This not only keeps you aligned properly, it also keeps those abs working, which eventually will result in a stronger, flatter stomach. In effect, you're helping create your own natural "belly buster."

• *The old "go for the burn" mentality isn't necessary and, in fact, may be harmful*—When you're doing exercises for specific muscles, you don't need to feel a burn. Just work the muscle.

• *Think when you exercise*—Concentrate on the muscles you are working. This helps you isolate the proper muscles and ensures that you're getting the most out of your exercise.

• *As with aerobics and weights, don't forget to stretch!*—This will relax the muscles you've worked, elongate them, and increase your flexibility.

Yoga, Tai Chi, and Other Mind-Body Exercises

More and more people are rediscovering yoga, tai chi, and other forms of Eastern exercise. These are an excellent choice for a woman in premature menopause. The benefits? The different postures and positions tend to have a lengthening effect on your muscles, making you look leaner. They are also designed to help energize your body by working on specific parts of your system, including your reproductive system, your thyroid, and your endocrine system, all of which are affected by premature menopause. In addition, these forms of exercise help make you more supple and flexible; they have a natural calming effect, and they're easy on your joints.

In fact, in many ways, yoga is a good all-round exercise, incorporating natural resistance work with stretching. This can trim and tone you, and can help you keep your bones strong. Power yoga, a newly popular form of yoga in which postures are changed rapidly, allowing you to get your heart rate up while exercising, even gives you an aerobic workout as well.

Most of all, however, yoga and tai chi are wonderful stress-relievers. By combining meditation, breathing, and exercise, you not only get a physical workout, you also get a mental workout. You can relax, destress, and calm yourself, helping to fight back against the emotional fallout of premature menopause.

A few general tips:

- *As with weight training, it's a good idea to take a class or watch a video to get a clear idea of how to exercise properly.* A picture is often too static to teach you how to do certain postures or positions well. By taking a class, you can learn exactly what to do and how to do it. Once you've learned, you can easily do it at home.
- *Take it very slowly.* Both tai chi and most forms of yoga are meant to be done mindfully, with all of your concentration. You shouldn't cram yoga into your day; set a time when you know you can relax and go through your program in an unrushed manner.

Conclusion

I wrote this book because I had so many questions that weren't being answered, and I wanted so badly to better understand and come to grips with premature menopause. This book has been a labor of love for me, and in many ways has helped me better understand this transition that I certainly never expected to be going through at this age. And I hope it has been a learning experience for you as well.

If you are going through premature menopause, I'm sure you have, as I had, hundreds of questions. And I hope this book has helped answer them and, perhaps most important, helped you realize that you aren't alone.

This is the most important lesson I've learned since I was diagnosed. There are millions of women like us out there, all asking questions, trying to cope with this unexpected change in our lives, and moving ahead with new acceptance.

But acceptance should never lead to passivity. I urge all of you to visit your doctor, to keep abreast of new research, and to take an active role in your condition. Knowledge is power. Remember, this is your body we're talking about, and you have it within you to take charge of that body. The resources listed in the Appendix can help you. Furthermore, if you need help in setting up a support group or establishing ties with other women going through premature menopause, or simply need someone to talk to who understands, feel free to contact me at petrask@aol.com, or by writing to me in care of the publisher.

One final note: as I've said dozens of times throughout this book, premature menopause does change aspects of our lives, but it doesn't have to be a totally negative change. By coping with this change and moving ahead to the rest of our lives, we can emerge stronger, more confident, and better able to handle the challenges that life tosses us.

Remember, premature menopause is just one fact of our lives. We are so much more than just our reproductive systems. We are people with capabilities, dreams, and strengths, and premature menopause does not have to hinder us. We can all learn from this experience and emerge better, wiser, more vital women—*whole* women!

Resource Listings

PREMATURE MENOPAUSE

Support Groups

Early Pausers
America Online's Early Menopause Support Group
AOL Keyword: Women Talk
>America Online's only support group for women in premature meno-
>pause (and the group I am very proud to be a member of). Operates
>a message board and on-line chats. AOL members can access the
>group by using the keyword: Women Talk. Once you reach the main
>Women's channel screen, click on message boards, then Wellness,
>then Health Central. The Early Menopause board is listed along with
>other women's health boards. (It seems complicated, but it's well
>worth the trouble!) An excellent source of support, members share
>information, vent about fears and problems, help one another in ad-
>justing to the physical and emotional changes that premature meno-
>pause brings, offer advice and a helping hand.

Premature Ovarian Failure (POF) support Group
PO Box 23643
Alexandria, VA 22304
703/913–4787
>National support group for women with POF; publishes quarterly
>newsletter, offers doctor referrals, holds conferences.

Web Sites

Early Menopause
www.earlymenopause.com
> *A web site I've set up that is specifically designed for women going through menopause years before they expected it—whether naturally, surgically, or due to cancer treatments. Includes general information about the causes of premature menopause, different treatment options, tables of hormone levels, news updates, and links to other useful resources and groups (including premature ovarian failure sites, infertility groups, ongoing research studies in premature menopause, osteoporosis information, and more)—and also has a message board for women to discuss their concerns, ask questions, and find support from other women coping with early menopause.*

Daisy Chain
www.daisychain.org
> *One of the few Web sites specifically dedicated to premature menopause, this is the site for Britain's premature menopause association, "Daisy Chain"; includes general information, doctors' articles on premature menopause. Good source for basic information.*

Premature Ovarian Failure Support Group (As Above) WEB Site
pofsupport.org
> *Includes current newsletter, downloadable pamphlet explaining POF, links to NICHD clinical studies; "Ask the Doctor" area in which three doctors will answer your questions on-line; operates listserv.*

Premature Menopause Support Group
www.members.aol.com/menochat
> *On-line support group and bulletin board; also operates chat room specifically for women in premature menopause.*

Note: Because there is so little information readily available for women about premature menopause, I've found certain medical sites on the Internet to be one of the best sources of articles, studies, and the like on this condition. Here are a few sites that

I've had the best luck with when using "premature menopause" or "premature ovarian failure" as a search term.

Healthgate
www.healthgate.com
Easy-to-use health search engine.

Medline
www.medline.com
(Also available through a number of other health-related Web sites, including Medscape and Healthgate.)
Considered one of the top medical sites on the Web; offers article abstracts from a wide range of medical and scientific journals. The only problem: since they're abstracts, not full-text articles, you don't always get all the information you'd like. You can order full-text articles, but this can get costly—about $25 an article. Even so, the abstracts often contain useful information and can help you begin researching premature menopause.

Medscape
www.medscape.com
Possibly the best source of medical information on-line; excellent site for finding full-text articles published in medical journals, including articles on premature menopause and/or premature ovarian failure, surgical menopause, HRT, and much more. One note: since the articles are from medical and scientific journals, they're sometimes extremely technical. Even so, this is a great place to find out about recent studies, promising research.

In addition to these, you may want to try a search on one of the major search engines (such as Lycos, Hotbot, Excite, Webcrawler) or on a metasearch engine that will search other search engines and return one list (such as metacrawler.com or infind.com). One drawback, though: when doing a search engine search, you may wind up with a lot of posts from message boards, not articles.

MENOPAUSE

These resources aren't specifically aimed at a woman in premature menopause, but most offer good general information about menopause and often do cover premature menopause (although usually only in passing). Even so, these are good sources of information about menopause basics such as HRT, herbs and vitamins, and so on. In addition, some of the associations offer doctor referrals.

Associations

American College of Obstetricians and Gynecologists
600 Maryland Ave., S.W.
Washington, DC 20024
202/638–5577
  Provides general information about menopause and doctor referrals.

American Menopause Foundation
350 Fifth Ave., Suite 2822
New York, NY 10118
212/714–2398

Natural Woman Institute
8539 Sunset Blvd., Suite 135
Los Angeles, CA 90069
800/4U WOMAN
  Organization that focuses on natural plant-derived HRT; offers doctor referrals.

North American Menopause Society (NAMS)
2074 Abington Rd.
Cleveland, OH 44106
216/844–3334
www.menopause.org
  Provides general information about menopause, as well as listings of doctors in your area who have registered with them as menopause specialists.

Web Sites

Menopause and Beyond
www.oxford.net/~tishy/asm.html
> *Excellent Web site that was the unofficial site for the menopause discussion group alt.support.menopause. Includes information on everything from menopausal symptoms to HRT to surgical menopause to herbs and vitamins; links; opinions and a "quack watch."*

American College of Obstetrics and Gynecology
www.acog.com
> *Includes on-line referral for member doctors; offers free pamphlets on range of women's health issues from menopause to hysterectomies to osteoporosis and more, which you can order on-line.*

Hotflash Listserv
> *listserv for women in perimenopause and menopause—generally aimed at older women, but may have younger women in premature menopause as participants. To subscribe, go to: http://www.onelist .com/subscribe.cgi/hotflash.*

Menopaus
www.howdyneighbor.com/menopaus
> *Another general menopause site that contains useful basic information as well as links to other sites. They also operate a mailing list/listserv that you can subscribe to to share information on menopause and related issues with other women. While most are older women in menopause, there are often younger women in the listserv as well. To join, E-mail listserv@maelstrom.stjohn.edu and put "Subscribe menopaus" (no e!) as a subject heading and include your name in the body of the letter.*

Menopause—Doctor's Guide to the Internet
www.pslgroup.com/menopause.htm
> *Site aimed at both doctors and patients; includes recent news articles, links to other related sites, general articles.*

Menopause Online
www.menopause-online.com
> *Good general site; includes news articles, general information on menopause, HRT, herbs, and vitamins.*

Women's Health—Menopause

www.ama-assn.org
General information on menopause from the AMA.

Menopause Clinics

These medical clinics specialize in the treatment of menopause and hormone disorders. One big plus is that because they're specialized treatment centers, many also are well versed in premature menopause and have numerous patients going through this.

Cleveland Menopause Clinic

Mt. Sinai Medical Center
29001 Cedar Rd., Suite 600
Lyndhust, OH 44124
216/442–4747
Offers comprehensive menopause care, including premature menopause.

The Climacteric Clinic, Women's Medical and Diagnostic Center

222 SW 36 Terrace, Suite C
University of Florida
Gainesville, FL 32607
904/372–5600

Columbia-Presbyterian Center for Menopause, Hormonal Disorders and Women's Health

16 E. 60th St., Suite 490
New York, NY 10022
212/332–8548
Specializes in a wide range of hormone disorders, including premature menopause.

Hormone Clinic/Mature Women's Clinic

Albert Einstein College of Medicine
1300 Morris Park Ave.

Bronx, NY 10461
718/430–3152
*In addition to general menopause, specializes in premature meno-
pause (premature ovarian failure) and operates an egg donation
program.*

Menopause Clinic
Brigham and Women's Hospital
Fertility, Endocrine & Menopause Unit
75 Francis St.
Boston, MA 02115
617/732–4220

Menopause Center at UCLA
Center for Health Sciences, Department of OB/Gyn
Room 22–117CHS
Los Angeles, CA 90024–1740
213/825–7755

UMDNJ-Robert Wood Johnson Medical School
Department of Obstetrics and Gynecology
1 Robert Wood Johnson Place, Cn19
New Brunswick, NJ 08903–0019
201/937–7633

Menopause Care Center
George Washington University
2300 I Street, NQ
Washington, DC 20037
202/994–5656

Menopause Clinic
Yale University School of Medicine
Physician's Building
Howard Ave.
New Haven, CT 06520
203/785–4708

Menopausal Section
Baylor Ob/Gyn
6550 Fannin St.
Houston, TX 77030
713/798–7500

Menopause Clinic
University of San Diego Medical Center
Department of Reproductive Endocrinology
225 Dickenson St.
San Diego, CA 92103
619/543–3210
619/453–3210 (hot line)
> *Educational/support group only; no hands-on care. Offers sessions on dealing with doctors; general menopause education. Can offer doctor referrals. Most participants are in their forties and fifties; no special expertise in premature menopause.*

Northwest Memorial Faculty Foundation
Department of Reproductive Endocrinology
680 N. Lakeshore Dr., Suite 810
Chicago, IL 60611
312/908–7269

Menopause Clinic
University of Illinois Hospital and Clinic
840 S. Wood, Room 13 Yello
Chicago, IL 60612
312/996–6870

SURGICAL MENOPAUSE

Hysterectomy Educational Resources and Services (Hers Foundation)
422 Bryn Mawr Ave.
Bala Cynwyd, PA 19004

610/667–7757
www.ccon.com/hers
www.dca.net/~hers

Offers wide range of support services including free information by mail, telephone counseling by appointment, physician referral for treatment options, medical articles, and more. Web site offers information about symptoms and conditions including cancer, prolapse, and osteoporosis, and different treatments, including HRT for postsurgery.

Sans Uteri Hysterectomy Forum

www.findings.net/sans-uteri.html

Internet resource offering information, resources, and more. Operates an Internet mailing list (a listserv) so you can share information, support, and so on with other women. Intends to begin operating actual support groups (not on-line) across the country.

The Gynecological Cancers On Line Support Group

www.tile.net.2001/lsts/gynonc.html
(also accessible through Sans Uteri site)

Operates a listserv (effectively, an on-line support group) for women who have dealt with gynecological cancers, including ovarian, uterine, and so on.

GENERAL WOMEN'S HEALTH

Sources of information about women's health in general, these resources often include good general information about menopause, surgical menopause, HRT, osteoporosis, and the like.

AMA Main Web Page

www.ama-assn.org

This home page for the American Medical Association provides links to its publication, JAMA, as well as other medical journals. Good for searching recent news articles and scientific studies on menopause-related issues. Operates a special Women's Health Information Center that includes articles about women's health culled from JAMA as well as other major medical journals.

Healthfinder
www.healthfinder.gov
> *A Web site operated by the government, this leads you to on-line sites, databases, support groups, and more, as well as government agencies.*

National Women's Health Resource Center
www.healthywomen.org
> *Offers information on a range of general women's health topics, including menopause in general, surgical menopause, osteoporosis, and so on from a wide variety of sources; also includes links to other sites.*

Nethealth.com
www.obgyn.com
> *Information on health issues.*

Obgyn Net
www.obgyn.net
> *Information for patients as well as doctors on wide range of gynecological topics, including menopause, hysterectomy and oophorectomy, breast cancer, fibroids, and so on.*

Women's Health Resources on the World Wide Web
www.cpmcnet.columbia.edu
> *Provides information and links on range of Web sites covering women's health.*

BREAST CANCER

National Breast Cancer Coalition
1707 L Street, NW, Suite 1060
Washington, DC 20036
202/296–7477

Y-Me National Breast Cancer Organization
212 West Van Buren St.
Chicago, IL 60607
312/986–8228
800/221–2141

OSTEOPOROSIS

National Osteoporosis Foundation
2100 M Street, NW, Suite 602
Washington, DC 20037
800/223–2226
Publishes information on osteoporosis, including pamphlets, as well as information on medication for osteoporosis. Also provides doctor referrals.

OVARIAN CANCER

National Cancer Institute
Bethesda, MD 20205
301/496–5583
800/4–CANCER

Society of Gynecologic Oncologists
401 N. Michigan Ave.
Chicago, IL 60611
312/644–6610

INFERTILITY

American Society for Reproductive Medicine
1209 Montgomery Highway
Birmingham, AL 35216–2809
205/978–5000
www.asrm.org
Association of doctors specializing in reproductive medicine; publishes information booklets.

The American Surrogacy Center
www.surrogacy.com
On-line group offering information, support, extensive resources for people interested in surrogacy and egg donation.

Child of My Dreams

www.child-dream.com

> *On-line resource offering information and support for infertile women; including articles, message boards, chat groups. Covers topics such as egg donation and also has a special area devoted to adoption.*

Inciid (The International Council on Infertility Information Dissemination)

PO Box 6836

Arlington, VA 22206

703/379–9178

FAX: 703/379–1593

www.inciid.org

> *The largest Internet site providing infertility information and support; includes message boards, articles, transcripts of guest speakers, links to other resources. The Immunological Issues area is of special interest to women with premature ovarian failure who are interested in exploring immunological suppression as a means of attempting pregnancy.*

Internet Health Resources

www.ihr.com/infertility

> *An excellent on-line source that offers information on infertility, surrogate services, and support groups. Also provides a listing of infertility clinics by region.*

Resolve, Inc.

1310 Broadway

Somerville, MA 02144–1779

617/623–1156

National Helpline: 617/623–0744

www.resolve.org

> *A national infertility association that provides information and support; puts out a newsletter and wide range of publications (including one on premature ovarian failure); offers doctor referrals. Local chapters also offer support groups and other assistance.*

ADOPTION

Associations

Adoptive Families of America, Inc.
3333 Highway 100 N.
Minneapolis, MN 55442
612/535-4829
800/372-3300
www.adoptivefam.org
   Provides information about adoption as well as resources; pub-
   lishes magazine. Offers support to adoptive parents and maintains
   200 regional support groups across the country.

American Academy of Adoption Attorneys
PO Box 33053
Washington, DC 20033-0053
202/832-2222
   Offers referrals for adoption attorneys.

Americans Adopting Orphans, Inc.
12345 Lake City Way, NE, #2001
Seattle, WA 98125-5401
www.orphans.com
   Licensed agency that also offers assistance for parents exploring
   private international adoption.

International Concerns Committee for Children
911 Cypress Dr.
Boulder, CO 80308-2821
303/494-8333
   Provides information about domestic and international children
   available for adoption, including photolist of international children,
   a report on foreign adoption.

Internet Adoption Registry
AOC 8640-M Guilford Rd., #211
Columbia, MD 21046

www.adoptiononline.com
> *Web resource that allows prospective adoptive parents to post a letter on-line seeking children.*

National Adoption Center
and
National Adoption Exchange
1500 Walnut Street, #701
Philadelphia, PA 19102–3523
215/735–9988
800/TO ADOPT
www.adopt.org/adopt
> *Excellent resource providing information for prospective adoptive parents. Includes help for parents at all stages of the adoption process.*

National Adoption Information Clearinghouse (NAIC)
PO Box 1182
Washington, DC 20013–1182
703/352–3488
888/251–0075
www.calib.com/naic
> *Another excellent source of information for prospective adoptive parents at all stages of the process. The Web site is a great place to begin researching adoption and contains numerous helpful articles, links, and other resources to explore.*

U.S. Department of State, Bureau of Consular Affairs
Office of Children's Issues
Room 4811, Department of State
Washington, DC 20520–4848
202/647–2688
www.travel.state.gov
> *Provides timely information on international adoption, including updates on adoption laws, practices, and so on in over 60 countries; information on visas and more.*

Book Publishers

Perspectives Press
PO Box 90318
Indianapolis, IN 46290–0318
317/872–3055
www.perspectivespress.com
Specializes in adoption and infertility.

Tapestry Books
PO Box 359
Ringoes, NJ 08551–0359
908/806–6695
800/765–2367
www.tapestrybooks.com
One of the leading publishers specializing in adoption (as well as infertility). Web site lists available books.

Publications

Beating the Adoption Odds: Using Your Head and Your Heart to Adopt
by Cynthia D. Martin and Dru Martin Groves
(Harcourt Brace & Company, 1998)
An excellent, compassionate, and information-packed book on every phase of the adoption process, from decision-making to preparing for adoption to the steps to take whether you're opting for a private or agency adoption, domestic or international.

ALTERNATIVE THERAPIES (HERBS, VITAMINS, ETC.)

Associations

The American Botanical Council
PO Box 201660
Austin, TX 78720

American Association of Naturopathic Physicians
601 Valley, #105
Seattle, WA 98109
206/298–0126
www.naturopathic.org
Licensing body for naturopathic physicians (N.D.s); offers referrals to licensed naturopathic doctors in your area.

American Holistic Medical Association
2002 Eastlake Ave. East
Seattle, WA 98102
206/322–6842
Provides doctor referrals.

The Herb Research Foundation
1007 Pearl St., Suite 200
Boulder, CO 80302
303/449–2265
303/449–7849
sunsite.unc.edu/herbs/hrfinfo.html
Provides information on herbs, including new research and studies.

National College of Naturopathic Medicine
11231 SE Market St.
Portland, OR 97216
503/255–4860
College for naturopathic physicians; offers referrals.

Healthworld Online
www.healthy.net
On-line source of information on complementary medicine— including herbs and vitamins (also includes access to Medline).

Compounding Pharmacies

These pharmacies specialize in compounding natural forms of HRT (such as natural micronized progesterone, tri-est cream, and so on) according to a doctor's prescription. If your doctor has prescribed natural HRT (non-brand-name) and you have trouble finding a compounding pharmacy in your area, first try contacting one of these.

International Academy of Compounding Pharmacists
PO Box 1365
Sugarland, TX 77487
713/933–8400
800/927–4227
   Helps you locate compounding pharmacies in your area.

The following compounding pharmacies fill prescriptions by mail order:

Bajamar Women's Healthcare Pharmacy
9609 Dielman Rock Island
St. Louis, MO 63132
800/255–8025

Belmar Pharmacy
8015 W. Alameda Ave., Suite 100
Lakewood, CO 80226
800/525–9473

Health Watchers Systems
13402 N. Scottsdale Rd., Suite B-150
Scottsdale, AZ 85254
800/321–6917

Professional and Technical Services, Inc.
621 SW Alder, Suite 900
Portland, OR 97205–3627
800/888–6814

Women's Health America Group (formerly Madison Pharmacy Associates)
429 Gammon Pl.
PO Box 9641
Madison, WI 53715
800/558–7046

Women's International Pharmacy
5708 Monona Dr.
Madison, WI 53716–3152
800/279–5708
800/525–9473

Selected Bibliography

Abraham, D., Carpenter, P.C. "Issues concerning androgen replacement therapy in postmenopausal women." *Mayo Clinic Proceedings* 1997; 72(11): 1051–1055.

Adlercreutz, H. "Phytoestrogens: Epidemiology and possible role in cancer protection." *Environmental Health Perspectives* 1995; 103(7): 103–112.

Albertazzi, P., Pansini, F., Bonaccorsi, G., Zanotti, L, Forini, E., De Aloysio, D. "The effect of dietary soy supplementation on hot flushes." *Obstetrics & Gynecology* 1998; 91(1).

Anasti, J.N., et al. "Bone loss in young women with karyotypically normal spontaneous premature ovarian failure." *Obstetrics & Gynecology* 1998; 91(1): 12–15.

Anasti, J.N. "Premature ovarian failure: An update." *Fertility and Sterility* 1998; 70(1): 1–15.

Anderson, J.J.B., Garner, S.C. "The effects of phytoestrogens on bone." *Nutrition Research* 1997; 17(10): 1617–1632.

Baber, R., Abdalla, H., Studd, J. "The premature menopause." *Progress in Obstetrics and Gynecology* 1993; 209–226.

Baird, David T. "Amenorrhoea." *The Lancet* 1997; 350(9073): 275–279.

Baird, D.D., Umbach, D.M., Lansdell, L., Hughes, C.L,. Setchell, K.D.R., Weinberg, C.R., Haney, A.F., Wilcox, A.J., McLachlan, J.A. "Dietary intervention study to assess estrogenicity of dietary soy among postmenopausal women." *Journal of Clinical Endocrinology and Metabolism* 1995; 80(5): 1685–1690.

Baker, A., Simpson, S., Dawson, D. "Sleep disruption and mood changes associated with menopause." *Journal of Psychosomatic Medicine* 1997; 43(4): 359–369.

Barrett-Connor, E. "Fortnightly review: Hormone replacement therapy." *British Medical Journal* 1998; 317(7156): 457–461.

Beckham, N. "Phyto-oestrogens and compounds that affect oestrogen metabolism." *Australian Journal of Medical Herbalism* 1995; 7(1): 10–16.

Brzezinski, A., Adlercreutz, H., Shaoul, R., Rosler, A., Shmueli, A., Tanos, V., Schenker, J.G. "Short term effects of phytoestrogen-rich diet on postmenopausal women." *Menopause: The Journal of the North American Menopause Society* 1997; 4(2): 89–94.

Burke, G.L. "The potential use of a dietary soy supplement as a post-menopausal hormone replacement therapy." *The Second International Symposium on the Role of Soy in Preventing and Treating Chronic Disease,* Belgium, September 1996.

Busacca, M., Fusi, F.M., Brigante, C., Doldi, N., Vignali, M. "Success in inducing ovulation in a case of premature ovarian failure using growth hormone-releasing hormone." *Gynecology and Endocrinology* 1996; 10 (4): 277–279.

Bywaters, P., Bond, M. "Rethinking the concept of compliance: Making decisions about hormone replacement therapy." *Social Sciences in Health: International Journal of Research and Practice* 1997; 3(2): 73–82.

Cassidy, A., Bingham, S., Setchell, K. "Biological effects of isoflavones in young women: Importance of the chemical composition of soya bean products." *British Journal of Nutrition* 1995; 74(4): 587–601.

Clarkson, T.B., Anthony M.S., Williams, J.K., Honore, E.K., Cline, J.M. "The potential of soybean phytoestrogens for postmenopausal hormone replacement therapy." *Proccedings of the Society for Experimental Biology & Medicine* 1998; 217(3): 365–8.

Colditz, G.A., Hankinson, S.E., Hunter, D.J., et al. "The use of estrogens and progestins and the risk of breast cancer in postmenopausal women." *New England Journal of Medicine* 1995; 332: 1589–93.

Conway, G.S., Kaltsas, G., Patel, A., Davies, M.C., Jacobs, H.S. "Characterization of idiopathic premature ovarian failure." *Fertility and Sterility* 1996; 65:2, 337–41.

Conway, Gerard S. "Premature ovarian failure." *Current Opinion in Obstetrics and Gynecology* 1997; 9 (3), 202–206.

Coulam, C.B., Adamson, S.C., Annegers, J.F. "Incidence of premature ovarian failure." *Obstetrics & Gynecology* 1986; 67: 604–606.

Cumnane, S.C. "Nutritional attributes of traditional flaxseed in healthy young adults." *American Journal of Clinical Nutrition* 1993; 69(2): 443–453.

Dalais, F.S., Rice, G.E., Bell, R.J., Murkies, A.L., Medley, G., Strauss, B.J.G., Wahlqvist, M.L. "Dietary soy supplementation increases vaginal cytology maturation index and bone mineral content in postmenopausal women." *The Second International Symposium on the Role of Soy in Preventing and Treating Chronic Disease,* Belgium, September 1996.

Dancer, Tina W., Cummins, Dosha. "Approaches to estrogen replacement therapy." *Drug Topics* 1998; 142(8):102–111.

Davidson, Nancy E. "Hormone replacement therapy—breast versus heart versus bone." *New England Journal of Medicine* 1995; 1638.

Davis, S.R. "Premature ovarian failure." *Maturitas* 1996; 23(1): 1–8.

Davis, S.R., Burger, H.G. "Use of androgens in postmenopausal women." *Current Opinion in Obstetrics and Gynecology* 1997; 9(3): 177–80.

Draper, C.R., Edel, M.J., Dick, I.M., Randall, A.G., Martin, G.B., Prince, R.L. "Phytoestrogens reduce bone loss and bone resorption in oophorectomized rats." *Journal of Nutrition* 1997; 127(9): 1795–1799.

Dwyer, J.T., Goldin, B.R., Saul, N., Gualtieri, L., Barakat, S., Adlercreutz, H. "Tofu and soy drinks contain phytoestrogens." *Journal of the American Dietetic Association* 1994; 94(7): 739–743.

Eden, J., Knight, D., Mackey, R. "Hormonal effect of isoflavones." *The Second International Symposium on the Role of Soy in Preventing and Treating Chronic Disease*, Belgium, September 1996.

"The emerging role of estrogen-androgen therapy in the postmenopausal patient." *The Fifteenth World Congress of Gynecology and Obstetrics*, August 7, 1997.

Fackelmann, Kathleen. "Early menopause for diabetic women." *Science News* July 5, 1997; 152(1): 15.

Farhi, J., Homburg, R., Ferber, A., Orvieto, R., Ben Rafael, Z. "Non-response to ovarian stimulation in normogonadotrophic, normogonadal women: A clinical sign of impending onset of ovarian failure pre-empting the rise in basal follicle stimulating hormone levels." *Human Reproduction* 1997; 12(2): 241–243.

Gelfand, M.M. "Estrogen-androgen hormone replacement therapy." *European Menopause Journal* 1995; 2(3): 22–26.

Genant, H.K., Lucas, J., Weiss, S., et al. "Low dose esterified estrogen therapy: Effects on bone, plasma estradiol concentrations, endometrium, and lipid levels." *Archives of Internal Medicine* 1997; 157: 2609–2615.

Gordeski, G.L. "Premature menopause." *Menopause Management* 1997; 10–17.

Gradstein, F., Stampfer, M., Manson, J.E., et al. "Postmenopausal estrogen and progestin use and the risk of cardiovascular disease." *New England Journal of Medicine* 1996; 335: 453–61.

Gradstein, F., Stampfer, M.J. "The epidemiology of coronary heart disease and estrogen replacement in postmenopausal women." *Progress in Cardiovascular Disease*, 1995; 38: 199–210.

Hallowell, N. " 'You don't want to lose your ovaries because you think 'I might become a man.' " Women's perceptions of prophylactic surgery as a cancer risk management option. *Psychooncology* 1998; 7(3): 263–275.

Harding, C., Morton, M., Gould, V., McMichael Phillips, D., Howell, A.,

Bundred, N.J., "Dietary soy supplementation is oestrogenic in menopausal women." *The Second International Symposium on the Role of Soy in Preventing and Treating Chronic Disease,* Belgium, September 1996.

Hargreave, T.B., Mills, J.A. "Investigating and managing infertility in general practice." *British Medical Journal* 1998; 316(7142): 1438–1441.

Hartmann, B.W., Kirchengast, S., Albrecht, A., Huber, J.C., Stregi, G. "Effect of hormone replacement therapy on growth hormone stimulation in women with premature ovarian failure." *Fertility and Sterility* 1997; 68(1): 103–107.

Hirata, J.D., Swiersz, L.M., Zell, B., Small, R., Ettinger, B. "Does Dong Quai have estrogenic effects in postmenopausal women: A double-blind, placebo controlled trial." *Fertility and Sterility* 1997; 68(6): 981–986.

Hoek, A., Schoemaker, J., Drexhage, H.A. "Premature ovarian failure and ovarian autoimmunity." *Endocrinology Review* 1997; 18 (1): 107–134.

"Hormone replacement therapy." *Clinicians Reviews* 1997; 7(9): 53–56, 59–60, 62, 65–66, 69–72.

"Impact of hormone replacement therapy on the risk of cardiovascular disease." *Medscape Cardiology* 1997.

Ingram, D., Sanders, K., Kolybaba, M., Lopez, D. "Case control study of phytoestrogens and breast cancer." *Lancet* 1997; 350(9083): 990–994.

Israel, D., Quinn Youngkin, E. "Herbal therapies for perimenopausal and menopausal complaints." *Pharmacotherapy* 1997; 17(5): 970–984.

Johannisson, E., Holinka, C.F., Arrenbrecht, S. "Transdermal sequential and continuous hormone replacement regimens with estradiol and norethisterone acetate in postmenopausal women: Effects on the endometrium." *International Journal of Fertility and Women's Medicine* 1997; 42 Suppl 2: 388–98.

Kardinaal, A.F.M., Waalkensberendsen, D.H., Arts, C.J.M. "Pseudo-oestrogens in the diet: Health benefits and safety concerns." *Trends in Food Science and Technology* 1997; 8(10): 327–333.

Kenemans, P. "Rick profile-based long-term hormone replacement therapy." *European Menopause Journal* 1995, 2(4): 3–4.

Khastgir, G., Studd, J. "Hysterectomy, ovarian failure, and depression." *Menopause* 1998; 5(2): 113–122.

Kim, J.G., Moon, S.Y., Chang, Y.S., Lee, J.Y. "Autoimmune premature ovarian failure." *British Journal of Obstetrics and Gynaecology* 1995; 21(1): 59–66.

Knight, D.C., Eden, J.A. "A review of the clinical effects of phytoestrogens." *Obstetrics & Gynecology* 1996; 87(5-pt.2): 897–904.

Kohlmeier, Lynn. "Osteoporosis risk factors, screening, and treatment." *The 50th Annual Meeting of the American Academy of Family Physicians Scientific Assembly,* September 16–20, 1998.

Kurzer, M.S., Xu, X. "Dietary phytoestrogens." *Annual Review of Nutrition* 1997; 17: 353–381.

Lampe, J., Messina, M. "Are phytoestrogens nature's cure for what ails us? A look at the research [interview by Nancy I. Hahn]." *Journal of the American Dietetic Association* 1998; 98(9): 974–6.

Langenberg, P., Kjerulff, K.H., Stolley, P.D. "Hormone replacement and menopausal symptoms following hysterectomy." *American Journal of Epidemiology* 1997; 146(10): 870–880.

Lieman, H., Santoro, N. "Premature ovarian failure: A modern approach to diagnosis and treatment." *The Endocrinologist* 1997; 7: 314–321.

Lien, L.L., Lien, E.J. "Hormone therapy and phytoestrogens." *Journal of Clinical Pharmacology and Therapeutics* 1996; 21(2): 101–111.

Lip, G.Y.H., Blane, A.D., Jones, A.F., Beevers, G. "Effects of hormone replacement therapy on hemostatic factors, lipid factors, and endothelial function in women undergoing surgical menopause: Implications for prevention of artherosclerosis." *American Heart Journal* 1997; 134(4):764–771.

Lu, L.J.W., Anderson, K.E., Grady, J.J., Nagamani, M. "Effects of soy consumption for one month in premenopausal women: Implications for breast cancer risk reduction." *Cancer Epidemiology, Biomarkers and Prevention* 1996; 5(1): 63–70.

Lydic, M.L., Liu, J.H., Rebar, R.W., Thomas, M.A. "Success of donor oocyte in in vitro fertilization-embryo transfer in recipients with and without premature ovarian failure." *Fertility and Sterility* 1996; 65(1): 98–102.

McIver, Bryan, Romanski, Susan A., Noppoldt, Todd B. "Evaluation and management of amenorrhea." *Mayo Clinic Proceedings* 1997; 72 (12) 1161–1172.

Menashe, Y., Pearlstone, A.C., Surrey, E.S. "Spontaneous pregnancies despite failed attempts at ovulation induction in a woman with iatrogenic premature ovarian failure." *Journal of Reproductive Medicine* 1996; 41(3): 207–210.

Merrill, Joan T., Dinu, Anca R., Lahita, Robert G. "Autoimmunity: The female connection." *Medscape Women's Health* 1996; 1(11).

Messina, M. "The role of soy products in reducing risk of cancer." *Journal of the National Cancer Institute* 1991; 83(7): 541–545.

Mizumuna, H., Okano, H., Soda, M., Kagami, I., Miyamoto, S., Tokizawa, T., Honjo, S., Ibuki, Y. "Prevention of postmenopausal bone loss with minimal uterine bleeding using low dose continuous estrogen/progestin therapy: A 2 year prospective study." *Maturitas* 1997; 27(1):69–76.

Mohyi, D., Tabassi, K., Simon, J. "Differential diagnosis of hot flashes." *Maturitas* 1997; 27(3): 203–14.

Muller, P., Botta, L., Ezzet, F. "Bioavailability of estradiol from a new matrix and a conventional reservoir-type transdermal therapeutic system." *European Journal of Clinical Pharmacology* 1996; 51(3–4): 327–30.

Murkies, A.L., Wilcox, G., Davis, S.R. "Clinical review 92: Phytoestrogens." *Journal of Clinical Endocrinology and Metabolism* 1998; 83(2): 297–303.

Murkies, A. "Phytoestrogens—what is the current knowledge?" *Australian Family Physician* 1998; 27(1): S47–51.

Nelson, L.M., Anasti, J.N., Flack, M.R. "Premature ovarian failure." *Reproductive Endocrinology, Surgery, and Technology* 1996; Chapter 71: 1394–1410.

Park, K.H., Song, C.H. "Bone mineral density in premenopausal anovulatory women." *British Journal of Obstetrics and Gynaecology* February 1995; 21(1): 89–97.

Nilsson, P., Muller, L., Koster, A., Hollnagel, H. "Social and biological predictors of early menopause: A model for premature aging." *Journal of Internal Medicine* 1997; 242(4): 299–305.

Parazzini, F., La Vecchia, C., Negri, E., Franceschi, S., Moroni, S., Chatenoud, L., Bolis, G. "Case-control study of estrogen replacement therapy and risk of cervical cancer." *British Medical Journal* 1997; 315 (7100): 85–8.

Partington, M.S., York Moore, D., Turner, G.M. "Confirmation of early menopause in fragile x carriers." *American Journal of Medical Genetics* 1996; 64 (2): 370–372.

"Premature natural menopause can be devastating." *Menopause News* 1995, 5 (4) 1.

"Raloxifene: The first selective estrogen receptor modulator for postmenopausal osteoporosis." *Drug & Therapy Perspectives* 1998; 12(7):1–5.

Reinli, K., Block, G. "Phytoestrogen content of foods: A compendium of literature values." *Nutrition and Cancer* 1996; 26(2): 123–148.

Sable, David B. "Good eggs, FSH levels and ovarian reserve: The egg factor." *InterNational Committee for Infertility Information Dissemination (INCIID) Web site* 1997.

Santoro, N., Banwell, T., Tortoriello, D., Lieman, H., Adel, T., Skurnick, J. "Effects of aging and gonadal failure on the hypothalamic-pituitary axis in women." *Journal of Obstetrics and Gynecology* 1998; 178(4): 732–741.

Sheehan, D.M. "Herbal medicines, phytoestrogens and toxicity: Risk-benefit considerations." *Proceedings of the Society for Experimental Biology and Medicine* 1998; 217(3): 379–385.

Siegel, Marc. "Gambling with time." *Discover* 1996; 17 (12): 120–122.

Singer, Dani, Hunter, Myra S. "Dealing with loss of fertility." *British Medical Journal* 1997; 315 (7099) 66.

Soffa, V.M. "Alternatives to hormone replacement for menopause." *Alternative Therapies in Health and Medicine* 1996; 2(2): 34–39.

"Soybeans show promise in cancer prevention." *Primary Care & Cancer* 1995; 15(3): 11–12.

Stampfer, M.J, Colditz, G.A., Willett, W.C., et al. "Postmenopausal estrogen therapy and cardiovascular disease: Ten-year follow-up from the Nurses Health Study." *New England Journal of Medicine* 1991; 325: 756–62.

Steinberg, K.K., Thacker, S.B., Smith, S.J., Stroup, D.F., Zach, M.M., Flanders, W.D., Berkelman, R.L. "A meta-analysis of the effect of estrogen replacement therapy on the risk of breast cancer." *Journal of the American Medical Association* 1991; 265: 1985.

Taylor, Maida. "Alternatives to conventional hormone replacement therapy." *Comprehensive Therapy* 1997; 23(8): 514–532.

Thacker, H. "Update on hormone replacement: Sorting out the options for preventing coronary artery disease and osteoporosis." *Medscape Women's Health* 1996; 1(6).

Tham, D.M., Gardner, C.D., Haskell, W.L. "Clinical review 97: Potential health benefits of dietary phytoestrogens: a review of the clinical, epidemiological, and mechanistic evidence." *Journal of Clinical Endocrinology and Metabolism* 1998; 83(7): 2223–35.

Thompson, L.U., Rickard, S.E., Cheung, F., Kenaschuk, E.O., Obermeyer, W.R. "Variability in anticancer lignan levels in flaxseed." *Nutrition and Cancer* 1997; 27(1):26–30.

Thompson, Sylvia. "When menopause arrives in your 20s." *Irish Times* July 13, 1998.

Wang, C., Kurzer, M.S. "Effects of isoflavones, flavanoids, and lignans on proliferation of estrogen-dependent and independent human breast cancer cells." *Proceedings of the American Association for Cancer Research* 1996; 37: 277.

Watts, N.B., Notelovitz, M., Timmons, M.C., et al. "Comparison of oral estrogen and estrogen plus androgen on bone mineral density, menopausal symptoms, and lipid and lipoprotein profiles in surgically menopausal women." *Obstetrics and Gynecology* 1995; 85(4): 529–537.

Wheatcroft, N.J., Rogers, C.A., Metcalfe, R.A., Lenton, E.A., Cooke, I.D., Weetman, A.P. "Is subclinical ovarian failure an autoimmune disease?" *Human Reproduction* 1997, 12 (2): 244–249.

Wheatcroft, N.J., Salt, C., Milford-Ward, A., Cooke, I.D., Weetman, A.P. "Identification of ovarian antibodies by immunofluorescence enzyme-linked immunosorbent assay or immunoblotting in premature ovarian failure." *Human Reproduction* 1997; 12(12): 2617–2622.

Whitten, P.L., Lewis, C., Russell, E., Naftolin, F. "Potential adverse effects of phytoestrogens." *Journal of Nutrition* 1995; 125 (3 Suppl S): S776.

Williams, K. (speaker), Sznake, P. (reporter). "Interactive effects of soy protein and estradiol on arterial pathobiology." *The 70th Annual Scientific Sessions of the American Heart Association,* November 9–12, 1997.

Woods, M.N., Senie, R., Kronenberg, F. "Effect of a dietary soy bar on menopausal symptoms." *The Second International Symposium on the Role of Soy in Preventing and Treating Chronic Disease*, Belgium, September 1996.

Wren, B.G. "Hormonal replacement therapy and breast cancer." *European Menopause Journal* 1995; 2(4): 13–19.

The Writing Group for the PEPI Trial. "Effects of estrogen or estrogen/progestin regimens on heart disease risk factors in postmenopausal women: The Postmenopausal Estrogen/Progestin Interventions (PEPI) Trial." *JAMA* 1995; 273: 199–208.

Wu, Ah, Ziegler, R.G., Hornross, P.L., Nomura, A.M.Y., West, D.W., Kolonel, L.N., Rosenthal, J.F., Hoover, R.N., Pike, M.C. "Tofu and risk of breast cancer in Asian-Americans." *Cancer Epidemiology, Biomarkers & Prevention* 1996; 5(11): 901–906.

Zava, D.T., Dollbaum, C.M., Blen, M. "Estrogen and progestin bioactivity of foods, herbs, and spices." *Proceedings of the Society for Experimental Biology & Medicine* 1998; 217(3): 369–78.

Index